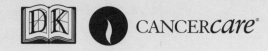 

# THE CANCER PATIENT'S WORKBOOK

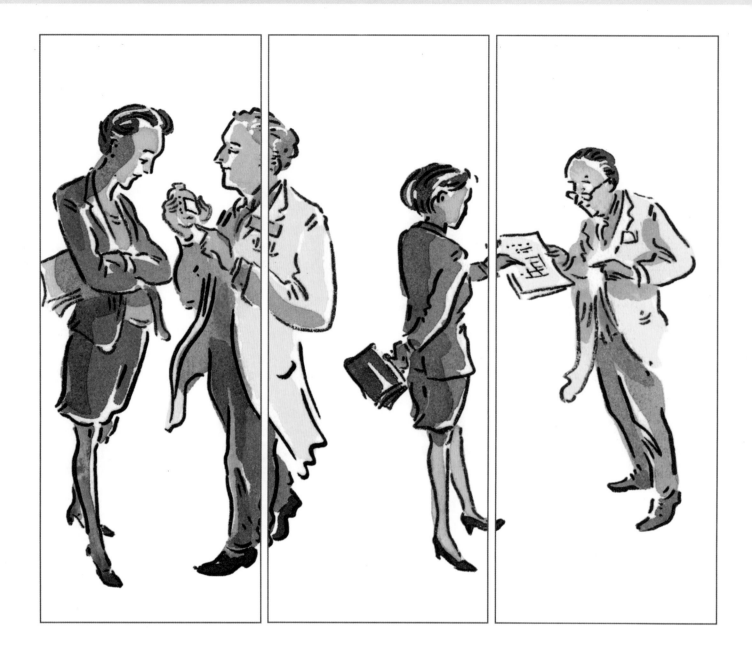

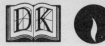

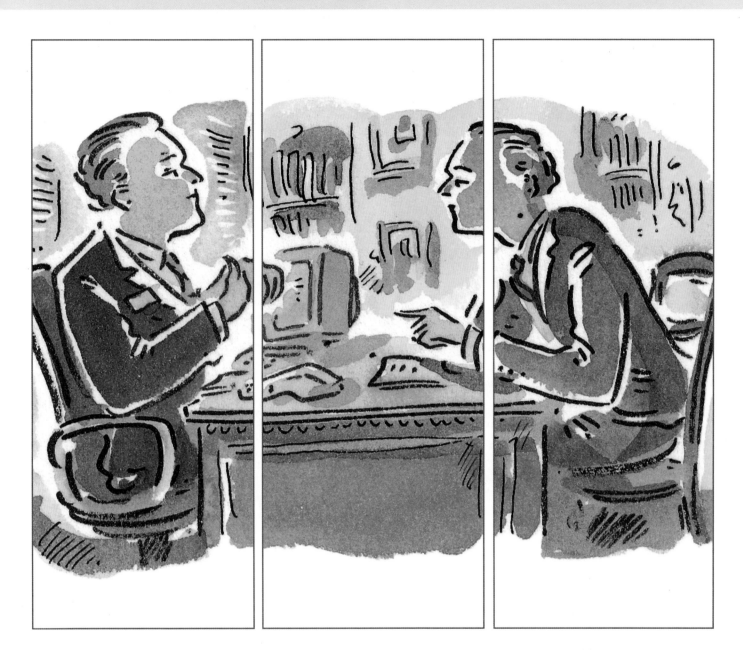

# THE CANCER PATIENT'S WORKBOOK

## EVERYTHING YOU NEED TO STAY ORGANIZED AND INFORMED

By Joanie Willis

London, New York, Sydney, Delhi,
Paris, Munich, Johannesburg

**Senior Editor:** Jill Hamilton
**Designer:** Diana Catherines
**Jacket Design:** Dirk Kaufman
**Senior Art Editor:** Mandy Earey
**Editorial Director:** LaVonne Carlson
**Art Director:** Tina Vaughan
**Publisher:** Sean Moore
**Production Director:** David Proffit

First American Edition, 2001
2 4 6 8 10 9 7 5 3 1
Published in the United States by
Dorling Kindersley Publishing, Inc.
95 Madison Avenue
New York, New York 10016

Dorling Kindersley Publishing, Inc. offers special discounts for
bulk purchases for sales promotions or premiums. Specific,
large-quantity needs can be met with special editions, including
personalized covers, excerpts of existing guides, and corporate
imprints. For more information, contact Special Markets
Department, Dorling Kindersley Publishing, Inc.,
95 Madison Avenue, New York, NY 10016 Fax: 800-600-9098.

Library of Congress Cataloging-in-Publication Data
Willis, Joanie.
    Cancer patient workbook/Joanie Willis.–1st American ed.
        p.        cm.
    Includes index
    ISBN 0-7894-6782-8 (alk. paper)
    1. Cancer–Popular works. 2. Cancer–Handbooks, manuals,
    etc. 3. Cancer–Miscellanea. I. Title.
RC263 W526 2001                    362.1'96994–dc21

Reproduced by Colourscan, Singapore
Printed and bound by Graphicom, srl in Italy

See our complete catalog at
**www.dk.com**

# Table of Contents

## 1 A PATIENT'S PRIVATE JOURNEY

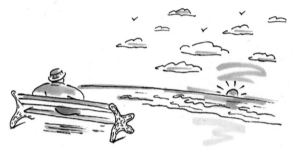

## 2 ON YOUR MARK, GET SET, GO...

## 3 NAVIGATING THE MEDICAL MAZE

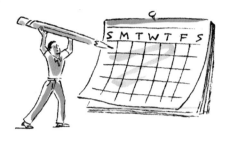

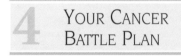

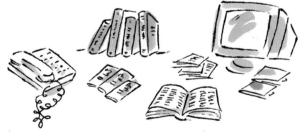

# Foreword

Cancer – once a word that was whispered among neighbors when a loved one became ill – has become one of the most critical public health issues facing Americans. Advances in the understanding, diagnosis, and treatment of cancer over the past few decades has enabled millions to survive what was once an almost certain death sentence. Today, over 8 million people in the United States are living with cancer, rather than dying from it.

But how exactly does one learn to live with cancer? In its 57-year history, Cancer Care has helped over 2 million people cope with the irreparable ways in which their lives have changed because of their cancer diagnosis or that of a loved one.

Through individual and group counseling, we help people with cancer, their loved ones and caregivers, to cope with the devastating effects of the disease. And through educational programs, financial assistance, and referrals to community resources, we provide practical help to tens of thousands of people each year so that they may live their lives while learning to live with cancer. The services we provide respond to the changing needs of people with cancer. No two people experience cancer in the same way, but several themes are critical in increasing one's chances of survival:

• being an educated consumer

• partnering with your healthcare team in determining your course of treatment

• continuing to work, whenever possible

• maintaining a positive attitude

• taking control of your life

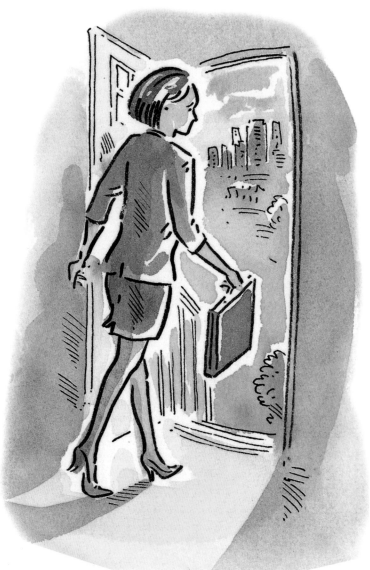

*And it is our vast experience that enables us to recognize what a tremendous resource the Cancer Patient's Workbook can be to people with cancer.*

*As the author of the workbook and a six-year survivor of Stage 4 lung cancer, Joanie Willis has used her experience to create a valuable tool that will prove indispensable to the person who is newly diagnosed. Her commitment and desire to help people with cancer has resulted in a comprehensive guide that will help you gather and retain important information; be an informed partner with your healthcare team when making decisions about your treatment, and serve as inspiration during what may be one of the most difficult times in your life – all with the ultimate goal of helping you focus your energy on getting well.*

*The complex emotions one feels after being diagnosed; the choices one must make – coupled with the physical demands of ongoing testing, treatment, and side-effects – can be overwhelming. With the support of the Cancer Patient's Workbook and organizations like Cancer Care, you can learn to cope with the challenges confronting you and learn to live with cancer.*

Diana Blum
Executive Director
Cancer Care, Inc

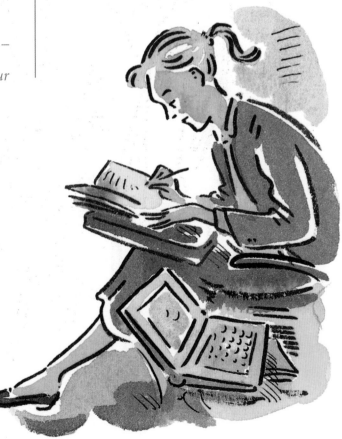

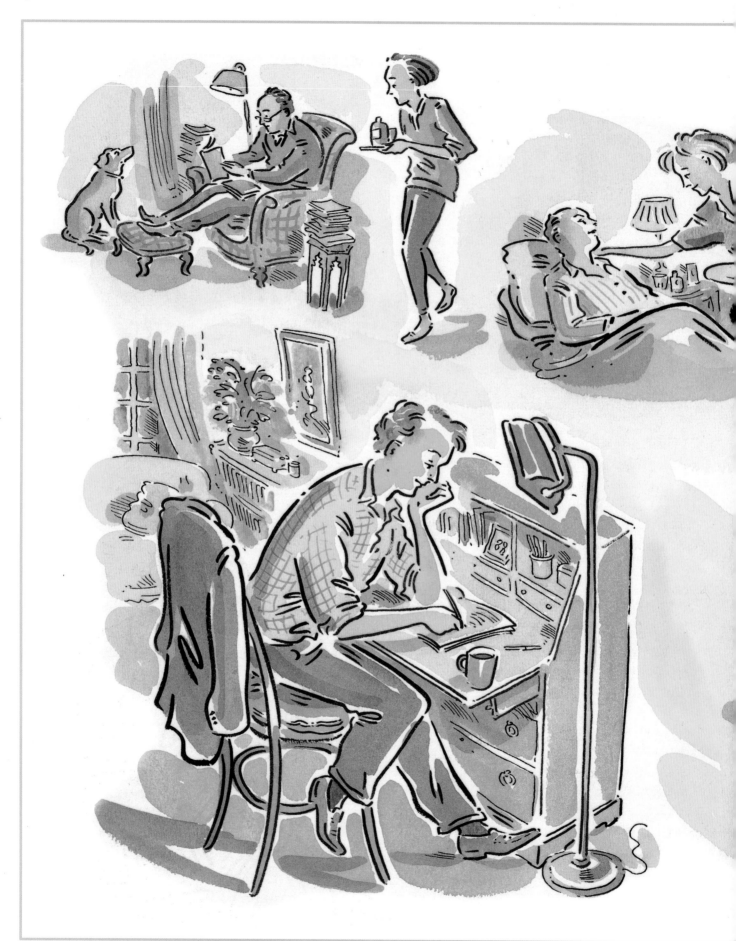

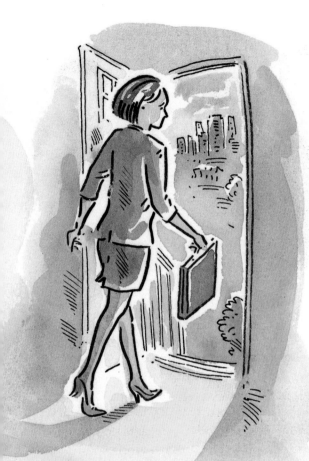

# A Patient's Private Journey

### Chapter 1

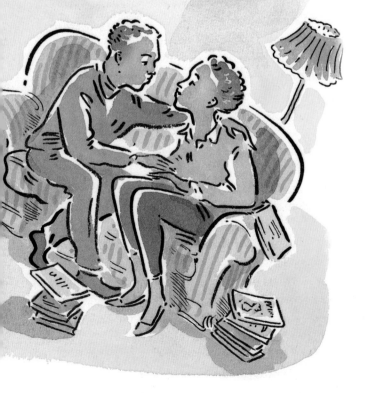

# My Personal Passage

It was the most surreal moment in my life. I was forty-four years old when I first heard the words "You have cancer." My doctors stood solemnly around my hospital bed after performing a biopsy and informed me that I had stage 4 lung cancer. The cancer had spread to my mediastinum area (wherever that was) and they would not be able to operate. I knew nothing about lung cancer, operations, or metastasis. The terminology was Greek to me, but I knew by the expressions on their faces that the circumstances were grim. It struck me like a thunderbolt. I had cancer and it just might kill me. If you have heard those words then you know how they impact your world. For me there was a heavy sensation of fear and terror, a sense of doom and sadness that was laced in a haze of disbelief. This was a betrayal of my body, a threatening situation I couldn't just walk away from. That reality overwhelmed me, and I felt trapped in panic.

The first week of diagnosis left me feeling unconnected and outside of myself. I really could not grasp that this was happening to me. My life had changed so completely in such a short time that I was left reeling. Days of testing replaced days of work. Light conversations were exchanged for life-and-death discussions, and the joy I had always taken for granted was long forgotten. I had bone scans, CT scans, MRIs, X rays, and blood tests. Doctors, nurses, and technicians swarmed in and out of my presence with so much information that I felt bewildered and confused. Phrases like "difficult case" and "we will do what we can" caused my heart to race madly. I wanted desperately to hear the words "cure," "remission," or "we are hopeful." I knew that I would never be the same again.

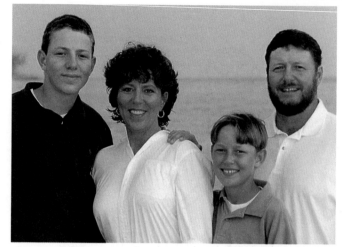

*Joanie Willis in 1999, five years after her first diagnosis of cancer, with sons, Andy and Mark, and husband, Jim.*

It wasn't only my life that was being altered, but my family's as well. My husband was placed in the position of providing for us financially, taking care of our sons, and being my primary caregiver. Our boys, Andy (age 12) and Mark (age 10), quickly realized that something was out of sync in their world. While I tried to put a positive spin on things for the kids' sake, they sensed, as kids do, that this was a serious situation. The day I came home from the hospital my son Andy asked me if I was going to die. I told him "No, I don't think so," to which he replied, "You didn't think it would be cancer either." It would be the first encounter my two boys would have with fear.

The nights were the worst for me. I had learned that I had about a four-percent chance of surviving my cancer and without fail I would awake each night in a drenching sweat, heart pounding, feeling total despair. I would sneak down to my boys' rooms and stand for hours at the foot of their beds watching them sleep, contemplating their lives and all that I would miss. For me, the thought of not being there to watch them play sports, graduate, get married, and have my grandchildren brought me physical pain. I could feel my heart break; I was devastated and sometimes beyond tears. I'd never given it a second thought that I wouldn't be there for them whenever they needed me, but now that was all I could think about. It was unbearable.

I don't remember the precise moment in time when my inner will to live manifested itself, but it did and for that I'm eternally grateful. I do remember a day when I stood

## FIGHTING FEAR

If you encounter moments of unsubstantiated fear, try one of the following:

- Listen to upbeat music.
- Watch a comedy.
- Call a friend – don't talk about cancer.
- Surf the Internet for fun things.
- Take a shower, get dressed, fix yourself up.
- Read a light, entertaining book.
- Go shopping.
- Pursue a hobby.
- Take a drive.
- Start exercising.
- Have lunch with a friend.
- Take a walk.
- Garden.

in my bedroom, all alone, and started repeating the word "NO" over and over again. No to feeling helpless, no to despair, no to depression, no to giving up, no to being a victim. I still felt sapped of emotional energy and physical strength and not capable of the most important fight of my life. However, the alternative for me was not only inconceivable but also quite simply unacceptable.

As silly as it sounds, I decided to make decisions. My first was to face the situation head on, get the facts no matter how disturbing, trust my own instincts, and act quickly. I liked my team of doctors and their willingness to treat me aggressively. I gave my medical team the approval for 36 radiation treatments to the chest and four sessions of three consecutive six-hour days of chemotherapy treatments. I embraced the radiation beams with the thought of burning out the cancer cells. I also made the choice to believe that the chemotherapy drugs were invading deep into the tumors and destroying them from within. It became my mental armor that the treatments were going to work and I fought doubt actively, as if it were a tangible enemy.

Experiencing all-consuming weakness and fatigue from my treatment, I determined to make use of the "down time" that I was forced to spend in bed. I obtained every book I could acquire on cancer, radiation, chemotherapy, vitamins, herbs, nutrition, exercise, and spiritual matters. It soon became apparent to me that my role in this fight needed to consist of a daily regimen to boost my immune system. I concluded that regardless of how many herbs and vitamins I had to take, how much I had to alter my present diet, and to whatever degree I had to change my life, I was willing to do so if it might enhance my chance of survival by even a few percentage points. I read, I researched, and I learned. Not to mention that I prayed, a lot.

Three years have passed since my original diagnosis. I have had more CT scans, MRIs, bone scans, and blood tests than I care to recall. I concentrate instead on the most recent CT scan, which was clear, and my last blood test, which was normal. In truth, I still have the desire for a brain scan every time I develop a headache rather then reacting normally by just taking an aspirin. I'm all too intimately acquainted with the fear that comes in the middle of the night when there is an unnerving twinge of inexplicable pain. I often feel as if I have been put out in the middle of a lake in a rowboat during an unrelenting thunderstorm with no oars. Know what I mean?

*Nevertheless, I make a point to live each day in joy, mindful of the fact that life is short. Colors seem more vibrant than ever before, and my children's laughter is the most important thing in my entire world.*

I go to lunch with my buddies and let the housework slide. I smile at strangers as if they were my best friends and laugh at others' mistakes almost as hard as I laugh at my own. I have let go of expectations, resentments, guilt, envy, uncertainty, high-maintenance people, animosity, and self-induced stress. I have embraced singing, alone time, laughter, pampering myself, yard work, helping others, family, friends, and the faith that has kept me going. Never have I been happier. I've changed.

*November, 1998*
*In March of 1998, I went for my routine six-month CT scan, secure in the knowledge that all would be well after nearly four years since my first bout with lung cancer. The nurses came to get me in the waiting room to show me a thickening of tissue where my original tumor had been. The doctors were optimistic that it was scar tissue forming. But I knew, I just did. The only thing I could do at that point was to pray for peace and strength. I was certain that I would need an abundance of it.*

*Not willing to take a wait-and-see approach, I flew to M.D. Anderson Cancer Center and met with a team of specialists. A biopsy was performed and I was diagnosed with recurrent lung cancer. Dr. Jack Roth decided to take out the section of lung that had the cancer in it, although it would be difficult due to scarring from previous radiation. I came back home to Florida, where I had four pre-op Taxol chemotherapy treatments. I really can't tell you how I felt going through the hair loss, the sickness, and the ordeal all over again. I just kept thinking that I'd been here and done this. I was so sad and numb. In a fog I flew back to Texas for lung surgery, and a week later I was home again to do six more chemotherapy treatments in order to wipe up any cancer cells that might have been left behind.*

# My Personal Passage, cont.

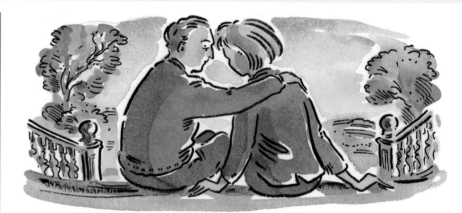

I'm now a week out from my last chemotherapy treatment. I look back on these eight months in almost total disbelief. My body is scarred, sore, and taking its time in healing. My thoughts run the scale of being ecstatic that the whole thing is over to fearing that the cancer is spreading throughout my body now that my chemotherapy treatments are done. It's a huge effort to put myself back together again. I feel like the first time I gave all I had to recover, but now I'm finding it difficult to scrape up enough courage and will to go through yet another day. There have been many moments lately when I've thought that I may never be the same. The despair, the helplessness, and the weakness seem to be who I have become and not necessarily a result of the suffering. I keep asking, "have I become my disease?"

✦

I heard myself laughing yesterday and, although the sound was foreign to me and the joy I felt was fleeting, I suddenly realized that my spirit hadn't died. That knowledge alone has brought with it hope, desire, and, most of all, determination. I am still here, I still have choices, and I am NOT cancer.

I am well aware that I am standing on the edge of a cliff where a strong wind could blow me over, but I choose, once again, to believe that my doctors have furnished the right treatment that has helped heal me. I believe that changing my diet and taking vitamins and herbs has helped heal me. I believe that being loved and cared for by my family and friends has helped heal me. I believe that once again my faith has been instrumental in healing me. I believe…

*October, 1999*
*It occurred to me just now, as I was reading the story of my diagnosis, just how hopeless my whole story sounds. It will be a year this month since my last treatment and I am not going to say that it has been easy. It hasn't. I have been through major depression and my body has been much slower healing this second time around. Most days I feel like I am just sleeping my life away and I'm sick and tired of living my life around the outcome of diagnostic tests. But, and this is a big "but," I am healing little by little every day, even if it's not as rapid as I would like it to be. I am still alive and I will do what I can to remain alive.*

For those of us who have cancer, life is precious and sweet. Never a day goes by that I am not thankful. Had I been given a choice I would not have chosen cancer as a life experience, but I can honestly say that the last five years has given me more than it has taken.

*Even in my darkest moments I never gave up and it's my fervent hope that you won't either. Like my mother used to say, "This too shall pass."*

---

### SIGNS OF DEPRESSION

- Insomnia
- Feeling of being overwhelmed
- Difficulty in relationships
- Feeling of stress.
- Panic attacks
- Worthless feelings
- Hopelessness
- Despair
- Exhaustion
- Crying easily
- Feelings of detachment
- Nervousness
- Difficulty communicating
- Thoughts of suicide

**It is not uncommon to experience varying degrees of depression during and after your treatments. DO NOT suffer in silence. Discuss your feelings, fears, and problems with your doctor. There are numerous antidepressant drugs now on the market. Your doctor may prescribe medication for you if he feels it could benefit you during this difficult period.**

# Working Your Workbook

During my initial bout with cancer I made it my mission to find new and practical information that I could utilize in my attempt to gain an advantage over my disease. My thought was that I would allow my doctors to treat me with their arsenal of drugs, radiation, surgery, and expertise, while I fought on another level using foods, exercise, clinical trials, vitamins, herbs, cancer support groups, late breaking research, and news. I wanted to be informed and stay informed but it was difficult since a great deal of the information

### THE CANCER PATIENT'S WORKBOOK

…is in no way intended to take the place of your efforts in researching your particular cancer and its treatment options. Rather, it is structured to enhance your research and give you:
• Step-by-step guidelines.
• Organizational lists and calendars.
• A sense of direction and control.
• A central location to keep your questions, answers, and information.
• A tool to use during doctor visits, hospital stays, and treatments.
• A complete source of organizations from which to obtain information.
In addition, each chapter includes:
• Recommended books to read.
• Helpful hints.
• Cancer facts.
• "Just for the fun of it" segments.
• Reminder messages.
• Lists or forms to complete.
• Enriching quotations.
Keep this workbook with you at all times and use a pencil.

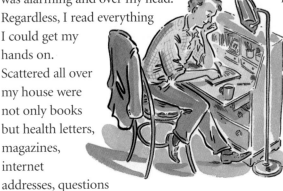

was alarming and over my head. Regardless, I read everything I could get my hands on. Scattered all over my house were not only books but health letters, magazines, internet addresses, questions to ask my doctor, journals, thank-you lists, documents, calendars, and bits and pieces of information scribbled hastily on scraps of paper. Not only was I frightened, bewildered, and exhausted from treatments, but the magnitude of data that accumulated overwhelmed and confused me. Never in my life had it been more important for me to retain and organize information. Never in my life was I more unable to do so.

Since I was managing to eke out an existence month by month and because my name was being passed around the cancer grapevine as someone currently surviving stage 4 lung cancer, I began receiving desperate calls from people who had recently heard the words "you have cancer." Many of the people who called me were frightened into total immobility, several were scrambling for answers, and still others had a fatalistic view of their chances without the benefit of ample knowledge. Nearly all those who called me felt they had no control over what was happening and their first question was always "what do I do now?"

Over the past five years I have tried to help cancer patients answer that question. I have come to the realization that there is a different answer for each individual person. I can't tell you what to do now and I don't believe anyone else can either. It's a matter of personal choice and conviction. What I can tell you is this: Knowledge is power and the more knowledge you have about your particular cancer, the easier it will be to make choices.

This workbook has been structured to assist you in gathering and retaining important information.

While there are sections designed to address the emotional aspects of having cancer, the workbook will also guide you in gaining a measure of control by way of being a pro-active participant in managing your health care. The workbook is just that, a workbook designed to take to doctors' offices, hospitals, and treatment centers. It is also a tool to give you direction, to motivate and organize you. Please take the time to read through the entire workbook now to familiarize yourself with it. My longing and desire for the last several years has been to help cancer patients. *The Cancer Patient's Workbook* is my best effort to do so.

*"Many things which cannot be overcome when they are together, yield themselves up when taken little by little."*

– Plutarch

# Your Personal Passage

_____

_____

_____

_____

_____

_____

_____

_____

_____

_____

_____

_____

_____

_____

_____

_____

_____

_____

_____

_____

## SURE CURE

Beware of the natural products and unproven methods that claim to replace standard therapy. Do not allow fear of surgery, radiation, and chemotherapy treatments to cloud your judgment. If you are considering an unproven treatment instead of a conventional one, ask the following questions:

- Do the marketing write-ups use scientific jargon without backing up their claims with independent medical research?
- Are they claiming that the medical profession is trying to keep this "cure" from the public?
- Is the treatment covered by your medical insurance?
- Is it provided at a hospital?
- Does it sound too good to be really true?
- Most important, how advanced will your cancer get during the delay of standard treatment and the risk really worth it?

## SEE YOU LATER, ALLIGATOR!

The treatments are finally over, your doctor doesn't need to see you for six weeks, you're free to go home, pick up the pieces, and move on. YAY! But wait, what's this? FEAR? You bet it is and you are not unique. Being cut loose after months of treatments and close observation often causes a patient to feel stranded, unprotected, and vulnerable. Take heart: with the passing of time will come the passing of persistent fear. Really!

# Your Poetry

**I Believe**

F
  A
    L
      L
        I
          N
            G

At the speed of life
You lift us up
The eagle and I
And with your light
You hold us there
I Believe…

*By Joanie Willis*

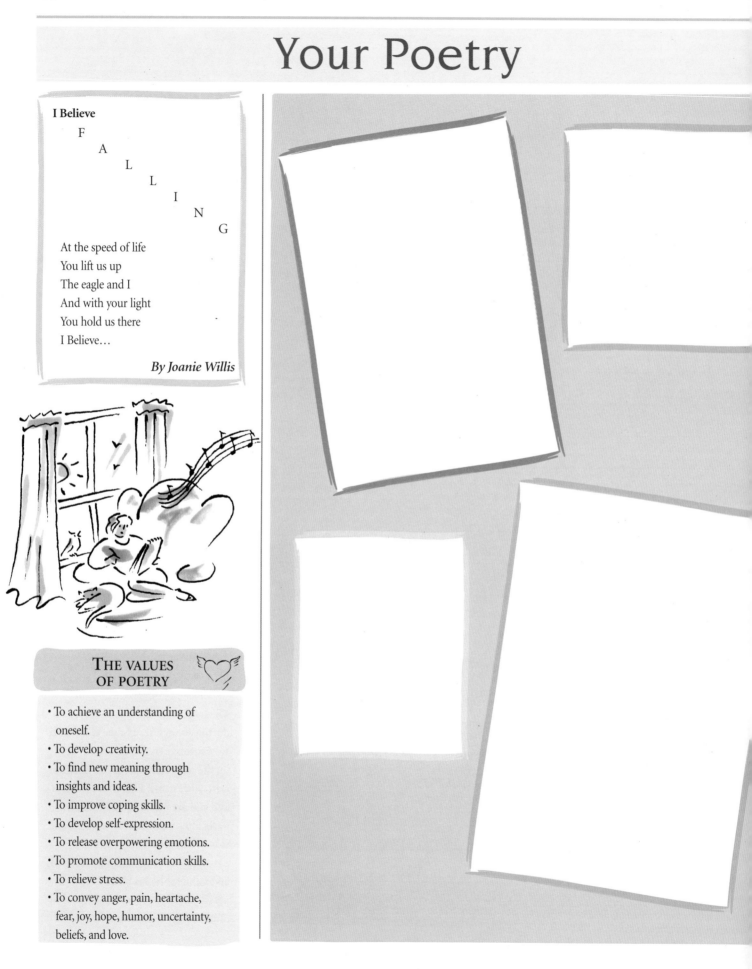

## THE VALUES OF POETRY

- To achieve an understanding of oneself.
- To develop creativity.
- To find new meaning through insights and ideas.
- To improve coping skills.
- To develop self-expression.
- To release overpowering emotions.
- To promote communication skills.
- To relieve stress.
- To convey anger, pain, heartache, fear, joy, hope, humor, uncertainty, beliefs, and love.

"Poetry is the
   response of our
   innermost being to
   the ecstasy, the agony and
   the all-embracing
   mystery of life.
   It is a song, or a sigh,
   or a cry,
   often all of them
   together."

*Charles Angoff (Lerner, 1994)*

## THE HEALING ASPECTS OF POETRY

Poetry, music, and journalism have been used for healing and personal growth since the beginning. It is often during periods of individual crisis when dealing with anger, fear, stress, sickness, and confusion that many people take pen to paper in an attempt to release their thoughts, frustrations, and emotions. For many, poetry is not an avenue we have used in the past for self-expression and self-examination. During this time in your life, however, poetry might provide a medium in which to convey your deepest thoughts. We have all heard of courageous people who have fought the disease of cancer and have emerged with newfound talents, passions, and gifts that they had not been aware they possessed. Give poetry a try; it might be your gift.

# Being In Need

Have you always thought of yourself as self-reliant, self-sufficient, self-assured, confident, determined, unrestricted, unhampered, unlimited, and free? Has receiving the diagnosis of cancer dramatically changed your self-image? Do you now sometimes feel helpless, defenseless, dependent, disabled, defective, invalid, weak, powerless, and unprotected?

Most of us are by nature an independent lot and cancer places us firmly on the foreign soil of the needy. Giving up control of our simple daily necessities and having to depend on others for every little thing can be nearly as devastating as the cancer itself – if you let it be.

*Your health must be your first consideration. Allowing your loved ones to "do for you" can be a major factor in your game plan toward achieving remission.*

If this takes an attitude adjustment on your part, then think of it this way. You are in control of enhancing your overall method and strategy for getting well by receiving treatments, learning about your cancer, eating healthy foods, taking vitamins, exercising, and looking into clinical trials. You can relieve stress and conserve energy if you allow others to nurture and care for you. It's just another component of your strategy.

Begin by forgetting the phrases "I'll get it myself," "I don't need a ride," "I'll make something to eat later," or "I don't need help." Never think of yourself as a burden and do not hesitate to let others take care of what you cannot. Remember that the cancer, the treatments, and the stress will leave you with a very limited supply of energy. You can deplete it attempting to do business as usual or you can spend it taking exceptional care of yourself. Never knowing how you will feel from one day to the next can cause upset and frustration for you if you don't make up your mind ahead of time as to what is important and what is not. What's it going to be? Are you going to mow the lawn and do the dishes or eat a salad and take a nap?

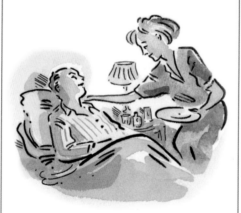

The most important helper roles to you at the moment are the patient advocate and principle caregiver. They may be one and the same. The caregiver is generally a family member (most likely your spouse, child, or sibling) who assumes caring for your immediate daily needs. The patient advocate can also be a family member or a friend who is in charge of organizing a workforce, or team if you will, that can provide occasional meals, do your shopping, furnish rides, and help with the periodic family. Don't fall into the trap of believing that the principal caregiver can do it all. Perhaps he or she can, but at what cost?

*Never let being in need distress you.*

Do for yourself whenever you can, communicate honestly with your caregivers as to when you need help and when you do not, and graciously accept the thoughtful acts of others. The concept is actually quite simple: you should embrace being loved.

# The Kind Acts of Others

The loving acts of your friends and family expressing their support for you during this time can be a healing component in your fight against cancer. Using the chart below, keep track of even the smallest thoughtful gesture. Not only will it encourage you to look back at all the wonderful things that others have done for you, but having it recorded will assist you in properly expressing your gratitude. Gifts of love come in all shapes and sizes. Don't forget things like visits, meals, rides, and shopping. You might want to take your address book and thank-you cards to your chemotherapy treatments; it's a perfect way to make the time go by.

DATE:_____

NAME:_____

GIFT OR DEED:_____

ACKNOWLEDGMENT:_____

_____


DATE:_____

NAME:_____

GIFT OR DEED:_____

ACKNOWLEDGMENT:_____

_____


DATE:_____

NAME:_____

GIFT OR DEED:_____

ACKNOWLEDGMENT:_____

_____


DATE:_____

NAME:_____

GIFT OR DEED:_____

ACKNOWLEDGMENT:_____

_____


DATE:_____

NAME:_____

GIFT OR DEED:_____

ACKNOWLEDGMENT:_____

_____


DATE:_____

NAME:_____

GIFT OR DEED:_____

ACKNOWLEDGMENT:_____

_____


DATE:_____

NAME:_____

GIFT OR DEED:_____

ACKNOWLEDGMENT:_____

_____


DATE:_____

NAME:_____

GIFT OR DEED:_____

ACKNOWLEDGMENT:_____

_____


DATE:_____

NAME:_____

GIFT OR DEED:_____

ACKNOWLEDGMENT:_____

_____

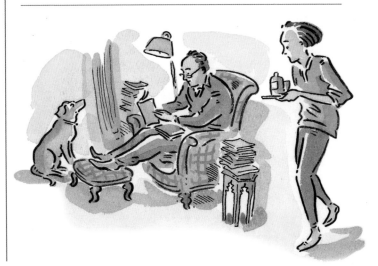

# Being Resilient Helps

Resilience is the ability to get through, get over, and thrive after trauma, trials, and tribulations. The National Cancer Institute has recently called for more study of resilient cancer patients – those who survive the worst-possible odds – to better understand what might work in treating the disease of cancer.

*"The people who are most resilient have a learning reaction, not a victim reaction, to bad events"*

– Al Siebert, Ph.D.

Adapted from *The Survivor Personality* by Al Siebert, Ph.D.

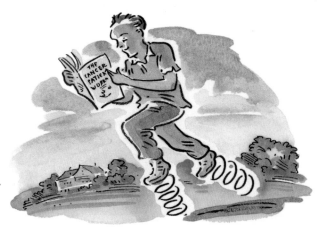

**From 1 to 5, rate how much each of the following applies to you (1= very little, 5= very much).**

**Circle one**

| | 1 | 2 | 3 | 4 | 5 |
|---|---|---|---|---|---|
| 1. Curious, ask questions, want to know how things work, experiment. | 1 | 2 | 3 | 4 | 5 |
| 2. Constantly learn from your experience and the experiences of others. | 1 | 2 | 3 | 4 | 5 |
| 3. Need and expect to have things work well for yourself and others. Take good care of yourself. | 1 | 2 | 3 | 4 | 5 |
| 4. Play with new developments, find the humor. Laugh at self, chuckle. | 1 | 2 | 3 | 4 | 5 |
| 5. Adapt quickly to change, highly flexible. | 1 | 2 | 3 | 4 | 5 |
| 6. Feel comfortable with paradoxical qualities. | 1 | 2 | 3 | 4 | 5 |
| 7. Manage the emotional side of recovery. grieve, honor, and let go of the past. | 1 | 2 | 3 | 4 | 5 |
| 8. Develop better self-esteem and self-confidence every year. Develop a conscious self-concept or professionalism. | 1 | 2 | 3 | 4 | 5 |
| 9. Listen well. Treat others, including difficult people, with empathy. | 1 | 2 | 3 | 4 | 5 |
| 10. Think up creative solutions to challenges, invent ways to solve problems. Trust intuitions and hunches. | 1 | 2 | 3 | 4 | 5 |
| 11. Anticipate problems and avoid difficulties. | 1 | 2 | 3 | 4 | 5 |
| 12. Expect tough situations to work out well, keep on going. Help others, bring stability to times of uncertainly and turmoil. | 1 | 2 | 3 | 4 | 5 |
| 13. Find the gift in accidents and bad experiences. | 1 | 2 | 3 | 4 | 5 |
| 14. Convert misfortune into good fortune. | 1 | 2 | 3 | 4 | 5 |

## SEVEN RESILIENT TRAITS ARE:

- Mental insight
- Intimate relationships
- Strong independence
- Express creativity
- Finding humor
- Taking charge
- Knowing morality

## SCORING YOURSELF

Add the numbers to get your total score.

- If you scored 60–70, you are highly resilient.
- If your score was 50–60, you're better than most people.
- If your score was 40–50, you are considered adequate.
- If your score was 30–40, then you are struggling.
- If your score was under 30, you might want to seek help.

**If your score was under 30, you might want to consider seeking professional help.**

**To improve your resilience, try practicing more of the traits above.**

# Before & After the Diagnosis

What are you willing to do to survive cancer? The commitment to becoming a survivor often requires sacrifice and change at a time in the patient's life when he or she barely has the energy and strength to get through the days. Don't kid yourself though; if you are not willing to give up unhealthy foods, drugs, relationships, habits, cigarettes, alcohol, and other stressful influences in your life, you are really stating that you are only willing to live as long as you don't have to change. Be honest with yourself. What areas need to change? List them below.

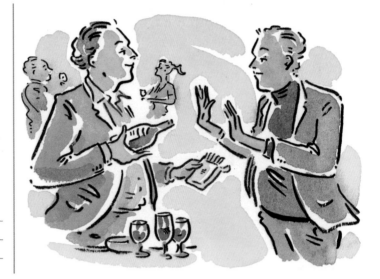

_____

_____

_____

## THE CANCER SURVIVOR TEST

**Check yes or no**

1. I'm unable to express my anger and disappointment.    yes_____  no _____
2. I feel isolated and lonely most of the time.    yes_____  no _____
3. I am not interested in intimacy.    yes_____  no _____
4. I will not consider giving up cigarettes or cigars.    yes_____  no _____
5. I drink heavily and I am not willing to stop.    yes_____  no _____
6. I don't want to put out my family or friends.    yes_____  no _____
7. I'm overweight and I don't care.    yes_____  no _____
8. I don't exercise and I don't plan to.    yes_____  no _____
9. I'm not interested in being proactive in this disease.    yes_____  no _____
10. I do illegal drugs and I don't intend to quit.    yes_____  no _____
11. I'm going to fight this disease with all my energy.    yes_____  no _____
12. I love my life.    yes_____  no _____
13. I will eliminate as much stress from my life as I can.    yes_____  no _____
14. I have long-term goals and dreams.    yes_____  no _____
15. I love my spouse, my children, and my family life.    yes_____  no _____
16. I am confident in my doctors and my treatments.    yes_____  no _____
17. I will take the vitamins and herbs I have researched and believe might be a benefit to my health.    yes_____  no _____
18. I will never miss a treatment if I can help it.    yes_____  no _____
19. I believe I will be one of the people who survives my particular cancer.    yes_____  no _____
20. I will make all the necessary changes in my lifestyle to increase my chances even by a small percent.    yes_____  no _____

## THE BENEFITS OF SCREENING

The American Cancer Society estimates that relative survival for nine screening-accessible cancer sites (breast, tongue, mouth, colon, rectum, cervix, prostate, testis, and melanoma) would increase from 80% to 95% if all Americans had regular cancer screenings.

## SCORING YOURSELF

Obviously questions 1–10 should be a "no" answer and questions 11–20 should be answered "yes." Are they? Make every effort to find help in any area of your life that could use direction and change. Cancer is never a good thing, but with the right attitude and determination valuable transformations can take place for you and your family. Most of us find that it is during trials and tribulations that we improve our lives, come to a deeper understanding of ourselves and others, and grow in uncharted territories.

**You won't be the same person when this experience is over so you might as well be a better one!**

# Goal Setting

*"Laughter solves a lot of problems because it gives you a more positive outlook. Change your outlook and you will change your life."*

– Robert H. Schuller

The process of defining and working toward goals is a popular route to achievement. The purpose of goal setting is to take a large objective and break it down into small tasks that are easy to focus on and accomplish. The success of completing your modest tasks will add up to accomplishing your larger goal. The objective can be anything; good health, a career change, education, retirement, vacation, spiritual renewal, or any dream you feel is meaningful. The significance of goal setting during your battle with cancer is an obvious one. You are looking to set targets for the future that you are determined to meet. Achieving my short-term goals (getting through treatments) has led me to have confidence that I will obtain my long-term goals (seeing my boys graduate from college). Your goals don't have to be elaborate. Sometimes just getting out of bed is task enough for the day.

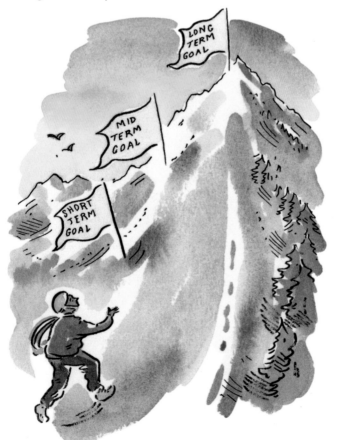

## SHORT-TERM

**Date:** *May, 1998*

**Short-term goal:** *Measure of normality during treatments & surgery.*

**Task #1:** *take a shower and get dressed every day.*

**Task #2:** *accomplish my exercise goals (page 106).*

**Task #3:** *do some kind of housework daily.*

**Task #4:** *eat at least twice a day, have 1 veggie drink.*

**Task #5:** *weekly "something special" with the kids.*

**Goal completed:** *Dec. '98, treatments over, I made it.*

## MID-TERM

**Date:** *May, 1998*

**Mid-term goal:** *Gain strength! Be back to work at least part-time.*

**Task #1:** *take vitamins and herbs three X's a day.*

**Task #2:** *increase my exercise goals (page 106).*

**Task #3:** *daily housework. Yard work once a week.*

**Task #4:** *gain at least 7 pounds.*

**Task #5:** *Twice-weekly "outing" with the kids.*

**Goal completed:** *Jan. 2001, I did it! Working 30 hrs.*

## LONG-TERM

**Date:** *May, 1998*

**Long-term goal:** *Do all those things I've always said I would.*

**Task #1:** *help cancer patients cope with the disease.*

**Task #2:** *see my sons graduate from college.*

**Task #3:** *redecorate our home.*

**Task #4:** *take a long family vacation.*

**Task #5:** *maintain a healthy diet.*

**Goal completed:**

## SHORT-TERM

Date: _____

Short-term goal: _____

_____

Task #1: _____

Task #2: _____

Task #3: _____

Task #4: _____

Task #5: _____

Goal completed: _____

## MID-TERM

Date: _____

Mid-term goal: _____

_____

Task #1: _____

Task #2: _____

Task #3: _____

Task #4: _____

Task #5: _____

Goal completed: _____

## LONG-TERM

Date: _____

Long-term goal: _____

_____

Task #1: _____

Task #2: _____

Task #3: _____

Task #4: _____

Task #5: _____

Goal completed: _____

## SHORT-TERM

Date: _____

Short-term goal: _____

_____

Task #1: _____

Task #2: _____

Task #3: _____

Task #4: _____

Task #5: _____

Goal completed: _____

## MID-TERM

Date: _____

Mid-term goal: _____

_____

Task #1: _____

Task #2: _____

Task #3: _____

Task #4: _____

Task #5: _____

Goal completed: _____

## LONG-TERM

Date: _____

Long-term goal: _____

_____

Task #1: _____

Task #2: _____

Task #3: _____

Task #4: _____

Task #5: _____

Goal completed: _____

# Goal Setting, cont.

## SHORT-TERM

Date: _____

Short-term goal: _____

_____

Task #1: _____

Task #2: _____

Task #3: _____

Task #4: _____

Task #5: _____

Goal completed: _____

## MID-TERM

Date: _____

Mid-term goal: _____

_____

Task #1: _____

Task #2: _____

Task #3: _____

Task #4: _____

Task #5: _____

Goal completed: _____

## LONG-TERM

Date: _____

Long-term goal: _____

_____

Task #1: _____

Task #2: _____

Task #3: _____

Task #4: _____

Task #5: _____

Goal completed: _____

## SHORT-TERM

Date: _____

Short-term goal: _____

_____

Task #1: _____

Task #2: _____

Task #3: _____

Task #4: _____

Task #5: _____

Goal completed: _____

## MID-TERM

Date: _____

Mid-term goal: _____

_____

Task #1: _____

Task #2: _____

Task #3: _____

Task #4: _____

Task #5: _____

Goal completed: _____

## LONG-TERM

Date: _____

Long-term goal: _____

_____

Task #1: _____

Task #2: _____

Task #3: _____

Task #4: _____

Task #5: _____

Goal completed: _____

# Lost & Found

Cancer, with its adverse effects and their aftermath, will not leave you as it found you. Your life and character had been based on being healthy, independent, and at liberty to live as you saw fit. Suddenly you realize that things have changed. Bits and pieces of your basic nature have been shed along the cancer trail and you wonder "who am I now?"

This ongoing process of grieving and yearning for the person you used to be can cause anxiety and distress. Do you miss who you were? Do you see who you've become? It is meaningful and healthy to keep tabs of the transformations in your life. Acknowledge what has ceased to exist and, just as important, the "new-sprung" qualities you have found. Bringing the ever-constant changes to light can dampen the overwhelming perception that you have lost control. Take inventory of yourself. You never know, it might encourage you to become better instead of bitter.

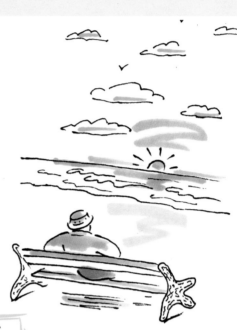

## LOST

Date: June, 1996          Lost: *I miss taking my health & body for granted.*

Date: _____          Lost: _____

Date: _____          Lost: _____

Date: _____          Lost: _____

Date: _____          Lost: _____

Date: _____          Lost: _____

Date: _____          Lost: _____

Date: _____          Lost: _____

Date: _____          Lost: _____

## FOUND

Date: August, 1996          Found: *I cherish the value I put on my days.*

Date: _____          Found: _____

Date: _____          Found: _____

Date: _____          Found: _____

Date: _____          Found: _____

Date: _____          Found: _____

Date: _____          Found: _____

Date: _____          Found: _____

Date: _____          Found: _____

### GRAB A WORD AND WORK WITH IT

| | |
|---|---|
| Miss | Odd |
| Gone | Abnormal |
| Absent | Improved |
| Ache | Better |
| Defeated | Stronger |
| Beaten | Exceed |
| Destroyed | Beat |
| Pain | Relieved |
| Suffer | Benefit |
| Grieve | Surmount |
| Torment | Fortunate |
| Confused | Joyful |
| Puzzled | Lucky |
| Toll | Successful |
| Damage | Committed |
| Soul | Devotion |
| Feelings | Passion |
| Tragic | Cherish |
| Unhappy | Forgive |
| Sad | Pity |
| Melancholy | Mercy |
| Depressed | Kindness |
| Pensive | Feelings |
| Altered | Character |
| Indifferent | Honor |
| Hate | Integrity |
| Remade | Change |

# Richard Bloch's *"Fighting Cancer"*

Richard A. Bloch, cofounder of the worldwide tax preparation company H & R Bloch, Inc., and his wife Annette are my heroes. Richard was diagnosed with "terminal" lung cancer in 1978 and in 1989 with colon cancer. After undergoing various treatments during both bouts with the disease, he and his wife Annette combined their experience and knowledge to write three wonderful, reliable, and comprehensive publications.

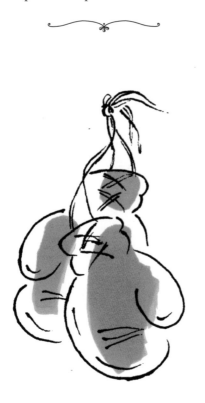

## FIGHTING CANCER CHECKLIST

**Carefully read each statement and place an "X" in the box if it is true.**

☐ I am starting off with a positive mental attitude.

☐ I do not compare myself with anyone else.

☐ I do not think of why I got cancer.

☐ I do not think of why I did not discover my cancer earlier.

☐ I do not think of what caused my cancer.

☐ I really have a strong desire to get well.

☐ I am having my cancer treated as promptly as possible.

☐ I have a doctor who is qualified to treat cancer.

☐ I have a doctor who says he can successfully treat me.

☐ I have a doctor who is totally honest with me.

☐ I have a doctor who takes time to explain everything about my cancer.

☐ I have a doctor who answers all my questions so that I understand.

☐ I appreciate the sacrifices others made so I may take treatments.

☐ I have a doctor who has my complete confidence.

☐ I have a doctor who is giving me a treatment I believe will be successful.

☐ I have gotten a qualified second opinion.

☐ I do not worry about hurting my doctor's feelings.

☐ I make lists of questions to ask my doctor.

☐ I am willing to do anything my doctor says I must.

☐ I take a friend or relative with me when I visit my doctor.

☐ I take a tape recorder when I visit my doctor.

☐ I make every effort to take each treatment on schedule.

☐ I have nothing that is important enough to postpone a cancer treatment for.

☐ I am taking the pain medication the way the doctor recommends.

☐ I am finding out all I can about my disease.

☐ I have called (800) 4-CANCER to find the state-of-the-art therapy on PDQ.

☐ I eat a well-balanced diet.

*More questions on the next page.*

## MORE HYPE THAN SUBSTANCE

Despite the recent popularity of shark cartilage, a study in the *Journal of Clinical Oncology* found that taking shark cartilage pills for 12 weeks had no effect on late-stage cancer patients.

## SIGNS & SYMPTOMS OF ANXIETY

- Faintness
- Twitching
- Sweating
- Dry mouth
- Rapid heart beat

- Muscle tension
- Hoarseness
- Headaches
- Sexual impotence
- Diarrhea

- Difficulty swallowing
- Trembling
- The feeling that something harmful is about to happen

## FIGHTING CANCER CHECKLIST, CONT.

- [ ] I make myself eat enough to maintain my weight.
- [ ] I do not smoke.
- [ ] I have a strong support group of family and/or friends.
- [ ] I let my support group know how much I appreciate and need them.
- [ ] I am happy to answer questions about how I feel.
- [ ] I confide in my support group.
- [ ] I am willing to discuss my problems with my family or friends.
- [ ] I ask my family or friends for help whenever I need it.
- [ ] I continuously state that I am going to do everything to beat this disease.
- [ ] I try to talk out anything that bothers me.
- [ ] I set aside time daily for my personal pleasure.
- [ ] I expose myself to humor and laugh whenever possible.
- [ ] I am being selfish in that I am doing what I believe is best for myself.
- [ ] I give in to myself and rest when I get tired.

- [ ] I lead a full life, trying to keep my activities as close to normal as possible.
- [ ] I exercise regularly.
- [ ] I have pleasant activities planned for whenever I may become depressed.
- [ ] I change my thoughts when I become depressed.
- [ ] I have goals to shoot for and projects to complete.
- [ ] I practice relaxation and imagery 3 times a day.
- [ ] I am finished with any emotional problems I may have had in the past.
- [ ] I believe the good things that have happened to me far outweigh the bad.
- [ ] I say a prayer at least daily.
- [ ] I am confident that when cancer is behind me, it will never come back.
- [ ] I am making plans for things to do when I am well.
- [ ] I am keeping busy and doing everything I am capable of doing.
- [ ] I feel I am in charge.
- [ ] I am doing everything I can to beat my cancer.

## R.A. BLOCH CANCER FOUNDATION, INC.

Over 8,416,080 Americans are alive today with a history of serious cancer because they didn't give up hope and fought their disease. For immediate online access to the three books that Mr. Bloch has written, go to:

**http://www.blochcancer.org/**

You may read the books on-line or print them out. Investigate their other links as well: • Information for patients • Information for supporters • Articles • Programs

---

*"Having cancer is bad enough! Not knowing what to do about it is even worse."*

### CUT, CURL, CANCER?

Hairdressers are at a higher risk of developing salivary gland cancer then the general population. Exposure to chemicals, fumes and spray may be the cause.

*Annuals of Epidemiology*

### FREE BOOKS

**Cancer...There's Hope** is a story of Richard and Annette's fight against his "terminal" lung cancer. **Fighting Cancer** is a step-by-step guide to assist cancer patients in fighting the disease. These two books are both available and may be obtained by calling the Cancer Hot Line at (800) 433-0464. Their latest book, **Guide for Cancer Supporters**, is written to help supporters exclusively and is also available by calling the Cancer Hot Line.

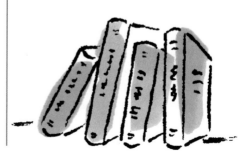

# The 10 Commandments for the Cancer Patient

As we all know, many years ago Moses stumbled down from the mountain with two stone tablets on which were engraved the ten commandments. Or was it Charlton Heston? In any event, new studies have examined the other side of tablet and, lo and behold, we now have the ten commandments for the cancer patient.

*– Edward T. Creagan, M.D.*

I  Thou shalt know thy diagnosis. This involves knowing the name of the cancer under the microscope, the size and grade of the cancer, and whether or not this is viewed as a slow-growing or as an angry process. Without knowing the name of the cancer, one cannot access information about the problem.

II  Thou shalt know thy treatment options. Traditionally, surgery has been the mainstay of treatment for most cancers. However, there is clearly a drift toward less invasive and less mutilating surgeries for cancer patients. Ask the physician about the pros and cons of less invasive techniques. For example, a generation ago, women with breast cancer were treated by a radical mastectomy. Today, the removal of several sugar cubes of breast tissue followed by radiation and chemotherapy provides results equal to or better than more aggressive treatments.

III  Thou shalt know all about chemotherapy. In general, these can be somewhat toxic regimens with significant side effects. What am I buying from chemotherapy? Now what does this mean? Doctors may state that survival is increased by 50 percent by the use of chemotherapy. Now for the bad news: If survival is increased from two months to four months and if those remaining eight weeks are associated with nausea, vomiting, weakness, and fatigue, that may not be a good bargain. Find out exactly what you are "buying" from chemotherapy.

IV  Thou shalt recognize the importance of a second opinion. No one institution and no one physician or healthcare provider can have complete information about all types of cancers. If there is a major cancer center or university that has a particular expertise in your cancer, it certainly makes good sense to seek out a second opinion; almost never will the local physician be offended and if he or she is, that is even more reason to seek out another opinion.

V  Thou shalt acknowledge the importance of a support system. Lots of studies show that friends, families, colleagues, and even pets can enhance the well-being of a cancer patient…and perhaps increase survival, although the latter point is somewhat controversial. A friend or confidante can be an anchor during some stormy times.

VI  Thou shalt acknowledge one's limitations. As a result of surgery, chemotherapy, and radiation, one's energy, vitality, and focus may well diminish. It is not reasonable to continue to work 50 hours a week, reshingle the roof, and put on a dinner party for the south of Iowa while dealing with serious cancer problems. Prioritize, make lists, acknowledge that there are limitations to one's stamina.

VII  Thou shalt know thy medication and previous treatment. It is astonishing that patients take "a little blue pill and a little white pill" and have no understanding about the name of the medications, who prescribed it, or why. This is not a good practice. Likewise, know dosages, schedules, and the names of previous chemotherapy. This will help the doctors provide the best care during a very difficult situation.

VIII  Thou shalt know about hospice programs. During the middle ages, hospices were inns along difficult journeys for the tired traveler. Today, a hospice program focuses on quality of life and comfort care for patients with advanced cancer. Some hospices are physical structures, others are programs taken directly into the patient's home. Ask the American Cancer Society in your neighborhood or your local physician about the importance of hospice programs.

IX  Thou shalt not look back with anger or regret. On Monday morning, everyone is an expert quarterback. This also applies to picking winning stocks! Energies need to be focused on today and not on past events. To ruminate over diagnostic tests or treatments that were not effective simply diffuses energies from the task at hand.

X  Thou shalt be realistic and spend one's time profitably. To fly all over the country and access 17 different opinions from a variety of cancer centers is bewildering, diffusing, and enormously expensive…not only in terms of dollars and cents but in terms of wasted time. One or possibly two confirmatory opinions at the most are more than adequate to provide some reasonable directions for cancer treatment.

## LAUGHTER IS THE BEST MEDICINE!

Research suggests that many systems in your body get a great workout with a boisterous laugh.

- **Respiratory system:** Whole-hearted laughing causes you to take frequent deep breaths and at times lung-cleansing coughs.
- **Immune system:** Laughter increases the number and activity of the natural killer cells that attack some types of cancer/ tumor cells.
- **Cardiovascular system:** When you laugh, both your heart rate and blood pressure go up much like they do during aerobic exercise.

- **Decreases in stress hormones:** Research has suggested that stress hormones responsible for constricting blood vessels and suppressing immune activity are decreased during bouts of laughter.
- **Skeletal-muscular system:** "Fall-down laughter" can be so intense that it makes you weak due to the relaxation of muscles.

> **STOP** If you haven't already done so, take the time right now to skim theentire workbook. Prior knowledge of the chapters will help you ask the right questions.

## JUST FOR THE FUN OF IT — THINGS TO THINK ABOUT

### MYSTERIES OF LIFE

- Why do you need a driver's license to buy liquor when you can't drink and drive?
- Why are there interstate highways in Hawaii?
- Why are there flotation devices under plane seats instead of parachutes?
- Have you ever imagined a world with no hypothetical situations?
- If 7–11 is open 24 hours a day, 365 days a year, why are there locks on the doors?
- You know how most packages say "Open here." What is the protocol if the package says "Open somewhere else"?
- Why do we drive on parkways and park on driveways?
- Why is brassiere singular and panties plural?
- You know that indestructible black box that is used on planes? Why can't they make the whole plane out of the same substance?
- Why is it when you're driving and looking for an address, you turn down the volume on the radio?

### ADVICE FROM THE YOUNG:

- Never trust a dog to watch your food. *Patrick, age 10*
- When your dad is mad and asks you, "Do I look stupid?" don't answer him. *John, 13*
- Never tell your mom her diet's not working. *Michael, 14*
- Don't pull dad's finger when he tells you to. *Emily, 10*
- When your mom is mad at your dad, don't let her brush your hair. *Taylia, 11*
- Don't sneeze in front of mom when you're eating crackers. *Mitchell, 12*
- Puppies still have bad breath even after eating a tic tac. *Andrew, 6*
- Never hold a dust buster and a cat at the same time. *Kyoyo, 10*
- You can't hide a piece of broccoli in a glass of milk. *Aimir, 9*
- If you want a kitten, start out by asking for a horse. *Naomi, 15*
- When you get a bad grade in school, show it to your mom when she's on the phone. *Alyesha, 11*

## COULD THESE BE REAL PRODUCT WARNING LABELS?

- On a cardboard windshield sun shade:
  "Warning: Do Not Drive With Sun Shield in Place."
- On a disposable razor:
  "Do not use this product during an earthquake."
- On a handgun: "Not recommended for use as a nutcracker."
- On a blender: "Not for use as an aquarium."

- On work gloves:
  "For best results, do not leave at crime scene."
- On a microscope:
  "Objects are smaller and less alarming than they appear."
- On a wet suit: "Capacity, 1."

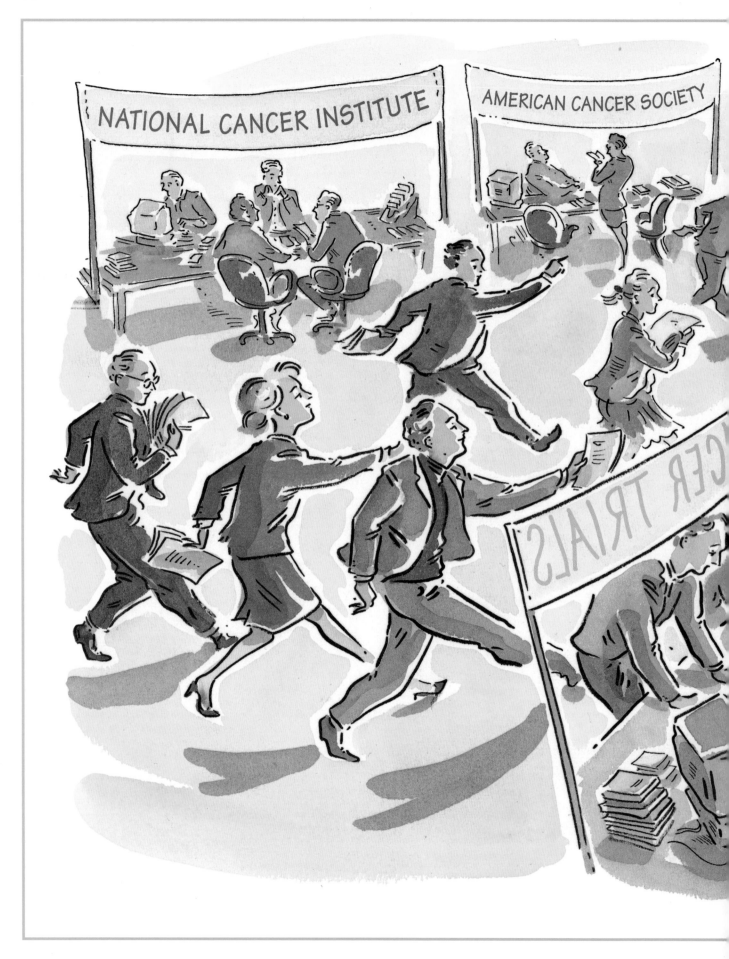

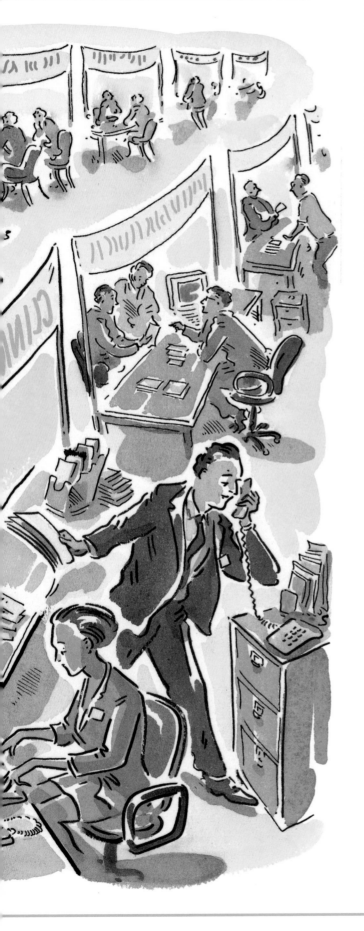

# On Your Mark, Get Set, Go...

*Chapter 2*

# Don't Ever Give Up

You're lying in bed, feeling lousy after treatments, reading this workbook, and wondering what kind of person would be pushing you so hard. Call this place, write that place, research your cancer, look for a clinical trial, make an effort to change what you eat, do this, do that. Surely I must not understand. What gives me the right to suggest such an undertaking?

I'm convinced that my experience with cancer gives me the privilege to encourage you to fight as hard as you can and to believe in the power of hope, will, and miracles. I wish I could be with you right now and tell you my story. I know it would encourage you in your moments of uncertainty. My circumstances were so grave six years ago that I thought of giving up all the time – I just never did.

For 16 years I had worked in a small, close-knit restaurant that had become my home-away-from-home. We were family; loving, supporting, and socializing with one another in and out of work. Our job was so much fun, the bosses so great, the employees so close, the money so good that we were the envy of the whole service industry in our town. No one ever quit. We really loved one another. For years the wisecrack in our community had been that someone "had to die" for a position to open up in our special restaurant.

## SHAKE IT OFF

There once was an old dog that fell into a farmer's well. The farmer sympathized with the dog but decided that neither the dog nor the well were worth the trouble of saving. Instead he decided to bury the old dog in the well and put him out of his misery. As the farmer began shoveling, the old dog became hysterical. But as the farmer continued shoveling and the dirt hit his back, it dawned on him that perhaps he should shake it off and step up. This he did, blow after blow. "Shake it off and step up, shake it off and step up!" he repeated to encourage himself. No matter how painful the blows or how distressing the situation seemed, the old dog fought panic and just kept shaking it off and stepping up. It was not long before the dog, battered and exhausted, stepped triumphantly over the wall of that well. What seemed as if it would bury him actually benefited him – all because of the way he handled his adversity.

## "DOWN TIME" STRETCH

No one wants to spend time in bed wasting the day away, but you may find that some days you feel you just have no other choice. Transform the day into a productive one with very little physical effort. Make a commitment to complete one or two pages in your workbook, place a few phone calls, order some free publications, do some research. Trust me, you'll feel better both about yourself and the day.

Janie Mullins, age 44, was our first coworker to be diagnosed with cancer, beginning a chain of events that few of us has ever really come to terms with. A few months later I was diagnosed with lung cancer. Shortly after, Dee Stewart, age 37, was told she had cancer, and a month or so later Jan Sutherland, age 34, was given her prognosis: cancer. Everyone was in shock. Our coworkers and employers provided the four of us with meals, money, and emotional support. Soon our small island became involved as they immersed themselves in an outpouring of sympathy and assistance for us and our families. Over the next several months our quiet island became stricken with grief as a young boy age 7 and five more women were diagnosed with various cancers. We underwent treatments together, visited one another in the hospital, supported each other on the phone, and comforted each other. One by one each beautiful person lost his or her private battle to cancer. Nine funerals, nine friends gone, nine families without their most precious loved ones. There just are no words to express my heartache and loss. I, of course, was sure that I'd be next.

I know what it is like to think that you might die. I have visited that doorstep hundreds of times. I know what it is to be sick and want to give up; I've been there too.

*The thing is, you just never know and you need to fight as long as there is even a small chance.*

These pages are full of people to call and things to do. It isn't busy work, it's important work and I believe that action is hope. When you feel discouraged and the odds seem stacked against you, think of me. I'm not special. I'm just like you. I just refused to give up...ever.

# Cancer Care, Inc.

Since 1944, Cancer Care has been dedicated to providing emotional support, information, and practical help to people with cancer and their loved ones. As the oldest and largest national nonprofit agency devoted to offering professional services, Cancer Care has helped over a million people nationwide through its toll-free counseling line – (800) 813-HOPE – and teleconference programs, its office-based services, and via the Internet. All services are provided free of charge.

Their staff of professional oncology social workers provides services to people of all ages, with all types of cancer, at any stage of the disease. Cancer Care's reach, including its cancer awareness initiatives, also extends to family members, caregivers, and professionals, providing vital information, assistance, and support.

### What services does Cancer Care offer?

**Counseling and emotional support:** Cancer Care has more than 45 professional oncology social workers on staff who can speak to you over the phone, work with you in a support group, or meet with you in private consultation. They provide emotional support, assist in coping with treatment and its side effects, help you communicate with healthcare providers, and guide you to additional resources.

**Information about cancer and treatment:** People often become overwhelmed when they learn they have cancer and are confused about the meaning of their diagnosis or the options that they have. The Cancer Care staff has extensive information about cancer, diagnosis, and treatment and can help you find even more.

**Referrals to other support services:** If you are calling from a small, rural town or visiting an agency office, Cancer Care will help you find resources in your community that can assist you with things like home care, child care, transportation to and from treatment, pain management, or entitlements. Their Helping Hand Resource Guide is available on their web site.

**Teleconferences, seminars, and workshops:** Cancer Care's teleconferences, seminars, and workshops help those who are facing cancer cope with the day-to-day challenges of the disease. These educational programs provide helpful information and practical assistance to people with cancer, their families, caregivers, and health professionals. (No phone charges apply to teleconferences.)

**Financial guidance:** Cancer can have a devastating impact on a person's financial well-being. Costs related to transportation to and from treatment, pain medication, child care, and home care can be overwhelming for patients and loved ones. Whether it's a referral to a local source of financial assistance, guidance provided in a financial planning workshop, or a stipend, Cancer Care works with patients and their loved ones to help ease the burden of these costs.

---

## HELP AND HOPE

**Cancer Care reaches a variety of populations on a host of cancer-related issues through these special programs:**

- Helping Children Cope
- Adolescent Outreach
- Breast Cancer Awareness and Support
- Prostate Cancer Awareness
- Older Adult

- Lung Cancer Support
- African-American Outreach
- Melanoma Initiative
- Hispanic Outreach Cancer Pain Initiative
- AIDS/HIV Patients with Cancer

- Heart and Soul Spirituality
- Cancer Survivors
- Bereavement Support
- Worksite Counseling and Consultation
- Patient Advocacy

**Cancer Care has over 30 briefs on its web site on the following topics:**

- Cancer, Treatment, and Side Effects
- How to Get Better Medical Care
- Where to Go for Other Kinds of Help
- Talking to Others/Caring for Yourself

- Prevention
- Concerns of People with Advanced Cancer
- Special Series on Lung and Colon Cancer

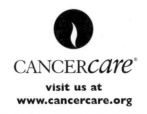

CANCER*care*®

**visit us at**
**www.cancercare.org**

# American Cancer Society

The American Cancer Society is a nationwide, community-based, voluntary health organization dedicated to eliminating cancer as a major health problem by preventing cancer, saving lives from cancer, and diminishing suffering from cancer through research, education, and service.

Millions of cancer patients have been helped either directly or indirectly by the programs, services, and research provided by the ACS. Some of their services are available nationwide, others only in some states or localities. In the box (right) are just a few of the many frontline services that are available to cancer patients and their families. Read through these carefully, write down any other needs or services you may require on the lines below, and then call your local ACS chapter for information and assistance.

In addition to the community programs offered by the American Cancer Society, they contribute other aid and types of assistance as well. There are a number of free pamphlets and brochures to help cancer patients understand and cope with their disease. Topics include: caring for the cancer patient at home, Sexuality and cancer, talking with your doctor, and many others. Call or visit your local ACS office to obtain the free pamphlets. Some ACS chapters also lend videotapes to patients. Furthermore, many ACS chapters provide funds, equipment, and other items. List other needs you have below and inquire if they can provide help in these areas.

1. _____
2. _____
3. _____

If the American Cancer Society cannot help you, it is likely that they will know who in

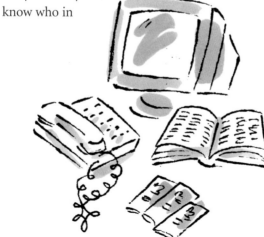

your community can. Write down the organizations and phone numbers they suggest of those able to assist you.

_____ TEL # ( )
_____ TEL # ( )
_____ TEL # ( )

## PROGRAMS AND SERVICES OF THE AMERICAN CANCER SOCIETY

Each ACS chapter differs slighty in what they offer. Call the national office – (800) 227-2345 – for the number of your local ACS chapter.

**Record your local ACS phone number:** ( )_____

**Road to Recovery:** Some ACS units have trained volunteers that transport cancer patients to and from medical treatments, appointments, and hospitals.

**CanSurmount:** Trained volunteers offer one-on-one support to people with cancer and their families.

**I Can Cope:** An educational program for people with cancer and their families. In a series of classes, healthcare providers present information on diagnosis, treatment, communication skills, community resources, and self-care strategies.

**Look Good Feel Better:** In partnership with the Cosmetic, Toiletry, and Fragrance Association Foundation and the National Cosmetology Association, this free public service program is designed to teach women cancer patients beauty techniques that will help restore their appearance and self-image during chemotherapy and radiation treatments.

**Reach to Recovery:** A program designed to help women with the physical, emotional, and cosmetic needs related to breast cancer. Trained volunteers who have experienced breast cancer themselves provide information and support.

**Man to Man:** An educational and support program for men with prostate cancer.

**Project Detect:** A mammogram program for indigent women to ensure that this essential screening is available to everyone who needs it.

**ACS College Scholarship Program:** Only available in Florida and California. The American Cancer Society's College Scholarship program offers college scholarships to qualified students with a history of cancer.

**Lodging Assistance:** For patients who must travel far from home to receive treatment, lodging assistance is sometimes available. In some areas, patients may stay at a Hope Lodge, the American Cancer Society's home-away-from-home for patients and a family member.

# National Cancer Institute

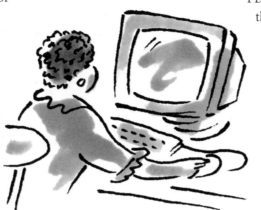

The National Cancer Institute (NCI), a division of the National Institutes of Health, is the federal government's principal agency for cancer research and training. The NCI supports a wide range of cancer research and information services, including the construction of laboratories and clinics; collection and dissemination of information; direction of a national network of cancer centers; support of clinical cancer trials; and coordination of research projects conducted by hospitals, universities, and research foundations through research grants and cooperative agreements. The National Cancer Program, coordinated by the NCI, also conducts and supports clinical research, training, the dissemination of health information, and other programs relating to the cause, diagnosis, prevention, and treatment of cancer, rehabilitation from cancer, and the continuing care of cancer patients and their families. The Cancer Information Service, with fourteen regional offices, is operated by the federal government and supported by the NCI. To request the latest information on state-of-the-art research, treatments, and clinical trials for your specific cancer, call the NCI at (800) 4-CANCER It only takes a few minutes and I think it's one of the most important steps you can take.

**Tell them:**
- Your name
- Your address
- Your age
- Your type of cancer

**Ask for any of the following information to be sent to you:**
- Information on your type of cancer
- Information on the latest treatments
- Information on clinical trials
- Information on financial aid
- Information on board-certified cancer specialists in your geographic region

## What Is PDQ?

PDQ is the computer service of the National Cancer Institute (NCI) designed specifically for the use of people who have been diagnosed with cancer, their families, and for doctors, nurses, and other healthcare professionals. PDQ gives up-to-date information on cancer and its prevention, detection, treatment, and supportive care, and provides information about doctors who treat cancer, research on new treatments (clinical trials), and hospitals with cancer programs. All PDQ cancer information summaries are peer-reviewed and updated monthly by five editorial boards of oncology specialists in the following areas: adult treatment, pediatric treatment, supportive care, screening and prevention, and cancer genetics. These specialists review current literature from more than 70 biomedical journals, evaluate its relevance, and synthesize it into clear summaries that are provided on their web site.

PDQ's Physician Directory includes the names, addresses, and telephone numbers of more than 22,000 physicians. These physicians are members of 30 professional societies, clinical investigators with protocols listed on the PDQ site, recipients of NCI grants, or members of clinical cooperative groups.

PDQ's Organization Directory includes a listing of healthcare organizations with cancer care programs, including NCI-designated comprehensive and clinical cancer centers; community clinical oncology programs; clinical trial groups; and members of the Association of Community Cancer Centers.

PDQ contains the world's most comprehensive cancer clinical trials database. It includes approximately 1,700 abstracts of trials that are open/active and approved for patient accrual (accepting patients), including trials for cancer treatment, diagnosis, supportive care, screening, and prevention.

# Clinical Trials

Clinical trials are studies that evaluate the effectiveness of new treatments for a wide range of medical conditions, including virtually every type of cancer. Each year, the National Cancer Institute works with 10,000 scientists and 20,000 patients enrolled in such research. Many successful treatments have emerged as the direct result of clinical trials. However, the misperception that clinical trials are simply scientific experiments results in only about five percent of cancer patients participating in research studies. In most cases, the new treatments that are being tested have already shown promise of being an improvement over the current therapy and are often being tested to see how much better they perform. Clinical trials may be a patient's best chance for survival.

**The potential benefits of participating in a clinical trial are as follows:**

• Your health care will be provided by the leading physicians in the field of cancer.
• You will have an active role in your own health care.
• You may be the first to benefit from a new treatment.
• You will be very closely monitored.
• You will be making a valuable contribution to the body of cancer research.

**The potential risks of participating in a clinical trial are as follows:**

• There may be unknown side effects or risks that doctors have not yet discovered.
• Side effects and results may be worse than with conventional therapy.
• The treatment may benefit many patients but possibly not you.
• Additional costs to the patient during the trial may not be covered by the insurance company. Research costs are covered by the organization conducting the study.

Promising drugs, gene therapy, immune vaccines, and new advances are underway in hospitals, clinics, cancer centers, pharmaceutical labs, physicians' offices, and military hospitals across the country. The good news is that research has begun to focus on unconventional approaches to treating cancer, replacing the traditional chemotherapy that kills all cells, whether healthy or ill.

*The latest therapies are proving effective and are less detrimental to the patient, causing fewer side effects and less damage to the body.*

I believe that everyone, without exception, should research the clinical trials that are being done for their type of cancer. You may locate a trial in which you absolutely believe and want to participate in rather than following the recommended therapy. Alternatively, you might find yourself in the tough situation of a previous therapy failing and requiring a new and different treatment, or you may decide that a vaccine or additional therapy following the conventional or recommended treatment would give you the peace of mind of future protection. Either way, it is important that you investigate all of the options available to you.

## CLINICAL TRIAL TERMINOLOGY

**Bias:** Patients joining a study are randomly chosen by computer as to which group they will be in so that no human bias will affect the results.

**Control group:** The group of patients receiving the standard treatment.

**Double blind study**: A trial in which neither the patients or the physicians know whether they are in the control or treatment group.

**Placebo:** Some studies compare a new drug with a pill that looks like the real drug but contains no active medication. Rarely used.

**Protocol:** Strict scientific guidelines prepared by the chief investigator for each trial is called a protocol. These guidelines include:

• How many participants will be in the study;
• Who is eligible;
• What drugs will be tested;
• What medical tests they will have and how often;
• What information will be collected.

**Randomization:** The process of being chosen by chance for the new intervention or the standard treatment.

**Treatment group:** The group of patients receiving the new intervention.

# Finding the Right Trial

The first step in finding a clinical trial should be to inquire of your cancer specialist whether or not he or she knows of a study that might benefit you. The second step is to begin a search on your own since no one doctor can possibly know of all the studies currently being done. Strive to locate at least two studies that look promising to you. Discuss the abstracts (brief summaries) with your doctor, who will be able to determine whether or not you meet the eligibility requirements and may want to contact the principle investigator to obtain more information about the trial. Call the Cancer Information Service or go online for abstracts of clinical trials (page 35).

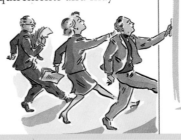

### TALKING ABOUT CLINICAL TRIALS

- **Rationale:** The explanation of why researchers are conducting the trial.
- **Purpose:** The description of what type of trial is being conducted, what treatment and tests will be preformed, and the reason for the study.
- **Eligibility:** The requirements (type and stage of cancer, age, health conditions, and previous therapy) for the patient to be admitted into the study.
- **Treatment summary:** A description of the type of treatment, how often it will be given, and how long it will last.
- **Investigator:** The person for you or your doctor to contact for information, answers, and enrollment in the trial.

---

Date: _____ Name of study: _____ Phase: _____

Participating organization/investigators: _____

Chair phone #: _____     Location of trial: _____

Principle investigator: _____     Phone #: _____

Eligibility for trial: 1} _____  2} _____  3} _____

4} _____  5} _____  6} _____

Rationale: _____

Purpose: _____

Treatment summary: _____

---

Date: _____ Name of study: _____ Phase: _____

Participating organization/investigators: _____

Chair phone #: _____     Location of trial: _____

Principle investigator: _____     Phone #: _____

Eligibility for trial: 1} _____  2} _____  3} _____

4} _____  5} _____  6} _____

Rationale: _____

Purpose: _____

Treatment summary: _____

# Questions to Ask *about a Clinical Trial*

Once you and your doctor have found a study you believe is suitable for you, call the principle investigator. The questions below will aid you in making your final decision. Write down your answers so that you will recall what has been discussed.

1   WHAT IS THE PURPOSE OF THIS STUDY?
_____
_____

2   HOW MANY PARTICIPANTS ARE IN THIS STUDY?
_____
_____

3   WHY DO YOU THINK THIS TREATMENT WILL BE EFFECTIVE?
_____
_____

4   WHAT WILL I HAVE TO DO IF I DECIDE TO PARTICIPATE?
_____
_____

5   HOW LONG WILL THE STUDY LAST?
_____
_____

6   HOW IS THE SAFETY OF THE PARTICIPANTS MONITORED?

## WHEN YOU TALK TO YOUR DOCTOR ABOUT CLINICAL CANCER TRIALS

**Remember to:**
- Take a family member or friend to help ask questions.
- Bring a tape recorder.
- Take a list of prepared questions, but if new questions come up during your discussion, don't hesitate to ask them.
- Write down the answers to your questions so that you can review them at a later date.
- Don't leave the office without all your questions answered.
- Be sure to ask your doctor for his or her gut reaction to the trial and the probability of it affecting your individual circumstances.

7   WHAT ARE THE RESULTS OF THE STUDY SO FAR?
_____
_____

8   WHAT ARE THE SIDE EFFECTS?
_____

9   WHAT ARE THE POSSIBLE SHORT-TERM RISKS?
_____

10   WHAT ARE THE POSSIBLE LONG-TERM RISKS?
_____

11   WHAT KIND OF THERAPIES WILL I HAVE DURING THE TRIAL?
_____

12   WHAT KIND OF PROCEDURES ARE INCLUDED IN THE TRIAL?
_____

13   WILL IT HURT AND, IF SO, FOR HOW LONG?
_____

14   WHERE WILL THE TESTS BE GIVEN?
_____

15   WHERE WILL I RECEIVE MY MEDICAL CARE?
_____

16   WHO WILL BE IN CHARGE OF MY CARE DURING THE STUDY?
_____

**HELP ONLINE:** The NCI has made searching for an ideal clinical trial fast, comprehensive, and downright easy.
**cnetdb.nci.nih.gov/trialsrch.shtml**

## BENEFITS VS. RISKS

Once you have found a study that you are seriously considering, ask about the potential benefits of this particular study:

1. _____
2. _____
3. _____
4. _____

Investigate the known risks that have been noted to date in this specific study. Weigh the risks listed below against the benefits.

1. _____
2. _____
3. _____
4. _____

**17** WHAT IS THEIR PHONE NUMBER?

_____

**18** WHO WILL BE IN CHARGE OF MY CARE AFTER THE STUDY?

_____

_____

**19** HOW WILL THIS STUDY AFFECT MY DAILY LIFE?

_____

_____

**20** WILL I HAVE TO PAY FOR ANY TESTS DURING THE STUDY?

_____

_____

**21** WILL I HAVE TO PAY FOR ANY DRUGS DURING THE STUDY?

_____

_____

**22** WHAT IS MY HEALTH INSURANCE LIKELY TO COVER?

_____

_____

**23** CAN THE TREATMENT BE ADMINISTERED TO ME LOCALLY OR WILL I NEED TO GO TO THE CANCER RESEARCH CENTER?

_____

_____

**24** WILL I HAVE TO TRAVEL?

_____

**25** WILL I BE HOSPITALIZED DURING THE TREATMENTS?

_____

_____

**26** IF SO, FOR HOW LONG?

_____

_____

**27** WILL I TAKE MY REGULAR MEDICATIONS DURING THE TRIAL?

_____

_____

**28** WHAT WILL MY FOLLOW-UP CARE BE?

_____

_____

**29** HOW WILL I KNOW IF THE TREATMENT WORKED?

_____

_____

**30** OTHER QUESTIONS

_____

## PHASES OF CLINICAL TRIALS

When research on a new drug has been completed in experimental laboratories, the study progresses to clinical trial phases involving humans. Each phase answers different questions for scientists.

**Phase I:** This is the first step in evaluating a new cancer treatment in patients. Phase 1 trials usually enroll a very small number of patients who would not be helped by other known treatments. Researchers look for the best way to administer the new treatment, the dosage, the timing, and the safety of the drug.

**Phase 2:** These trials focus on the new treatment's anticancer effects, its safety, and how the drug works.

**Phase 3:** Studies that have moved into phase 3 testing have generally shown promise. This phase typically involves a large number of participants. The patients who are receiving the new treatment are compared with those who are receiving the standard conventional therapy. The study concentrates on which patients have the better survival rates and fewer side effects.

**OTHER CLINICAL TRIALS:** This is a very complete site of other clinical trials throughout the country.
**www.oncolink.upenn.edu/clinical_trials/other_info.html**

# Insurance Information

There are some 58 million HMO members, 91 million PPO members, 39 million Medicare members, and 34 million Medicaid members. There are Cobra Plans, Medigap, Disability Income Insurance, POS Plans, Longterm Care Plans, MedSupp, group and individual policies. Had enough? Even on a good day insurance can be confusing. In a healthcare crisis it is invaluable to understand your coverage. If you have questions, don't hesitate to call your insurance agent.

*"Most people cower in front of insurance companies – I want them to clamor for their rights."*

*– Dorthy Cantor, Psy.d., a psychologist in Westfield, NJ and past president of the American Psychology Society*

Membership effective date: _____

Name of insurance company: _____

Local phone #: _____

Toll-free phone #: _____

Name of agent: _____

Type of policy (HMO, PPO): _____

Group/contract holder #: _____

Subscriber/insured number: _____

Is it a group or individual policy?_____

Claim number: _____

Total monthly premium: $ _____

Deductible: $_____

## OUTPATIENT BENEFITS

$ _____    co-pay or % co-insurance per office visit for your primary care physician.

$ _____    co-pay or % co-insurance per office visit for your specialist physician.

$ _____    co-pay or % co-insurance per office visit for outpatient rehabilitation.

$ _____    co-pay or % co-insurance per hospital outpatient visit.

$ _____    co-pay or % co-insurance per diagnostic testing.

$ _____    co-pay or % co-insurance per office visit for outpatient emergency services.

$ _____    co-pay or % co-insurance per office visit for mental health visits.

$ _____    co-pay or % co-insurance for ambulance service.

$ _____    co-pay or % co-insurance per office visit for outpatient surgery.

$ _____    co-pay or % co-insurance for wellness care (includes annual eye exam, physical, etc.)

$ _____    co-pay or % co-insurance for dental care.

What % do I pay after my deductible is met? _____%

What are my total costs (out-of-pocket expenses) for the calendar year? (co-pays are not included)$ _____

What is the maximum lifetime benefit/cap (if any)? $ _____

## COMMON REASONS CLAIMS ARE DENIED

**1: Doctor error:** Doctors can mistakenly write in wrong codes or make other errors on the insurance forms.

**2: Out of network:** Some companies will deny your claim if you get medical treatment from a doctor or hospital that is "out" of your insurance plan "network."

**3: Not medically necessary:** An insurance claims processor can deny your claim, ruling that the procedure or service was not "medically necessary."

**4: Preexisting conditions:** Some policies use the term "preexisting" to describe a condition that was diagnosed and treated before the insurance policy went into effect. Other policies state that just having the symptoms prior to the plan's effective date constitutes a preexisting condition.

**5: Non-covered benefit:** Your insurance policy includes a list of services that are NOT covered. Most plans have an appeals process that both you and your doctor can use if you disagree with the plan's findings. Do not pay medical bills until you feel the insurance company has paid everything it should.

## INPATIENT BENEFITS

$ _____ co-pay or % co-insurance for acute care/inpatient hospital care.

$ _____ co-pay or % co-insurance for hospice care.

$ _____ co-pay or % co-insurance for a skilled nursing facility.

$ _____ co-pay or % co-insurance for acute care/inpatient hospital care.

## PRESCRIPTION DRUGS

$ _____ co-pay or % co-insurance for brand-name prescription drugs.

$ _____ co-pay or % co-insurance for generic prescription drugs.

Each prescription is limited to a _____ day supply.

THE DETAILED DIFFERENCE BETWEEN ONE INSURANCE PLAN AND ANOTHER CAN ONLY BE UNDERSTOOD BY CAREFUL READING OF THE POLICY AND MATERIALS PROVIDED TO YOU ABOUT YOUR COVERAGE. TAKE THE TIME TO COMPREHEND YOUR POLICY. DOING SO WILL NOT ONLY SAVE YOU HEADACHES BUT MAY SAVE YOU MONEY AS WELL.

## ODDS & ENDS

How much more will I pay to use a doctor outside my plan's network? _____

Do I need a referral or preauthorization for specialized health care and treatment? _____

Are second opinions covered? _____

What hospitals in my area are covered by my plan?

_____

Will home health care be provided if needed? _____

_____

If so, what is the $ _____ co-pay or % co-insurance.

If I decide on a clinical trial, what, if anything, will my insurance plan cover? _____

How do I file claims? _____

_____

## INSURANCE CORRESPONDENCE

Date: _____

Time: _____

Name of phone contact: _____

Question, issue, dispute, or problem being discussed:

_____

_____

_____

Outcome: _____

_____

_____

Date: _____

Time: _____

Name of phone contact: _____

Question, issue, dispute, or problem being discussed:

_____

_____

_____

Outcome: _____

_____

_____

## BE SURE YOU KEEP A WRITTEN RECORD OF

• **All correspondence with your insurance company.**

• **Claims forms and copies of bills.**

• **Phone conversations – the date and time, the people you speak with, and the nature of each call.**

Contact the member services division of your plan for information or for a grievance. If you have a dispute, you may decide to bring the matter to the attention of your employee benefits manager, your state insurance commissioner, your state department of health, or the legal system. If you are a Medicare or Medicaid beneficiary, there are additional ways to file a grievance. For information, contact your state's Medical Peer Review Organization or State Medicaid Program.

# Recording Medical Expenses

The next several pages are designed for you to keep track of all your medical expenses during the calendar year. Begin keeping records as soon as you possibly can. If you do not have all of your receipts for the year, simply call your doctors and pharmacies and ask that your current patient history expense sheet be mailed to you. Knowing what you've spent in healthcare costs in one year can save you money in tax returns, insurance reimbursements, and insurance annual caps. Keep records for tax purposes if you don't have insurance.

## Tax Deductions:

The intention of this section is to inform you of the basics of medical tax deductions and to organize your records of what you have spent in a given calendar year. You can include all medical expenses, mental illness costs, transportation to medical care, the portion of medical insurance you pay, prescription drugs, medical supplies and equipment, and dental expenses. You cannot include medical expenses that were paid by your insurance company or other sources, and you must deduct all

reimbursements paid to you by your insurance company. You can deduct only the amount of your medical and dental expenses that exceeds 7.5 percent of your adjusted gross income. Example: Your adjusted gross income is $40,000, 7.5 percent of which is $3,000. You paid $1,600 after deducting insurance reimbursements. You cannot deduct any of your medical expenses because they are less than 7.5 percent of your adjusted gross income. Write everything down, keep all receipts together, and call the IRS if you have questions.

### TRAVEL EXPENSES

Save gas, toll, hotel, meal, and airline receipts for expenditures getting to and from medical care. Total your receipts monthly and enter the paid out amount below.

January: _____   Amount $ _____

February: _____   Amount $ _____

March: _____   Amount $ _____

April: _____   Amount $ _____

May: _____   Amount $ _____

June: _____   Amount $ _____

July: _____   Amount $ _____

August: _____   Amount $ _____

September: _____   Amount $ _____

October: _____   Amount $ _____

November: _____   Amount $ _____

December: _____   Amount $ _____

**Date:** _____   **Yearly total paid:** _____

### INSURANCE PREMIUM PAYMENTS

Record only the amount of money you pay toward your insurance policy and no more. What your employer pays does not go toward your tax deduction because it is considered an employment benefit.

Date:_____   Amount $_____
Premium paid to _____

Date:_____   Amount $_____
Premium paid to _____

Date:_____   Amount $_____
Premium paid to _____

Date:_____   Amount $_____
Premium paid to _____

Date:_____   Amount $_____
Premium paid to _____

Date:_____   Amount $_____
Premium paid to _____

Date:_____   Amount $_____
Premium paid to _____

Date:_____   Amount $_____
Premium paid to _____

Date:_____   Amount $_____
Premium paid to _____

Date:_____   Amount $_____
Premium paid to _____

Date:_____   Amount $_____
Premium paid to _____

## ANNUAL DEDUCTIBLE

Some policies state that you owe an annual deductible (such as $500) before the insurer starts paying. After you have met the deductible, most plans begin to pay a percentage of what they consider the "Usual and customary" charge for covered services. If you have a deductible, record the expenditures below, being attentive to when your deductible is met.

Date: _____ Policy deductible: $ _____

Date: _____ Doctor: _____

Reason for visit: _____

Amount paid:_____

Date: _____ Doctor: _____

Reason for visit: _____

Amount paid:_____

Date: _____ Doctor: _____

Reason for visit: _____

Amount paid:_____

Date: _____ Doctor: _____

Reason for visit: _____

Amount paid:_____

Date: _____ Doctor: _____

Reason for visit: _____

Amount paid:_____

Date: _____ Doctor: _____

Reason for visit: _____

Amount paid:_____

Date: _____ Deductible met: $ _____

## CO-INSURANCE

The portion of the covered medical expenses you pay is called co-insurance. Most policies state that once the patient's annual deductible is met the insurance company will reimburse the doctors at 80% of the "Usual and customary" costs and you pay the other 20% (known as co-insurance). If the doctor/provider charges more than the "Usual and customary" rate, you will have to pay both the co-insurance and the difference. Be sure to record all of your medical expenditures.

Date: _____ Doctor: _____

Reason for visit: _____

Amount paid:_____

Date: _____ Doctor: _____

Reason for visit: _____

Amount paid:_____

Date: _____ Doctor: _____

Reason for visit: _____

Amount paid:_____

Date: _____ Doctor: _____

Reason for visit: _____

Amount paid:_____

Date: _____ Doctor: _____

Reason for visit: _____

Amount paid:_____

Date: _____ Doctor: _____

Reason for visit: _____

Amount paid:_____

Date: _____ Doctor: _____

Reason for visit: _____

Amount paid:_____

Date: _____ Doctor: _____

Reason for visit: _____

Amount paid:_____

Date: _____ Doctor: _____

Reason for visit: _____

Amount paid:_____

Date: _____ Doctor: _____

Reason for visit: _____

Amount paid:_____

Date: _____ Doctor: _____

Reason for visit: _____

Amount paid:_____

Date: _____ Doctor: _____

Reason for visit: _____

Amount paid:_____

Date: _____ Subtotal paid out $_____

Date: _____ Yearly total paid out $ _____

# Recording Medical Expenses, cont.

## CO-PAYS

Your co-payment is a predetermined flat fee that you pay for your healthcare services in addition to what your insurance pays for your treatment. For example, your co-payment may be $10 for a primary doctor visit, $25 for a diagnostic test, $5 for a prescription, and so on. Keep an account of all monies you have paid out.

Date: _____ Doctor: _____ Reason for visit: _____ Co-pay paid: $ _____

Date: _____ Doctor: _____ Reason for visit: _____ Co-pay paid: $ _____

Date: _____ Doctor: _____ Reason for visit: _____ Co-pay paid: $ _____

Date: _____ Doctor: _____ Reason for visit: _____ Co-pay paid: $ _____

Date: _____ Doctor: _____ Reason for visit: _____ Co-pay paid: $ _____

Date: _____ Doctor: _____ Reason for visit: _____ Co-pay paid: $ _____

**Date:** _____ **Subtotal paid out: $** _____

Date: _____ Doctor: _____ Reason for visit: _____ Co-pay paid: $ _____

Date: _____ Doctor: _____ Reason for visit: _____ Co-pay paid: $ _____

Date: _____ Doctor: _____ Reason for visit: _____ Co-pay paid: $ _____

Date: _____ Doctor: _____ Reason for visit: _____ Co-pay paid: $ _____

Date: _____ Doctor: _____ Reason for visit: _____ Co-pay paid: $ _____

Date: _____ Doctor: _____ Reason for visit: _____ Co-pay paid: $ _____

**Date:** _____ **Subtotal paid out: $** _____

Date: _____ Doctor: _____ Reason for visit: _____ Co-pay paid: $ _____

Date: _____ Doctor: _____ Reason for visit: _____ Co-pay paid: $ _____

Date: _____ Doctor: _____ Reason for visit: _____ Co-pay paid: $ _____

Date: _____ Doctor: _____ Reason for visit: _____ Co-pay paid: $ _____

Date: _____ Doctor: _____ Reason for visit: _____ Co-pay paid: $ _____

Date: _____ Doctor: _____ Reason for visit: _____ Co-pay paid: $ _____

**Date:** _____ **Yearly total paid out: $** _____

## PRESCRIPTION CHARGES

Insurance policies differ in the coverage of outpatient prescription drugs. You may have a co-pay or co-insurance fee for your medications. Document all co-pays and co-insurance charges for your drugs.

Date: _____ Doctor: _____

Reason for prescription: _____

Amount paid: _____

Date: _____ Doctor: _____

Reason for prescription: _____

Amount paid: _____

Date: _____ Doctor: _____

Reason for prescription: _____

Amount paid: _____

**Date:** _____ **Subtotal paid out $** _____

Date: _____ Doctor: _____

Reason for prescription: _____

Amount paid: _____

Date: _____ Doctor: _____

Reason for prescription: _____

Amount paid: _____

Date: _____ Doctor: _____

Reason for prescription: _____

Amount paid: _____

**Date:** _____ **Yearly total paid out $** _____

*4.56*  *16.95*  *4.52*  *8.57*

## YEARLY OUT-OF-POCKET

Most insurance policies have an "out-of-pocket" annual maximum. This means that once your total medical expenses have reached a certain amount in a given calendar year, the "Usual and customary" fee for covered benefits will be paid in full by the insurer and you will no longer pay the co-insurance. Periodically total your "out-of-pocket" expenditures to make sure that your insurance company begins to pick up 100% of your medical bills once you have reached your maximum.

"Out of pocket" annual maximum:     $ _____

Annual policy deductible paid out: $ _____

Annual co-insurance paid out:     $ _____

Annual co-pay paid out:     $ _____

Annual prescription charges:     $ _____

Miscellaneous:     $ _____

Total "out-of-pocket" paid out:     $ _____

**If you have any doubts or questions, call the Internal Revenue Service at (800) 829-1040.**

## REIMBURSEMENTS

A reimbursement is the money that you personally receive back from your insurance provider for the money you have paid out in medical care. The total amount of the reimbursements that your insurance company pays will be deducted from your yearly medical expenses for tax purposes. Record them below.

Date: _____ Reimbursement amount $ _____

Date: _____ Reimbursement amount $ _____

Date: _____ Reimbursement amount $ _____

Date: _____ Reimbursement amount $ _____

Date: _____ Reimbursement amount $ _____

Date: _____ Reimbursement amount $ _____

Date: _____ Reimbursement amount $ _____

**Date: _____ Total received: _____**

Keep your medical receipts together. When requested by the IRS you must be able to substantiate your deductions with a statement or itemized invoice showing the nature of the expense, for whom it was incurred, the amount paid, and the date of payment.

## COVERED MEDICAL SERVICES

- Inpatient hospital services
- Outpatient surgery
- Physician hospital visit
- Doctors' office visits
- Skilled nursing care
- Medical & lab tests
- Prescription drugs
- Mental health care
- Drug and alcohol abuse treatment
- Home health care
- Rehabilitation care
- Physical therapy
- Speech therapy
- Hospice care
- Maternity care
- Chiropractic services
- Preventive care and checkups
- Dental care
- Lodging ($50 a night) & meals while out of town for medical care
- Home improvements for the disabled
- Eyeglasses & contacts
- Hearing aids
- Oxygen
- Special care equipment
- Ambulance
- Acupuncture
- Artificial limbs
- Nursing home care

## MEDICAL DEDUCTIONS

**For the year of** _____

Go back through pages 40–45 and record the totals for money paid out in the spaces provided below.

Premium payments total paid:     $ _____

Travel expenses total paid:     $ _____

Annual insurance deductible:     $ _____

Co-insurance total paid:     $ _____

Co-pay total paid:     $ _____

Prescription charges total paid:     $ _____

Total:     $ _____

Subtract reimbursements paid:     $ _____

**Yearly total paid out:**     $ _____

**Yearly gross income:**     $ _____

x 7.5% $ _____

If the money that you have paid out after reimbursements is more than 7.5% of your yearly gross income, you can use the entire amount as a tax deduction.

# Phone & Fax Numbers

Throughout your treatments and follow-up visits you will be required to supply certain phone and fax numbers to the medical facilities performing diagnostic tests and offering clinical trials. For your convenience, record these important numbers in the space provided below.

## FAMILY DOCTOR

Name: _____

Phone #: _____

Fax #: _____

## ONCOLOGIST

Name: _____

Phone #: _____

Fax #: _____

## SURGEON

Name: _____

Phone #: _____

Fax #: _____

## RADIATION ONCOLOGIST

Name: _____

Phone #: _____

Fax #: _____

## PHARMACY

Name: _____

Phone #: _____

Fax #: _____

## PHYSICAL THERAPIST

Name: _____

Phone #: _____

Fax #: _____

## HOME HEALTH CARE

Name: _____

Phone #: _____

Fax #: _____

## INSURANCE COMPANY

Name: _____

Phone #: _____

Fax #: _____

## MEDICARE/MEDICAID

Name: _____

Phone #: _____

Fax #: _____

## CANCER SUPPORT GROUP

Name: _____

Phone #: _____

Fax #: _____

## HEALTH FOOD STORE

Name: _____

Phone #: _____

Fax #: _____

## HOPE HOSPICE

Name: _____

Phone #: _____

Fax #: _____

## POLICE

Name: _____

Phone #: _____

Fax #: _____

## AMBULANCE

Name: _____

Phone #: _____

Fax #: _____

## FIRE DEPARTMENT

Name: _____

Phone #: _____

Fax #: _____

You will no doubt end up with many different cards over the next few months associated with your health care. Many cancer centers and clinics give patients an ID number and card. Note the ID numbers for each of the following, just in case you misplace the cards themselves or neglect to bring them with you to an appointment. Do not, however, record your credit card numbers in this workbook in case you lose or misplace it.

Oncologist patient #: _____

Radiation oncologist patient #: _____

Surgeon patient #: _____

Cancer center patient #: _____

Clinical trial patient #:_____

Prescription card #: _____

Insurance card #: _____

## CANCER CENTERS BY GEOGRAPHIC REGION

Even though you could be eligible for numerous clinical trials in different parts of the country, you may decide that one of the most important factors to participating in a clinical trial is staying close to home. If this is the case, consider starting your clinical trial search by looking first in the geographical region where you live. If little is available in your region, then expand your search to areas where family and friends live. The NCI provides a map online that shows NCI-sponsored Cancer Centers.

**http://cancertrials.nci.nih.gov/finding/centers/ html/map.html**

If you lose this workbook you will want it returned to you as soon as possible. Complete your medical history on page 77; this will serve as a useful reference whenever you visit a new doctor as well.

**STOP**

## JUST FOR THE FUN OF IT

**These are actual excerpts from student science exam papers:**

- The theory of evolution was greatly objected to because it made man think.
- Three kinds of blood vessels are arteries, vanes, and caterpillars.
- The process of turning steam back into water again is called conversation.
- A magnet is something you find crawling all over a dead cat.
- The Earth makes one resolution every 24 hours.
- To collect fumes of sulfur, hold a deacon over a flame in a test tube.
- Parallel lines never meet, unless you bend one or both of them.
- Algebraical symbols are used when you do not know what you are talking about.
- Geometry teaches us to bisex angles.
- A circle is a line which meets its other end without ending.

- The pistol of a flower is its only protection against insects.
- The moon is a planet just like the Earth, only it is even deader.
- English sparrows and starlings eat the farmers grain and soil his corpse.
- A super-saturated solution is one that holds more than it can hold.
- Blood flows down one leg and up the other.
- The hookworm larvae enters the human body through the soul.
- When you haven't got enough iodine in your blood you get a glacier.
- It is a well-known fact that a deceased body harms the mind.
- For fractures: to see if the limb is broken, wiggle it gently back and forth.
- For dog bite: put the dog away for several days. If he has not recovered, then kill it.

- For nosebleed: put the nose much lower than the body.
- For drowning: climb on top of the person and move up and down to make artificial perspiration.
- To remove dust from the eye, pull the eye down over the nose.
- For head colds: use an agonizer to spray the nose until it drops in your throat.
- For asphyxiation: apply artificial respiration until the patient is dead.
- Before giving a blood transfusion, find out if the blood is affirmative or negative.
- Bar magnets have north and south poles, horseshoe magnets have east and west poles.
- When water freezes you can walk on it. That is what Christ did long ago in wintertime.
- When you smell an odorless gas, it is probably carbon monoxide.

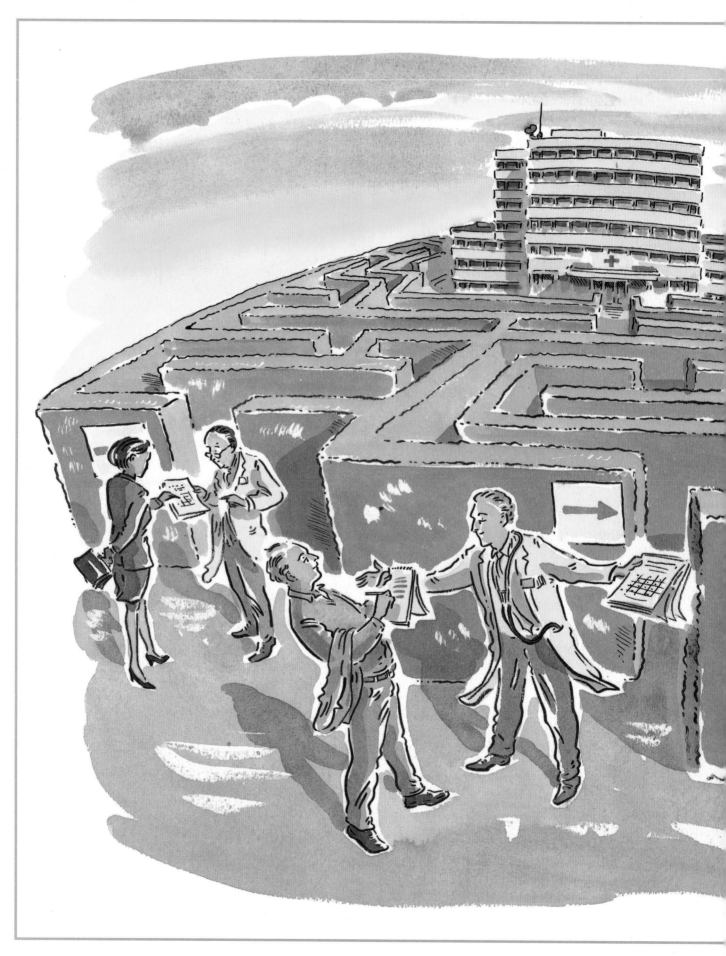

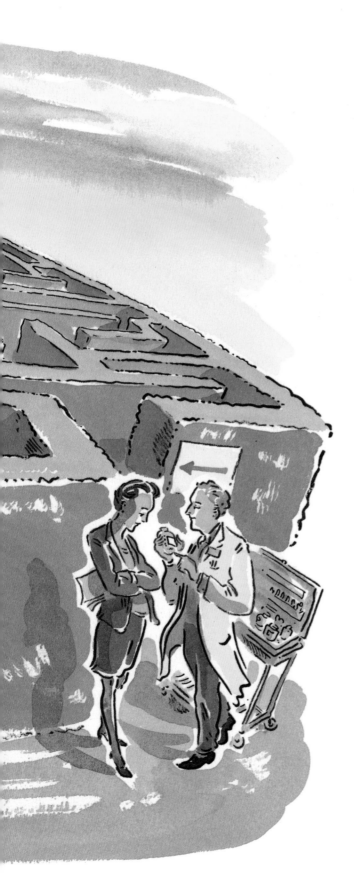

# Navigating the Medical Maze

## Chapter 3

# Keeping Things Straight

You have received a call from your physician's office. The results of your tests are back and the receptionist schedules an appointment for you for the next day. Now you are left to wrestle with the fears, the questions, and the "what ifs" overnight. The following day, your physician enters the examining room and begins to discuss your diagnosis. He or she tells you what type of cancer you have, the normal course of treatments, their side effects, future tests that you will need, the best surgeons in town, and so on and so forth. You came to this appointment with more than thirty questions, but at the moment you can recall only ten. You inquire about these of course, but since your mind keeps bounding ahead anticipating the next questions, the answers you receive seem hazy and later elude you altogether. As a matter of fact, less than twenty-four hours after the consultation with your physician, you can only remember bits and pieces of the conversation and you're feeling frustrated that you have more questions than ever before. Sound familiar?

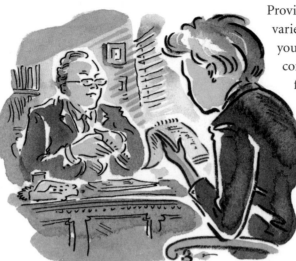

These consultations are one of the most significant aspects of your health care. It is here where information will be shared, decisions made, fears expressed, and issues resolved. Your first office visit is generally the longest and the most substantial one. Ordinarily, 45 minutes to an hour will be set aside for your first consultation. Your following checkup visits will be approximately 20 minutes long, adequate time to ask roughly five questions, so select them carefully. The subsequent pages have been designed to suggest crucial questions at every juncture, keep track of medication, describe pain, and provide an appointment calendar. All of it is designed to aid you in keeping things straight during this tumultuous period.

❖

It is important to keep concise records and notes on all medical appointments so that you can track your progress and keep your specialists informed and up-to-date.

Provided in this chapter are a variety of questionnaire pages for you to complete during major consultations and to use for future reference. Use a pencil throughout this chapter, and if you believe you might need more question forms, medication charts, or pain diagrams, photocopy them before you fill in the pages.

You should also keep track of certain basic information that is usually measured at each appointment. On page 62, you will notice a section to be completed with the doctor's name, the date, and your weight. Request the data on your red blood count (HGB) white blood count (WBC), and platelet count (PLT). In addition, record the results of your tumor marker number, if your particular cancer has a marker.

## MAKE AN IMPRESSION IN YOUR DOCTORS' OFFICES!

Be known for your kindness – score points by learning the name of the staff at each of your doctors' offices and go on a first-name basis.

### ONCOLOGIST

Dr._____

Tel #:_____

Receptionist's name:_____

Nurse's name:_____

### RADIATION ONCOLOGIST

Dr._____

Tel #:_____

Receptionist's name:_____

Nurse's name:_____

### SURGEON

Dr._____

Tel #:_____

Receptionist's name:_____

Nurse's name:_____

# Rating Your Doctor

He (or she) is knowledgeable, rushed, worried, compassionate, hopeful, overwhelmed, caring, baffled, distant, sensitive, brusque, intelligent, understanding, sorry for your circumstances, gentle, impatient, sympathetic, and proficient. He has a family, friends, and a life of his own. He can help you but not necessarily cure you, and he is influenced every day by the suffering and circumstances of his patients. He has moods, dreams, fears, problems, and desires. He's your doctor and he's human. The key is "Do you like this person and feel you can communicate with and trust him?"

One of the most critical decisions you will make is choosing "your team" and which doctor should lead it. The choice is yours and depends on what you consider important during this time. Ultimately, you are responsible for your health care and you give the authorization for any treatments you will receive.

*Choosing a doctor with whom you have a good rapport is invaluable and within your control.*

Do you care more about a doctor's bedside manner than his or her knowledge of treatments? Are you looking for a doctor who is aggressive or conventional? Would you rather your doctor be conveniently located or affiliated with a large cancer center, with all of its innovative equipment? What's important is up to you. Take the "Rate Your Doctor" test and determine how your doctor fares.

The first visits with your oncologist are likely to be lengthy. The doctor generally blocks out an ample amount of time, knowing that you will have many questions and will need a significant amount of information about your cancer. It is at this time that your doctor will outline the chosen treatment for you. You will learn what this treatment will

---

## RATE YOUR DOCTOR

**My doctor is: (circle)**
1. Easy to communicate with.
2. Trustworthy.
3. Specializes in my type of cancer.
4. Involved in new treatment studies.
5. Board-certified.
6. Easy to reach.
7. Allows office visits to be taped.

**My doctor has a: (circle)**
1. Clean, efficient office.
2. Teaching affiliation.
3. Convenient location.
4. Accounting department that submits insurance documents.
5. Well-trained and helpful staff.
6. Payment plan.
7. Good reputation.

**Score one point for each number that you circled. Your doctor should score a minimum of 11.**

---

## GET IT ON TAPE

Take a tape recorder with you to your doctor's appointment to record the conversation. Later, when it is convenient, document the answers in your workbook. Doing so furnishes you with all the questions and answers at your fingertips.

---

entail, whether surgery, radiation therapy, chemotherapy, or a combination of these. Ask the questions NOW. The more you understand about your cancer and the treatments, the less likely you are to be anxious and fearful. Your doctor can eliminate many false impressions you may have about cancer and the treatments, and this insight will give you a sense of stability. There are many questions on the following pages for you to read and consider. Decide before your initial doctor's visit which questions you want answered. Be prepared and methodical when you go for your consultations. One word of caution: Do not ask the question if you are not prepared to hear the answer. I didn't ask several of these questions until after my treatments were over and I was recovering emotionally and physically. In fact, there are some questions I have never asked.

# Simply Speaking

*"You have stage-four adenocarcinoma to the right upper apex of the lung that has metastases to the mediastinum region."*

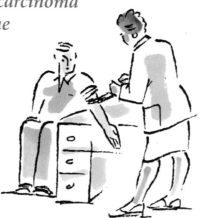

What?! Welcome to the world of big words you don't understand. This simple glossary will provide the basics in cancer terminology. Read through it and familiarize yourself with the terms so that you can comprehend and communicate with your doctor. Remember, no question is to stupid too ask.

### BLOOD COUNTS

- A low red blood cell count (HGB) can cause a tired and listless feeling.
- A low white blood cell count (WBC) can increase your risk of infection.
- A low platelet count (PLT) can put you at risk for bruising and bleeding.

*"It eliminates the guesswork if you bring a medical diary that has your medications, diagnoses, and family history."*

**– Richard W. Honsinger, MD, internist and allergist in Los Alamos, NM.**

### SIMPLY SPEAKING: *Remember, no question is too stupid to ask*

- **Adjuvant therapy:** Treatment used in addition to and following the primary treatment to cure, reduce, or control the cancer.
- **Alopecia:** Partial or complete loss of hair, often caused by chemotherapy.
- **Analgesic:** A drug that relieves pain.
- **Anemia:** A deficiency of red blood cells. Symptoms include fatigue, shortness of breath, and weakness.
- **Antibodies:** Proteins produced by the immune system to fight infection.
- **Aspiration:** Removal of fluid or tissue, usually with a needle or tube.
- **Barium enema:** A liquid barium mixture given to a patient before an X ray of the digestive system.
- **Benign:** A tumor that does not have the tendency to grow. Not cancerous.
- **Biopsy:** The removal of a piece of tissue to see if it is malignant.
- **Bone scan:** A test performed by injecting a tracer radioactive substance and, a few hours later, taking pictures as you lie on a table. "Hot spots" on the scan could be an indication of cancer. The test does not hurt.

- **Brachytherapy:** The use of a radioactive "seed" that is implanted directly into a tumor.
- **Carcinoma:** A form of cancer that develops in the tissue or lining of the body such as the breast, lung, skin, or uterus. More than 80% of all cancers are carcinomas.
- **CT scan:** A specialized type of X ray that produces cross-sectional scans of your body. The test does not hurt but you may get an injection of a radioactive substance.
- **CEA:** A "tumor marker" that may be in your blood indicating the presence of cancer. CEA is monitored to assess the progress of your treatment.
- **Chemotherapy:** Drugs that are used to stop or slow down the growth of cancer cells.
- **Clinical trial:** The final testing of experimental new cancer treatments that is performed on people.
- **Colonoscopy:** A procedure to inspect the rectum and colon with a long fiberoptic telescope. It is mostly done on an outpatient basis after administration of a local anesthesia.

- **Endoscope:** A flexible lighted instrument that enables examination within the organs.
- **Fine needle aspiration:** A simple and almost always painless way to get a sample of tissue for diagnosis.
- **Grading:** One means of classifying a tumor depending on whether the cells are differentiated.
- **Hope:** What living with cancer demands. To expect with confidence, and to remember that every cancer, at every stage, has been survived by someone.
- **Hormonal therapy:** Treatment that prevents cancer cells from growing by taking advantage of the hormonal needs of these cells.
- **Hospice:** A very special care program that provides medical, spiritual, and psychological care to patients and their families when life expectancy is very short.
- **Immune system:** The components of the body that are responsible for fighting and resisting infection; primarily white blood cells but also antibodies and the lymphatic system.

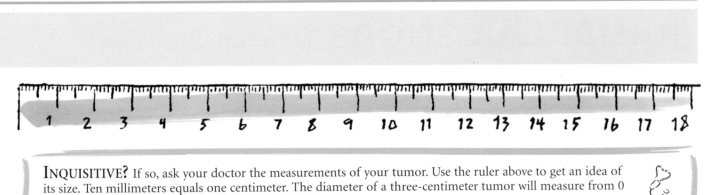

**INQUISITIVE?** If so, ask your doctor the measurements of your tumor. Use the ruler above to get an idea of its size. Ten millimeters equals one centimeter. The diameter of a three-centimeter tumor will measure from 0 to 3. A one-centimeter tumor contains over 1 billion cells.

## GRADE, STAGE, AND THE TNM SYSTEM

Once a cancerous tumor has been detected, the pathologists and physicians will use grading, staging, and/or the TNM system to determine how the cancer can best be treated.

- **Grade:** If the tumor cells resemble healthy, normal cells, they are said to be differentiated. If they do not, then they are undifferentiated. A Grade I tumor is 75–100% differentiated, while a Grade IV tumor is less than 25% differentiated.

- **Stage:** A cancer is staged based on the size of the primary tumor and on whether or not it has spread. A Stage I cancer is localized, small, and easily treatable; a Stage IV cancer has spread to other organs and surgery is no longer an option.

- **TNM system:** A system that looks at three aspects, the size and invasiveness of the tumor, whether the lymph nodes are involved, and whether the cancer has spread (metastasized).

## SIMPLY SPEAKING, CONT.

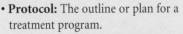

- **In-situ:** An early stage of cancer that is localized in one area.
- **Interferon:** Proteins that activate the immune system. Used to fight cancer as a "biological therapy."
- **Invasive cancer:** A stage of cancer in which the cancer cells have spread to other parts of the body.
- **Lobectomy:** Partial removal of the lung.
- **Lumpectomy:** Removal of a cancerous breast lump without removing the entire breast.
- **Lymph nodes:** Pea-sized organs that are located throughout the body. They filter out cancer cells and other foreign substances and produce infection-fighting antibodies.
- **Lymphedema:** Swelling in the arms or legs as a result of blocked lymphatic vessels.
- **Malignant:** Cancerous with a tendency to spread to other organs.
- **Mastectomy:** Surgical removal of the breast as a treatment of cancer.
- **Metastasis:** Spread of cancer from one part of the body to another.

- **MRI (Magnetic Resonance Imaging):** A test using magnetic fields to produce structural images of the inside of the body. This test doesn't hurt, but some people may feel claustrophobic or be affected by the loud noise of the machine.
- **Nadir:** The lowest point to which your platelets and white cells drop after chemotherapy.
- **Neoadjuvant chemotherapy:** Chemotherapy given before surgery or radiation therapy.
- **Neuropathy:** Numbness or tingling sometimes caused by anticancer drugs.
- **Oncologist:** A doctor whose specialty is cancer and its treatments.
- **Palliative treatment:** Medical treatment to relieve pain or symptoms when a cure is no longer the object.
- **Platelets:** One of three types of blood cells. Platelets promote blood clotting.
- **Prognosis:** The attempt to predict the outcome of the disease.
- **Primary tumor:** The place where the cancer first started to grow. Also known as the "place of origin."

- **Protocol:** The outline or plan for a treatment program.
- **Radiation therapy:** The use of a beam of energy to kill cancer cells.
- **Red blood cells:** The blood cells that carry oxygen from the lungs throughout the body.
- **Remission:** The decrease or disappearance of the disease.
- **Thrombosis:** Formation of a blood clot.
- **TNM classification:** A complex system doctors use to describe the stage of development of most cancers.
- **Tumor:** An abnormal tissue growth or mass that can be benign or malignant.
- **Tumor marker:** Proteins and other substances in the blood that indicate the presence of cancer cells somewhere else in the body.
- **Ultrasound:** A testing technique that uses sound waves to make pictures of the inside of the body.
- **White blood cells:** A general term for the cells in the body that play a major role in battling infection.

# Initial Questions *for Your Oncologist*

**1** SPECIFICALLY WHAT TYPE OF CANCER HAS BEEN DIAGNOSED?

_____

**2** WHAT STAGE AM I IN?

_____

**3** WHAT IS MY PROGNOSIS?

_____

**4** HAS THE CANCER SPREAD TO ANY OTHER SITE?

_____

**5** IF SO, WHERE?

_____

**6** WHAT OTHER SITES HAVE BEEN CHECKED FOR CANCER AND FOUND CANCER-FREE?

_____

**7** IS THERE A TUMOR MARKER YOU ARE TRACKING IN MY PARTICULAR CASE?

_____

**8** IF SO, WHAT IS IT AND WHAT IS CONSIDERED NORMAL?

(NORMAL) _____

(MINE) _____

**9** HOW OFTEN WILL I HAVE BLOOD AND TUMOR MARKER TESTS?

_____

**10** WILL I BE GETTING ANY OTHER TESTS FOR DIAGNOSTIC PURPOSES?

_____

**11** WHY?

_____

**12** WHAT WILL THOSE TESTS ENTAIL?

_____

**13** WHAT IS YOUR RECOMMENDED CHOICE OF TREATMENT?

_____

**14** HAVE YOU HAD SUCCESS WITH THIS TREATMENT?

_____

**15** WHAT ARE THE SHORT-TERM RISKS?

_____

**16** WHAT ARE THE LONG-TERM RISKS?

_____

**17** ARE THERE OTHER ALTERNATIVES?

_____

**18** WHAT ARE THEY?

_____

**19** DO YOU SUGGEST SURGERY?

_____

**20** CAN YOU RECOMMEND A GOOD SURGEON?

_____

**21** WHAT ARE THE CHANCES THAT SURGERY WILL REMOVE ALL THE CANCER?

_____

**22** HOW LONG WILL MY RECUPERATION PERIOD BE?

_____

**23** WILL THERE BE ANY LONG-TERM EFFECTS?

_____

## EVER ONLINE, DOC?

Ask your doctor if he has an e-mail address where you can contact him. If so: put his address here:

_____

Don't be surprised if he doesn't give it to you; not many doctors will.

*"Kindness is produced by kindness."*
— Marcus Tullius Cicero

**24** WILL I RECEIVE CHEMOTHERAPY?
_____

**25** WHAT CHEMOTHERAPY DRUGS WILL BE USED?
_____

NAME OF DRUG
_____

SIDE EFFECTS
_____

**26** HOW MANY TREATMENTS WILL I RECEIVE?
_____

**27** HOW WILL I FEEL AFTER EACH TREATMENT?
_____

**28** WHAT WILL THE LONG-TERM SIDE EFFECTS BE?
_____

**29** HOW WILL I KNOW IF THE TREATMENTS ARE WORKING?
_____

**30** WILL I NEED A PORT, SHUNT, OR CATHETER TO RECEIVE THESE TREATMENTS?

IF SO, COULD YOU EXPLAIN MORE ABOUT THAT?
_____

**31** WHO SHOULD I CONSULT IF I EXPERIENCE ANY PROBLEMS WITH SIDE EFFECTS OF TREATMENTS?
_____
_____

**32** WILL I RECEIVE RADIATION THERAPY?
_____

WHY?
_____

**33** CAN YOU RECOMMEND A RADIATION ONCOLOGIST?
_____

**34** HAS RADIATION THERAPY BEEN PROVEN EFFECTIVE FOR THIS TYPE OF CANCER?
_____

**35** WHAT ARE THE OTHER OPTIONS FOR TREATING THIS TYPE OF CANCER?
_____

**36** WOULD YOU SUGGEST A SECOND OPINION?
_____

**37** WOULD YOU SUGGEST THAT I GO TO A CANCER RESEARCH HOSPITAL THAT SPECIALIZES IN MY TYPE OF CANCER?
_____

**38** CAN THE CANCER SPREAD WHILE I AM BEING TREATED WITH CHEMOTHERAPY?
_____

**39** CAN THE CANCER SPREAD WHILE I AM BEING TREATED WITH RADIATION THERAPY?
_____

**40** WHAT SIGNS SHOULD I LOOK FOR THAT THE CANCER IS COMING BACK?
_____

**41** WHAT IS MY RED BLOOD COUNT (HGB)?

WHAT IS NORMAL?
_____

## STARVING CANCER CELLS

February 17, 1998

Researchers at Johns Hopkins have found evidence that some cancer cells are such incredible sugar junkies that they'll self-destruct when deprived of glucose, their biological sweet of choice.

# More Questions

*"Truth is the most valuable thing we have."*

— Mark Twain

**42** WHAT IS MY WHITE BLOOD COUNT (WBC)?

_____

WHAT IS NORMAL?

_____

**43** I AM HAVING TROUBLE SLEEPING. CAN YOU PRESCRIBE SOMETHING THAT WILL HELP ME SLEEP?

_____

**44** WHAT KIND OF TREATMENT OR MEDICATION CAN YOU PRESCRIBE FOR MY PAIN?

_____

**45** WHAT DO I DO IF MY PAIN WORSENS?

_____

**46** WHO WILL ADVISE ME ABOUT NUTRITION AND PROBLEMS I MIGHT HAVE EATING?

_____

_____

**47** HOW WILL MY PROGRESS BE MONITORED?

_____

**48** ARE THERE ANY DANGER SIGNS I SHOULD LOOK FOR?

_____

_____

**49** WHAT IS THE BEST WAY TO GET IN TOUCH WITH YOU?

_____

_____

## GOOD NEWS!

HOW MANY SURVIVE? MORE THAN EVER! IN THE 1930'S, LESS THAN ONE IN FIVE LIVED FIVE YEARS BEYOND TREATMENT. BY THE 1960'S, ONE IN THREE SURVIVED FIVE YEARS. TODAY, TWO OUT OF FIVE PATIENTS WHO GET CANCER THIS YEAR WILL STILL BE ALIVE FIVE YEARS AFTER THEIR DIAGNOSIS.

**Source: American Cancer Society**

## HORMONAL TREATMENT

For some cancers, such as prostate cancer, taking daily hormones will be part of your treatment. Other cancers that are promoted by hormones will necessitate a medication designed to deplete your body of hormones. If your doctor suggests this, the following questions will help get the information you need.

**50** WILL I NEED HORMONAL THERAPY?

_____

IF SO, WHAT IS THE NAME OF THE MEDICATION?

_____

**51** WHAT IS THE REASON FOR THE MEDICATION?

_____

**52** WILL THERE BE SIDE EFFECTS?

_____

**53** ARE THERE RISKS?

_____

**54** HOW LONG WILL I NEED TO STAY ON THIS MEDICATION?

_____

**55** DOES THIS THERAPY WORK WELL FOR EVERYONE?

_____

## PITCH THE PACK !

Cigarette smoke contains more than 4,000 different chemicals, many of which are proven carcinogens.

FRESHSTART is a no-nonsense quit-smoking program put on by the American Cancer Society. It consists of four one-hour sessions held during a two-week period. For smokers who wish to quit but don't want to attend FRESHSTART, or who want to do it on their own, Simon & Schuster has made the program available on video and audiocassette. Entitled "The American Cancer Society's Freshstart: 21 Days to Stop Smoking," the cassettes are available at many bookstores and retail outlets.

# Odds & Ends

Following are questions to review throughout your treatments and follow-up care. Look through these questions before your visits with your oncologist and decide which ones you want answered.

**1** Are there any exercises that I should or should not be doing at this time?

_____

_____

**2** How much exercise should I be getting and would a physical therapist help?

_____

_____

**3** I'm having the following symptoms. Are they normal?

_____

_____

**4** Should I have a blood test to see if I am now in menopause?

_____

_____

**5** My {family member} has a cold. Does this put me at any additional risk?

_____

**6** Should I have a flu shot?

_____

**7** Is there anything that I can do for this constipation/diarrhea?

_____

_____

**8** Is there anything I can take for my indigestion?

_____

_____

**9** Are there any foods I should or should not eat during my treatments?

_____

_____

**10** Is it safe for me to drink alcohol with the medications I am taking?

_____

_____

**11** Does alcohol affect my immune system?

_____

How?

**12** Can I get costly tests done before the end of the year so that my insurance will pay for it, since I have met my deductible for this year?

_____

**13** Would I be better off working or would my chances of benefitting from the treatment increase if I took time off from work?

_____

**14** How will you know if this treatment is working?

_____

_____

**15** If this treatment does not work as you hope it will, are there any clinical trials being done that you think may be appropriate for me?

_____

**16** How do I go about looking into different clinical trials? (See also pages 36–39)

_____

**17** Other questions:

_____

_____

_____

_____

# Questions to Ask *Your Oncologist*

You will have a series of appointments with your oncologist during the course of your treatments. I have provided two forms for the questions you will want to ask at these visits, but you will want to photocopy these pages to provide additional blank forms.

**During treatments:**

1 HOW AM I PROGRESSING?

2 IS THIS MORE OR LESS THAN YOU EXPECTED?

3 I AM EXPERIENCING {LESS PAIN, NEW PAIN, OR THE SAME PAIN} IN THESE AREAS:

IS THIS NORMAL?

WHY?

4 IS THERE ANYTHING WE CAN DO TO LESSEN THE PAIN?

5 ARE YOU SATISFIED WITH THE RESULTS OF MY BLOOD TESTS?

6 I AM HAVING THESE SIDE EFFECTS FROM MY TREATMENTS:

7 IS THERE ANYTHING THAT CAN MINIMIZE THE SIDE EFFECTS?

DR.

HAS GIVEN ME A PRESCRIPTION FOR THE DRUG

I AM TO TAKE IT ————— TIMES A DAY

FOR ————— DAYS.

8 WILL THIS INTERFERE WITH OTHER MEDICATIONS I AM TAKING?

HOW?

9 THE FOLLOWING THINGS CONCERN ME; PLEASE COMMENT:

PROBLEM:

DR.'S COMMENT:

PROBLEM:

DR.'S COMMENT:

PROBLEM:

DR.'S COMMENT:

*"Since everything is in our heads, we had better not lose them."*

– Coco Chanel

## During treatments:

**1**  HOW AM I PROGRESSING?

_____
_____
_____

**2**  IS THIS MORE OR LESS THAN YOU EXPECTED?

_____
_____
_____

**3**  I AM EXPERIENCING {LESS PAIN, NEW PAIN, OR THE SAME PAIN} IN THESE AREAS:

_____

IS THIS NORMAL?  _____

_____

WHY? _____

_____

**4**  IS THERE ANYTHING WE CAN DO TO LESSEN THE PAIN?

_____
_____

**5**  ARE YOU SATISFIED WITH THE RESULTS OF MY BLOOD TESTS?

_____
_____
_____
_____

**6**  I AM HAVING THESE SIDE EFFECTS FROM MY TREATMENTS:

_____
_____
_____

**7**  IS THERE ANYTHING THAT CAN MINIMIZE THE SIDE EFFECTS?

_____
_____
_____
_____

DR. _____

HAS GIVEN ME A PRESCRIPTION FOR THE DRUG _____

I AM TO TAKE IT _____TIMES A DAY

FOR _____ DAYS.

**8**  WILL THIS INTERFERE WITH OTHER MEDICATIONS I AM TAKING?

_____

HOW? _____

_____
_____

**9**  THE FOLLOWING THINGS CONCERN ME; PLEASE COMMENT:

PROBLEM: _____

_____

DR.'S COMMENT: _____

_____

PROBLEM: _____

_____

DR.'S COMMENT: _____

_____

PROBLEM: _____

_____

DR.'S COMMENT: _____

# Questions to Ask *Your Oncologist*

You will have a series of appointments with your oncologist after treatments are finished. Photocopy these pages to provide more blank forms.

**Following treatments:**

**1** HOW AM I PROGRESSING?
_____
_____
_____

**2** IS THIS MORE OR LESS THAN YOU EXPECTED?
_____
_____
_____

**3** I AM EXPERIENCING {LESS PAIN, NEW PAIN, OR THE SAME PAIN} IN THESE AREAS:
_____
IS THIS NORMAL?_____
WHY?_____
_____

**4** IS THERE ANYTHING WE CAN DO TO LESSEN THE PAIN?
_____
_____
_____

**5** ARE YOU SATISFIED WITH THE RESULTS OF MY BLOOD TESTS?
_____
_____
_____

**6** ARE THERE ANY SIGNS THAT I SHOULD BE LOOKING FOR THAT WOULD INDICATE CANCER?
_____
_____
_____

**7** WHEN ARE MY NEXT TESTS AND WHAT WILL THEY BE?
_____

**8** THE FOLLOWING THINGS CONCERN ME; PLEASE COMMENT:

PROBLEM: _____
DR.'S COMMENT: _____
_____

PROBLEM: _____
DR.'S COMMENT: _____
_____

PROBLEM: _____
DR.'S COMMENT: _____
_____

PROBLEM: _____
DR.'S COMMENT: _____
_____

PROBLEM: _____
DR.'S COMMENT: _____
_____

PROBLEM: _____
DR.'S COMMENT: _____
_____

PROBLEM: _____
DR.'S COMMENT: _____
_____

PROBLEM: _____
DR.'S COMMENT: _____
_____

*"I have no idea where I will go on this journey, but I know I must take it."*

– Martin Luther King Jr.

**Following treatments:**

**1** How am I progressing?

_____

_____

_____

**2** Is this more or less than you expected?

_____

_____

_____

**3** I am experiencing {less pain, new pain, or the same pain} in these areas:

_____

Is this normal? _____

Why? _____

_____

_____

**4** Is there anything we can do to lessen the pain?

_____

_____

_____

**5** Are you satisfied with the results of my blood tests?

_____

_____

_____

**6** Are there any signs that I should be looking for that would indicate cancer?

_____

_____

_____

**7** When are my next tests and what will they be?

_____

_____

_____

**8** The following things concern me; please comment:

Problem: _____

Dr.'s comment: _____

_____

_____

Problem: _____

Dr.'s comment: _____

_____

_____

Problem: _____

Dr.'s comment: _____

_____

_____

Problem: _____

Dr.'s comment: _____

_____

_____

Problem: _____

Dr.'s comment: _____

_____

_____

Problem: _____

Dr.'s comment: _____

_____

_____

Problem: _____

Dr.'s comment: _____

_____

_____

# This Year Counts

There are no hard and fast rules, but ordinarily you will be monitored closely after your treatments have been completed. This period can be a particularly frightening time for some people. While the surgery, chemotherapy, and radiation therapy have been no picnic, you may have had a feeling of security that at the very least the treatments were keeping your cancer at bay. When they stop, the fear often intensifies. You will receive different diagnostic tests on a regular basis. If your particular type of cancer has a tumor marker, your blood tests may become important to you. You will not always have a doctor's appointment each time you have a blood test. Provided below is a sheet to monitor your blood tests throughout the year. Copy this chart if you want to monitor the blood tests over a longer period.

Date:_____
Doctor:_____
Weight:_____
HGB:_____
WBC:_____
PLT:_____
Tumor marker:_____

Date:_____
Doctor:_____
Weight:_____
HGB:_____
WBC:_____
PLT:_____
Tumor marker:_____

Date:_____
Doctor:_____
Weight:_____
HGB:_____
WBC:_____
PLT:_____
Tumor marker:_____

Date:_____
Doctor:_____
Weight:_____
HGB:_____
WBC:_____
PLT:_____
Tumor marker:_____

Date:_____
Doctor:_____
Weight:_____
HGB:_____
WBC:_____
PLT:_____
Tumor marker:_____

Date:_____
Doctor:_____
Weight:_____
HGB:_____
WBC:_____
PLT:_____
Tumor marker:_____

Date:_____
Doctor:_____
Weight:_____
HGB:_____
WBC:_____
PLT:_____
Tumor marker:_____

Date:_____
Doctor:_____
Weight:_____
HGB:_____
WBC:_____
PLT:_____
Tumor marker:_____

Date:_____
Doctor:_____
Weight:_____
HGB:_____
WBC:_____
PLT:_____
Tumor marker:_____

Date:_____
Doctor:_____
Weight:_____
HGB:_____
WBC:_____
PLT:_____
Tumor marker:_____

Date:_____
Doctor:_____
Weight:_____
HGB:_____
WBC:_____
PLT:_____
Tumor marker:_____

Date:_____
Doctor:_____
Weight:_____
HGB:_____
WBC:_____
PLT:_____
Tumor marker:_____

# One Month at a Time

Contrary to what most people believe, not all chemotherapy treatments carry the high price of serious side effects. Unfortunately, however, many chemotherapy drugs do and some of these effects can be long-lasting. After all of your treatments are completed, you may experience various distressing health problems for a long period of time. It is helpful to write down how you feel in general terms about once a month. Not only will this assist you in communicating with your doctor but it will also give you a barometer by which to measure your progress. Use the chart below to track your fatigue, body aches and pains, and all other problems you are experiencing.

Date: _____ How I feel: _____
_____
_____
_____

Date: _____ How I feel: _____
_____
_____
_____

Date: _____ How I feel: _____
_____
_____
_____

Date: _____ How I feel: _____
_____
_____
_____

Date: _____ How I feel: _____
_____
_____
_____

Date: _____ How I feel: _____
_____
_____
_____

Date: _____ How I feel: _____
_____
_____
_____

Date: _____ How I feel: _____
_____
_____
_____

Date: _____ How I feel: _____
_____
_____
_____

Date: _____ How I feel: _____
_____
_____
_____

# Questions *for Your Surgeon*

Surgery is used most often for the treatment of cancer. It can also be used in prevention and diagnosis and to relieve pain. Choose a board-certified surgeon who has performed your type of surgery many times. Make sure that your surgeon is easy to talk with and is part of a group or hospital-based. Verify with the hospital before surgery that your insurance is accepted. Always get a second opinion before surgery.

## Before the surgery:

**1** WHAT IS THE PURPOSE OF THIS SURGERY?

_____

_____

**2** IS THERE ANY OTHER OPTION TO SURGERY?

_____

_____

**3** WHY DO YOU FEEL SURGERY IS THE BEST CHOICE FOR ME IN THIS CASE?

_____

_____

**4** WHAT ARE THE CHANCES THAT YOU WILL BE ABLE TO SURGICALLY REMOVE ALL OF THE CANCER?

_____

_____

**5** WHAT ARE THE DANGERS OF THIS SURGERY?

_____

_____

**6** WHAT COMPLICATIONS OR SPECIAL CIRCUMSTANCES ARE COMMON WITH THIS TYPE OF SURGERY?

_____

_____

**7** HOW LONG WILL THE OPERATION TAKE?

_____

**8** WILL I HAVE SPECIAL CONCERNS, SUCH AS DRAINS OR CATHETERS TO TAKE INTO ACCOUNT?

**9** HOW LONG WILL I BE IN THE HOSPITAL?

_____

_____

**10** WILL I HAVE SPECIAL DIETARY REQUIREMENTS?

_____

_____

**11** WILL I HAVE ANY DISFIGUREMENT?

_____

_____

**12** WHERE WILL THE SCAR BE AND WHAT WILL IT LOOK LIKE?

_____

_____

**13** WHAT TYPE OF PAIN WILL I EXPERIENCE?

_____

_____

**14** WHAT TYPES OF PAIN CONTROL WILL YOU USE?

_____

_____

**15** HOW LONG WILL IT TAKE FOR ME TO RECUPERATE FULLY?

_____

_____

**16** WHAT WILL MY FOLLOW-UP CARE BE?

_____

_____

**17** OTHER QUESTIONS:

_____

_____

_____

_____

_____

_____

*"It is not because things are difficult that we do not dare. It is because we do not dare that things are difficult."*

– Seneca

### After the surgery:

Remember that surgeons are busy and do early-morning hospital rounds. Write down questions ahead of time since it's difficult to think clearly at 5:30 in the morning.

**1** HOW DO YOU FEEL THE SURGERY WENT?
_____
_____

**2** WERE YOU SUCCESSFUL IN REMOVING ALL OF THE CANCER?
_____
_____

**3** IF NOT, WHAT CANCER REMAINS?
_____
WHERE? _____

**4** WHAT IS MY PROGNOSIS?
_____

**5** WILL I REQUIRE FURTHER SURGERY?
_____

**6** WHAT IS YOUR OPINION OF WHAT I SHOULD DO NEXT?
_____
_____

**7** WHEN WILL I BE RELEASED FROM THE HOSPITAL?
_____

**8** ARE thkjshkjsjere any special instructions to follow at lkh
ARE THERE ANY SPECIAL INSTRUCTIONS TO FOLLOW AT HOME?
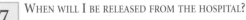
_____

**9** IS MY WOUND HEALING NORMALLY?
_____

**10** WHEN WILL YOU REMOVE THE STITCHES?
_____

## GENE THERAPY
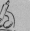

Research is being done in universities and hospitals throughout the United States involving cancer vaccines. The mutated P53 , RAS, and Her-2Nu gene are among a few. Ask your doctor to test your tumor cells for these and any other genes that may be mutated and promoting your cancer. Follow up by researching clinical trials {more information on pages 36–39} being conducted on the particular mutated gene you tested positive for. Arrange the details for participating in the clinical trial while you are undergoing conventional treatment.

**11** WHAT SYMPTOMS DO I NEED TO CALL YOU ABOUT?
_____

**12** WHAT ACTION ON MY PART CAN HELP PREVENT THESE SYMPTOMS?
_____

**13** I HAVE THESE SYMPTOMS; ARE THEY NORMAL?

SYMPTOM: _____
DR.'S COMMENT: _____

SYMPTOM: _____
DR.'S COMMENT: _____

**14** HOW SOON SHOULD I RESUME WORK? HOW SOON CAN I RESUME SPORTS ACTIVITIES? SEXUAL INTERCOURSE?
_____
_____

**15** OTHER QUESTIONS:
_____
_____
_____

*"Simplicity and straightforwardness are...in the power of all of us."*

– Henry Allford

# Initial Questions *for Your Radiation Oncologist*

Radiation therapy is used to kill cancer cells, shrink tumors before surgery, control pain, and in conjunction with chemotherapy and surgery to treat the patient. New forms and high-tech equipment have made radiation therapy, in some cases, the most effective arsenal we have against specific cancers. Make certain your radiation oncologist is certified by the American Board of Therapeutic Radiology, is well aquainted with your type of cancer, is easy to talk to, and has an efficient and well-equipped office.

### RADIATION TREATMENTS

- Wear clothing that is easy to take off and put on.
- Don't wash the location ink marks off.
- Each session takes 15 to 30 minutes.
- Treatments are painless.
- Don't hold your breath.
- Remain very still.
- The machines are large and move during treatments.
- See pages 68–69 for more information.

**1** WHAT DO YOU HOPE TO ACCOMPLISH WITH RADIATION?
_____

**2** HAVE YOU HAD SUCCESS WITH TREATING MY KIND OF CANCER WITH RADIATION BEFORE?
_____
_____

**3** ARE THERE OTHER OPTIONS?
_____
_____

**4** DO YOU HOPE TO COMPLETELY SHRINK THE TUMOR?
_____

**5** WILL IT STOP THE SPREAD OF CANCER?
_____

**6** WHAT ARE THE CHANCES OF THAT HAPPENING?
_____
_____

**7** WILL I BE RECEIVING RADIATION THERAPY AND CHEMOTHERAPY AT THE SAME TIME?
_____
_____

**8** IS THERE A BENEFIT IF I DO?
_____

**9** WHAT KIND OF RADIATION THERAPY WILL I RECEIVE?
_____

**10** COULD YOU EXPLAIN THE PROCEDURE TO ME?
_____
_____

**11** HOW MANY TREATMENTS WILL I HAVE?
_____

**12** WHEN DO YOU WANT TO BEGIN?
_____

**13** WHEN WILL IT END?
_____

**14** WHAT SIDE EFFECTS AM I LIKELY TO EXPERIENCE?
_____
_____

**15** ARE THERE SHORT-TERM RISKS?
_____
_____

**16** ARE THERE LONG-TERM RISKS?
_____

**17** OTHER QUESTIONS:
_____
_____
_____

*"Courage is fear that has said its prayers."*

– Unknown

*"It takes courage to live – courage and strength and hope and humor."*

– Jerome Fleischman

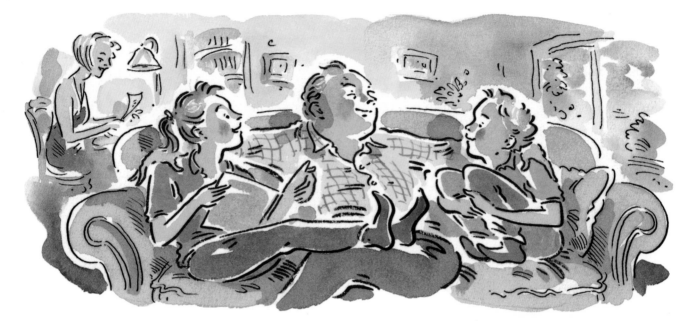

## THE GAMMA KNIFE®

A high-dose beam of radiation precisely focused on tumors or lesions in the brain is delivered by the Gamma Knife. The procedure carries less risk than conventional brain surgery due to surrounding tissue remaining untouched. It is less expensive, generally safe, performed under local anesthesia, and only a one-day treatment. Approximately 70,000 patients have been successfully treated with the Gamma Knife. If you have brain cancer, ask your radiation oncologist if this treatment could benefit you. For more information contact: The San Diego Gamma Knife Center.
Tel #: (800) 92-GAMMA

**http://www.sdgkc.com/**

## EXTRA OXYGEN REDUCES NAUSEA AFTER COLON SURGERY

November 27, 1999  NEW YORK (Reuters Health) – Boosting the amount of oxygen given to patients during surgery of the colon can significantly reduce the chance of nausea and vomiting afterward, an international research team reports.

## RELAY FOR LIFE

This event is designed to mobilize communities throughout the country to celebrate cancer survivors, remember loved ones, and raise money for the fight against cancer. On the day of the event, teams of people gather at schools, football fields, fairgrounds, or parks, and take turns walking, jogging, or running laps. Teams are organized by friends, relatives, local businesses, hospitals, schools, churches, service clubs, and other organizations. If you have any other questions about Relay for Life, contact your local American Cancer Society office or call (800) ACS-2345.

## PROSTATE CANCER SURVIVORSHIP

A report published in the *Journal of the American Medical Association* revealed that, in a study of men diagnosed with prostate cancer, the chance of being alive 10 years after surgery depended on the severity of their disease, and ranged from 60 to 97%. To arrive at their findings, lead investigator Dr. Arnon Krongrad and his colleagues reviewed data from 3,636 men with an average age of 65 who had prostate-removal surgery in nine different regions of the United States.

# Questions to Ask *Your Radiation Oncologist*

## During treatments:

Most cancer patients will receive radiation treatments every day (except Saturdays and Sundays) for an average of six weeks. During this period of time you will likely have weekly doctor's visits that are designed to allow your radiation oncologist to examine you, assess your progress, and give you the opportunity to ask any questions. Keep a record of these weekly visits using the following questions.

**1** HOW ARE MY TREATMENTS PROGRESSING?
_____
_____

**2** IS THAT MORE OR LESS THAN YOU EXPECTED?
_____
_____

**3** IS THERE ANY MARKED IMPROVEMENT IN MY X RAYS?
_____
_____

**4** WHAT FURTHER TESTS WILL YOU CONDUCT TO TRACK MY PROGRESSION?
_____
_____

**5** HOW CAN I ALLEVIATE THESE PROBLEMS?
EXHAUSTION _____
APPETITE _____
SKIN PROBLEMS _____

**6** HOW LONG WILL THESE SIDE EFFECTS LAST?
_____

**7** OTHER QUESTIONS:
_____
_____
_____
_____

**1** HOW ARE MY TREATMENTS PROGRESSING?
_____
_____

**2** IS THAT MORE OR LESS THAN YOU EXPECTED?
_____
_____

**3** IS THERE ANY MARKED IMPROVEMENT IN MY X RAYS?
_____
_____

**4** WHAT FURTHER TESTS WILL YOU CONDUCT TO TRACK MY PROGRESSION?
_____
_____

**5** HOW CAN I ALLEVIATE THESE PROBLEMS?
EXHAUSTION _____
APPETITE _____
SKIN PROBLEMS _____

**6** HOW LONG WILL THESE SIDE EFFECTS LAST?
_____

**7** OTHER QUESTIONS:
_____
_____
_____
_____
_____

DON'T BE EMBARRASSED BY PERSONAL QUESTIONS. THE INFO YOU HOLD BACK COULD BE CRITICAL TO YOUR TREATMENT.

*Nieca Goldberg, MD, chief of the Women's Heart Program at Lenox Hill Hospital in New York City*

## AMERICA'S BEST HOSPITALS

**For a complete list of the best hospitals, go online:**
http://www.usnews.com/usnews/nycu/health/hosptl/tophosp.htm

1. University of Texas, MD Anderson Cancer Center, Houston, TX
2. Memorial Sloan-Kettering Cancer Center, New York, NY
3. Johns Hopkins Hospital, Baltimore, MD
4. Mayo Clinic, Rochester, MN
5. Duke University Medical Center, Durham, NC
6. University of Chicago Hospitals, IL
7. Massachusetts General Hospital, Boston, MA
8. UCLA Medical Center, Los Angeles, CA
9. Roswell Park Cancer Institute, Buffalo, NY
10. Clarian Health Partners, Indianapolis, IN
11. University of Washington Medical Center, Seattle, WA
12. Hospital of the University of Pennsylvania, Philadelphia, PA
13. Stanford University Hospital, Stanford, CA
14. Fox Chase Cancer Center, Philadelphia, PA
15. University of Michigan Medical Center, Ann Arbor, MI
16. University of Pittsburgh Medical Center-Presbyterian, Pittsburgh, PA
17. Cleveland Clinic, Cleveland, OH
18. University of Kentucky Hospital, Lexington, KY
19. University of Virginia Health Sciences Center, Charlottesville, VA
20. F.G. McGaw Hospital, Loyola University, Maywood, IL

---

**1** HOW ARE MY TREATMENTS PROGRESSING?
_____
_____

**2** IS THAT MORE OR LESS THAN YOU EXPECTED?
_____
_____

**3** IS THERE ANY MARKED IMPROVEMENT IN MY X RAYS?
_____
_____

**4** WHAT FURTHER TESTS WILL YOU CONDUCT TO TRACK MY PROGRESSION?
_____
_____

**5** HOW CAN I ALLEVIATE THESE PROBLEMS?
EXHAUSTION_____
APPETITE_____
SKIN PROBLEMS_____

**6** HOW LONG WILL THESE SIDE EFFECTS LAST?
_____

**7** OTHER QUESTIONS:
_____
_____
_____

---

**1** HOW ARE MY TREATMENTS PROGRESSING?
_____
_____

**2** IS THAT MORE OR LESS THAN YOU EXPECTED?
_____
_____

**3** IS THERE ANY MARKED IMPROVEMENT IN MY X RAYS?
_____
_____

**4** WHAT FURTHER TESTS WILL YOU CONDUCT TO TRACK MY PROGRESSION?
_____
_____

**5** HOW CAN I ALLEVIATE THESE PROBLEMS?
EXHAUSTION_____
APPETITE_____
SKIN PROBLEMS_____

**6** HOW LONG WILL THESE SIDE EFFECTS LAST?
_____

**7** OTHER QUESTIONS:
_____
_____
_____

# Questions to Ask *Your Radiation Oncologist*

**Following treatments:**

You will have several follow-up office visits with your radiation oncologist after your treatments have been completed. These appointments will give your doctor the opportunity to examine you and to schedule future tests. The effects of your treatments are cumulative and long-lasting, so make the most of these visits by discussing any problems and concerns you might have. Keep records for future reference.

**1** HOW AM I PROGRESSING?
_____

**2** IS THAT MORE OR LESS THAN YOU EXPECTED?
_____

**3** I AM EXPERIENCING (LESS PAIN, NEW PAIN, OR THE SAME PAIN) IN THESE AREAS:
_____

**4** IS THIS NORMAL?
_____

**5** WHAT FURTHER TESTS WILL YOU CONDUCT TO TRACK MY PROGRESSION?
_____

**6** WHAT PROBLEMS SHOULD I REPORT TO YOU?
_____
_____

**7** DO YOU HAVE ANY SUGGESTIONS AS TO HOW I CAN ALLEVIATE THESE PROBLEMS?

EXHAUSTION_____
APPETITE_____
SKIN PROBLEMS_____

**8** OTHER QUESTIONS:
_____
_____
_____
_____

---

### SMOKING MAY HASTEN SPREAD OF BLADDER CANCER

NEW YORK (Reuters Health) – Bladder cancer patients who continue to smoke after they have been diagnosed tend to be younger than nonsmokers diagnosed with the disease. In addition, patients with bladder cancer who smoke are at increased risk of faster disease recurrence than nonsmokers, report researchers.

**1** HOW AM I PROGRESSING?
_____

**2** IS THAT MORE OR LESS THAN YOU EXPECTED?
_____

**3** I AM EXPERIENCING {LESS PAIN, NEW PAIN, OR THE SAME PAIN} IN THESE AREAS:
_____

**4** IS THIS NORMAL?
_____

**5** WHAT FURTHER TESTS WILL YOU CONDUCT TO TRACK MY PROGRESSION?
_____

**6** WHAT PROBLEMS SHOULD I REPORT TO YOU?
_____

**7** DO YOU HAVE ANY SUGGESTIONS AS TO HOW I CAN ALLEVIATE THESE PROBLEMS?

EXHAUSTION_____
APPETITE_____
SKIN PROBLEMS_____

**8** OTHER QUESTIONS:
_____
_____
_____
_____

## WANT MORE INFORMATION ON HOSPITALS?

The book *America's Best Hospitals* is a complete list of all the best hospitals in the United States and much more. Want to know how to get into a hospital if it's not part of your health plan network? What if your doctor wants you to go to a hospital that doesn't score high?

How about emergency care? The book is based on analysis by the National Opinion Research Center at the University of Chicago and edited by *U.S. News* Assistant Managing Editor Avery Comarow. *America's Best Hospitals* costs $19.95 in bookstores. It can be ordered for

$25.95, including shipping and handling, by calling (800) 836-6397, ext. 1700, or by sending a check to: America's Best Hospitals US News Specialty Marketing Department 1700M P.O. Box 2284 South Burlington, VT 05407-2284.

**1** HOW AM I PROGRESSING?
_____

**2** IS THAT MORE OR LESS THAN YOU EXPECTED?
_____

**3** I AM EXPERIENCING {LESS PAIN, NEW PAIN, OR THE SAME PAIN} IN THESE AREAS:
_____
_____

**4** IS THIS NORMAL?
_____

**5** WHAT FURTHER TESTS WILL YOU CONDUCT TO TRACK MY PROGRESSION?
_____
_____

**6** WHAT PROBLEMS SHOULD I REPORT TO YOU?
_____
_____

**7** DO YOU HAVE ANY SUGGESTIONS AS TO HOW I CAN ALLEVIATE THESE PROBLEMS?

EXHAUSTION_____
APPETITE_____
SKIN PROBLEMS_____

**8** OTHER QUESTIONS:
_____
_____
_____

**1** HOW AM I PROGRESSING?
_____

**2** IS THAT MORE OR LESS THAN YOU EXPECTED?
_____

**3** I AM EXPERIENCING {LESS PAIN, NEW PAIN, OR THE SAME PAIN} IN THESE AREAS:
_____
_____

**4** IS THIS NORMAL?
_____

**5** WHAT FURTHER TESTS WILL YOU CONDUCT TO TRACK MY PROGRESSION?
_____
_____

**6** WHAT PROBLEMS SHOULD I REPORT TO YOU?
_____
_____

**7** DO YOU HAVE ANY SUGGESTIONS AS TO HOW I CAN ALLEVIATE THESE PROBLEMS?

EXHAUSTION_____
APPETITE_____
SKIN PROBLEMS_____

**8** OTHER QUESTIONS:
_____
_____
_____

# Questions to Ask *Before an* MRI, *an* X ray, *or a* CT *scan*

**G**ood news: For the most part, these tests don't hurt. MRIs, X rays, and CT scans are diagnostic tests for all parts of the body. Generally you will be required to lie on a table as the test is given. You may be given an intravenous contrast solution, or asked to drink a chalky, mint-flavored drink before the test, but often you won't have to do either. One word of caution: The MRI scanners are very noisy and if you have claustrophobia, alert the nurse. If you are nervous, ask your doctor for something to relax you beforehand. You will probably have many such scans over the coming months, and will speak to your doctor about each test before and after it is performed. Questions you might want to ask your doctor at each point are suggested on pages 72–76; photocopy these pages to provide more blank forms.

| | |
|---|---|
| **1** WHY AM I HAVING THIS TEST? | **1** WHY AM I HAVING THIS TEST? |
| **2** WHERE WILL I BE GIVEN THIS TEST? | **2** WHERE WILL I BE GIVEN THIS TEST? |
| **3** HOW LONG WILL THE TEST TAKE? | **3** HOW LONG WILL THE TEST TAKE? |
| **4** WHEN WILL I GET THE RESULTS FROM THIS TEST? | **4** WHEN WILL I GET THE RESULTS FROM THIS TEST? |
| **5** DO I NEED TO RESTRICT MY DIET? | **5** DO I NEED TO RESTRICT MY DIET? |
| **6** OTHER QUESTIONS: | **6** OTHER QUESTIONS: |

## POSITRON EMISSION TOMOGRAPHY

Also known as the Pet scan, the Positron Emission Tomography is the newest in diagnostic tools available to your doctor. To receive a Pet scan you will be injected with a small dosage of a chemical radionuclide, combined with glucose. Because malignant tumors grow at a faster rate than normal cells, they will absorb more of the glucose with the radionuclide attached to it. The Pet scan will then use the measurements of glucose to produce a picture of your body. The heavy concentration of glucose in one area denotes cancer activity. Receiving a Pet scan does not hurt.

**O**NLINE list of Pet Facilities in each state:  HYPERLINK
**http://www.nuc.ucla.edu/html_docs/PET/petcenters.html**

# Questions to Ask *After an MRI, an X ray, or a CT scan*

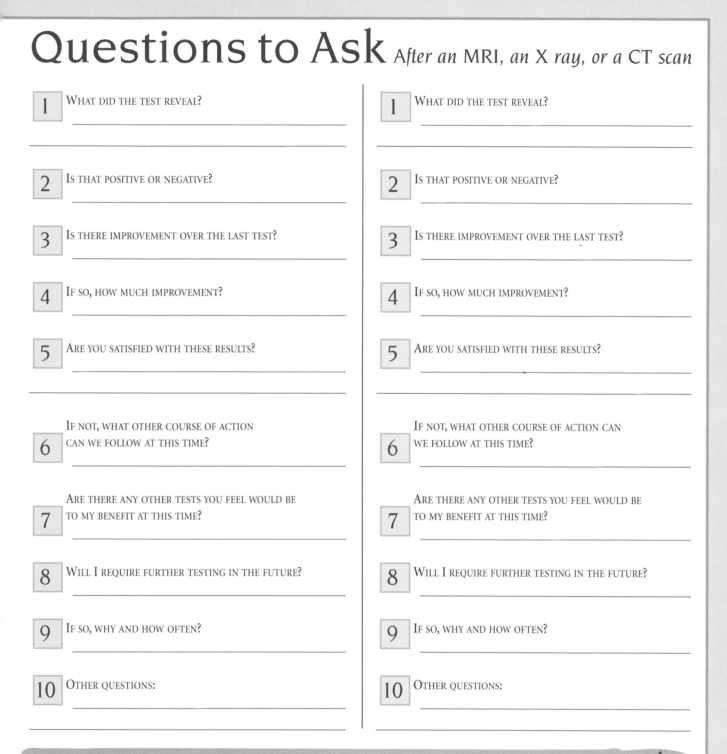

| 1 | WHAT DID THE TEST REVEAL? |

| 2 | IS THAT POSITIVE OR NEGATIVE? |

| 3 | IS THERE IMPROVEMENT OVER THE LAST TEST? |

| 4 | IF SO, HOW MUCH IMPROVEMENT? |

| 5 | ARE YOU SATISFIED WITH THESE RESULTS? |

| 6 | IF NOT, WHAT OTHER COURSE OF ACTION CAN WE FOLLOW AT THIS TIME? |

| 7 | ARE THERE ANY OTHER TESTS YOU FEEL WOULD BE TO MY BENEFIT AT THIS TIME? |

| 8 | WILL I REQUIRE FURTHER TESTING IN THE FUTURE? |

| 9 | IF SO, WHY AND HOW OFTEN? |

| 10 | OTHER QUESTIONS: |

---

| 1 | WHAT DID THE TEST REVEAL? |

| 2 | IS THAT POSITIVE OR NEGATIVE? |

| 3 | IS THERE IMPROVEMENT OVER THE LAST TEST? |

| 4 | IF SO, HOW MUCH IMPROVEMENT? |

| 5 | ARE YOU SATISFIED WITH THESE RESULTS? |

| 6 | IF NOT, WHAT OTHER COURSE OF ACTION CAN WE FOLLOW AT THIS TIME? |

| 7 | ARE THERE ANY OTHER TESTS YOU FEEL WOULD BE TO MY BENEFIT AT THIS TIME? |

| 8 | WILL I REQUIRE FURTHER TESTING IN THE FUTURE? |

| 9 | IF SO, WHY AND HOW OFTEN? |

| 10 | OTHER QUESTIONS: |

## THE IMPORTANCE OF A SECOND OPINION

BALTIMORE (Johns Hopkins) – A study of more than 6,000 patients by researchers at Johns Hopkins found that one or two out of every 100 people who come to larger medical centers for treatment following a biopsy arrive with a diagnosis that's "totally wrong." The results suggest that second-opinion pathology exams not only prevent errors but also save lives and money.

Patients who fail to receive a second pathologist's exam of their biopsied tissue at the incoming hospital or elsewhere "have a small but significant risk of getting the wrong treatment, including surgery or chemotherapy," says pathologist Jonathan L. Epstein, MD, who led a Hopkins research team. The study appears in the December 1999 issue of the journal *Cancer*.

# Questions to Ask *Before and After an MRI, an X ray, or a CT scan*

## Before the test:

**1** WHY AM I HAVING THIS TEST?
_____
_____
_____
_____

**2** WHERE WILL I BE GIVEN THIS TEST?
_____
_____
_____
_____

**3** HOW LONG WILL THE TEST TAKE?
_____
_____
_____
_____

**4** WHEN WILL I GET THE RESULTS FROM THIS TEST?
_____
_____
_____
_____

**5** DO I NEED TO RESTRICT MY DIET?
_____
_____
_____
_____

**6** OTHER QUESTIONS:
_____
_____
_____
_____
_____
_____

## After the test:

**1** WHAT DID THE TEST REVEAL?
_____

**2** IS THAT POSITIVE OR NEGATIVE?
_____

**3** IS THERE IMPROVEMENT OVER THE LAST TEST?
_____

**4** IF SO, HOW MUCH IMPROVEMENT?
_____

**5** ARE YOU SATISFIED WITH THESE RESULTS?
_____

**6** IF NOT, WHAT OTHER COURSE OF ACTION CAN WE FOLLOW AT THIS TIME?
_____

**7** ARE THERE ANY OTHER TESTS YOU FEEL WOULD BE TO MY BENEFIT AT THIS TIME?
_____

**8** WILL I REQUIRE FURTHER TESTING IN THE FUTURE?
_____

**9** IF SO, WHY AND HOW OFTEN?
_____

**10** OTHER QUESTIONS:
_____

ROUGHLY 175,000 NEW CASES OF INVASIVE BREAST CANCER AND NEARLY 40,000 IN SITU BREAST CANCERS WILL BE DIAGNOSED THIS YEAR. A RECENT STUDY CONDUCTED BY THE NCI SUGGESTS WOMEN AGE 65 AND OLDER STILL HAVE MANY MISCONCEPTIONS ABOUT THE NEED FOR MAMMOGRAPHY. THE REPORT SUGGESTS THAT EFFORTS SHOULD FOCUS ON OLDER WOMEN.

## THALIDOMIDE MAY AID CANCER PATIENTS

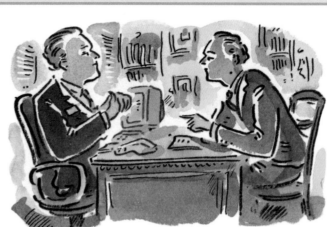

*The Associated Press*

Thalidomide, the drug infamous for causing ghastly birth defects during the 1960s, appears to be effective against a highly lethal form of bone cancer, even in patients in advanced stages of the disease. A study of 84 patients with multiple myeloma found that all signs of the disease disappeared in 10% of those getting thalidomide, and most of the others improved somewhat.

## Before the test:

**1** WHY AM I HAVING THIS TEST?

_____
_____

**2** WHERE WILL I BE GIVEN THIS TEST?

_____
_____

**3** HOW LONG WILL THE TEST TAKE?

_____
_____

**4** WHEN WILL I GET THE RESULTS FROM THIS TEST?

_____
_____

**5** DO I NEED TO RESTRICT MY DIET?

_____
_____

**6** OTHER QUESTIONS:

_____
_____
_____

## After the test:

**1** WHAT DID THE TEST REVEAL?

_____

**2** IS THAT POSITIVE OR NEGATIVE?

_____

**3** IS THERE IMPROVEMENT OVER THE LAST TEST?

_____

**4** IF SO, HOW MUCH IMPROVEMENT?

_____

**5** ARE YOU SATISFIED WITH THESE RESULTS?

_____

**6** IF NOT, WHAT OTHER COURSE OF ACTION CAN WE FOLLOW AT THIS TIME?

_____

**7** ARE THERE ANY OTHER TESTS YOU FEEL WOULD BE TO MY BENEFIT AT THIS TIME?

_____

**8** WILL I REQUIRE FURTHER TESTING IN THE FUTURE?

_____

**9** IF SO, WHY AND HOW OFTEN?

_____

**10** OTHER QUESTIONS:

_____
_____

# Questions to Ask *Before and After an MRI, an X ray, or a CT scan*

**Before the test:**

1 WHY AM I HAVING THIS TEST?
_____
_____
_____

2 WHERE WILL I BE GIVEN THIS TEST?
_____
_____
_____

3 HOW LONG WILL THE TEST TAKE?
_____
_____
_____

4 WHEN WILL I GET THE RESULTS FROM THIS TEST?
_____
_____
_____

5 DO I NEED TO RESTRICT MY DIET?
_____
_____
_____

6 OTHER QUESTIONS:
_____
_____
_____
_____
_____

**After the test:**

1 WHAT DID THE TEST REVEAL?
_____
_____

2 IS THAT POSITIVE OR NEGATIVE?
_____
_____

3 IS THERE IMPROVEMENT OVER THE LAST TEST?
_____

4 IF SO, HOW MUCH IMPROVEMENT?
_____

5 ARE YOU SATISFIED WITH THESE RESULTS?
_____

6 IF NOT, WHAT OTHER COURSE OF ACTION CAN WE FOLLOW AT THIS TIME?
_____

7 ARE THERE ANY OTHER TESTS YOU FEEL WOULD BE TO MY BENEFIT AT THIS TIME?
_____

8 WILL I REQUIRE FURTHER TESTING IN THE FUTURE?
_____

9 IF SO, WHY AND HOW OFTEN?
_____

10 OTHER QUESTIONS:
_____
_____
_____
_____

# Your Medical History

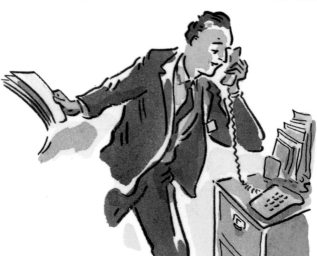

**M**any factors affect your cancer diagnosis and treatment, and it is important to be able to provide a complete and accurate picture of your medical history for your current specialists as well as any new ones who might join your cancer team or be called upon to provide a second opinion. The questions on this page are the ones that a doctor's office will ask you. Write in the answers now so that you will have the information available whenever you see a new doctor.

## PATIENT INFORMATION

*Name:* _____

*Age:* _____ *Blood type:* _____

*Date of birth:* _____

*Social Security #:* _____

*Home address:* _____

_____

*Home phone #:* _____

*Work phone #:* _____

*Nearest of kin:* _____

*Allergies (including allergies to any medications):* _____

_____

## PREVIOUS SURGERY

*Date:* _____

*Procedure:* _____

*Date:* _____

*Procedure:* _____

*Date:* _____

*Procedure:* _____

## MEDICAL HISTORY

**Check all that apply:**

- [ ] Alcoholism
- [ ] Alzheimer's
- [ ] Arthritis
- [ ] Asthma
- [ ] Cardiovascular disease
- [ ] Diabetes
- [ ] Emphysema
- [ ] Endometriosis
- [ ] Hepatitis
- [ ] High blood pressure
- [ ] HIV/AIDS
- [ ] Hypoglycemia
- [ ] Kidney or bladder problems
- [ ] Myocardial infarction
- [ ] Osteoporosis

## CANCER HISTORY

*Diagnosis:* _____

_____

_____

_____

*Treatment:* _____

_____

_____

_____

_____

*Chemotherapy drugs I have received:* _____

_____

_____

_____

_____

_____

## OTHER MEDICAL CONDITIONS

*Please explain:* _____

_____

_____

_____

_____

*Other medications:* _____

_____

_____

_____

# Medications

You may end up with three or four different doctors by the time your internist, oncologist, radiation oncologist, and surgeon are involved. Don't worry, they will contact each other and formulate an overall plan for your treatment. However, the issue with medications is tricky and can get out of hand. It is possible that your surgeon may prescribe a painkiller, your radiation oncologist a steroid, and your oncologist a sleeping aid. It is important to inform each doctor of the other prescriptions you are taking and why. Also, you will want to track each medication and the effect it has on you, alerting your doctors of adverse effects. The following chart will assist you in this process.

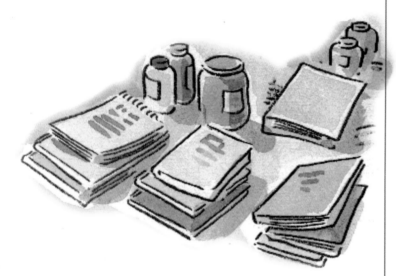

**Example of prescription chart**

Medication: *Compazine*

Date prescribed: *1-1-98*

Prescribing doctor: *Dr. Smith*

Doctors informed of new prescription: *Dr. Jones, Dr. Clark*

Reason for prescription: *Nausea*

Prescription instructions: *1 every 4 hours*

Side effects/results: *I get sleepy; works well on nausea*

## PRESCRIPTION CHART

Medication: _____

Date prescribed: _____

Prescribing doctor: _____

Doctors informed of new prescription: _____

Reason for medication: _____

Prescription instructions: _____

Side effects/result: _____


Medication: _____

Date prescribed: _____

Prescribing doctor: _____

Doctors informed of new prescription: _____

Reason for medication: _____

Prescription instructions: _____

Side effects/result: _____


Medication: _____

Date prescribed: _____

Prescribing doctor: _____

Doctors informed of new prescription: _____

Reason for medication: _____

Prescription instructions: _____

Side effects/result: _____


Medication: _____

Date prescribed: _____

Prescribing doctor: _____

Doctors informed of new prescription: _____

Reason for medication: _____

Prescription instructions: _____

Side effects/result: _____


Medication: _____

Date prescribed: _____

Prescribing doctor: _____

Doctors informed of new prescription: _____

Reason for medication: _____

Prescription instructions: _____

Side effects/result: _____

## SIGNS FOR CONCERN

- Abdominal tenderness
- Bleeding
- Balance disturbances
- Bone fractures
- Cough or fever
- Infection
- Rapid heart beat
- Shortness of breath
- "Tight collar" feeling
- Vomiting

## INSURANCE INFORMATION

*Name on policy:* _____

*Insurance company:* _____

*Policy number:* _____

*Doctors' co-pay:* _____

*Annual deduction:* _____

*Insurance agent's name:* _____

*Insurance agent's telephone #:* _____

*Insurance agent's fax #:* _____

*Procedure verification #:* _____

## MEDICATION CHART

It's important to keep a medication chart with the date, medication you received, the time the medication is taken, results, and reactions, if any. If you are required to take your pulse and temperature (also known as vital signs), do so at the time of medication administration. Carefully charting your medications and vital signs is especially important if there is more than one caregiver. You may need plenty of these charts, so you should make several photocopies of this page.

| MEDICATION | TIME | VITAL SIGNS | DOSAGE | RESULTS | REACTION/ SIDE EFFECTS |
|---|---|---|---|---|---|
|  |  |  |  |  |  |
|  |  |  |  |  |  |
|  |  |  |  |  |  |
|  |  |  |  |  |  |

# Pain Management

Many people think that the words cancer and pain automatically go together. That is NOT necessarily true. Having cancer does not always mean having pain. For example, pain is rarely a symptom of early cancer. Even patients with advanced cancers do not always have pain; however, if pain does occur, there are many ways to relieve or reduce it. Do not be afraid to ask your doctor for pain medication and, if the one prescribed for you isn't knocking it out, ask for something stronger. Pain is not something that you need to "learn to live with" so you should insist on good pain management from your medical team. Many people are afraid of becoming addicted, but that is highly unlikely and certainly the least of your

problems, I would think. Pain can cause depression, stress, loss of appetite, irritability, loss of sleep, and a feeling of hopelessness. Understanding that the vast majority of all cancer pain can be managed and controlled is essential to the patient. Today, pain relief techniques are geared toward restoring the quality and normalcy to the patient's life. Communication becomes the challenge on the part of the patient to accurately describe the pain, its severity, its location, and any recent changes. The physician's role is to assess all the information and to implement a pain management plan that is effective in relieving cancer discomfort and

pain. The following pages are designed to assist you in communicating to your doctor all aspects of your pain. If you experience new pain that you have not discussed with your doctor, observe it carefully for a week. Using

## NATURAL APPROACHES TO RELIEVING PAIN

- Acupuncture
- Cold
- Exercise
- Heat
- Hypnosis
- Imagery
- Massage
- Meditation
- Prayer
- Reflexology
- Relaxation
- Tai chi
- Yoga

• Stay ahead of pain and take the medication on time to prevent pain from starting.
• Try cold packs, rest, distracting activities, massages, and over-the-counter pain medications to help alleviate pain.
• Note carefully the activities that aggravate or increase your pain and avoid them when possible.
• Make use of prayer, meditation, and relaxation techniques.

## WORDS TO ASSIST YOU IN DESCRIBING YOUR PAIN

| | |
|---|---|
| aching | numbing |
| annoying | pounding |
| agonizing | pulsing |
| blinding | pressing |
| cold | pinching |
| cutting | penetrating |
| crushing | radiating |
| dull | rasping |
| distressful | sharp |
| frightful | suffocating |
| flickering | sore |
| freezing | spreading |
| gnawing | shooting |
| grueling | tender |
| hurting | taut |
| intense | tight |
| jumping | tingling |
| lacerating | throbbing |
| miserable | unbearable |
| nagging | vicious |
| nauseating | weak |

## PAIN SCALE

Doctors and nurses generally use one of two different pain scales in rating the pain of their patient. Ask your doctor whether he uses the 0 to 5 scale or the 1 to 10 scale.

My doctor uses the 0–5 scale _____     My doctor uses the 1–10 scale _____

Once you know your doctor's preference concerning the pain scale, use it consistently throughout your treatment and care.

**0–5 Pain scale**   0: no pain   1: slight discomfort   2: moderate pain   3: distressful pain   4: severe pain   5: grievous pain

| 1–10 Pain scale | 1 | 2 | 3 | 4 | 5 | 6 | 7 | 8 | 9 | 10 |
|---|---|---|---|---|---|---|---|---|---|---|
| | | Slight pain | | | | Medium pain | | | Worst pain | |

the body chart, keep track of when the pain started, its intensity, how it feels, the location, and its expansion, if any. Also take care to follow the pain medication you are taking and the effects it has on your new pain.

## INFORMATION TO GIVE YOUR DOCTOR WHEN YOU CALL

Be completely prepared when you call the doctor's nurse regarding your pain or side effects to treatment. Most likely you will not speak with your doctor directly, so make a concise, informative statement that the nurse can relay to your doctor, enabling him to make the right decision regarding your care. Of course, if it's an emergency, you must make the nurse aware of that immediately.

- When it started.
- Specifically where it is located.
- Describe the pain.
- Rate the pain on the pain scale.
- Explain what makes the pain better.
- Explain what makes the pain worse.
- What pain medication you are on now.
- How it is working.
- Side effects to pain medication.
- Any complications you are experiencing.

### WHAT IS BREAKTHROUGH PAIN?

Cancer patients may experience one of two types of chronic pain: persistent (continuous) pain and breakthrough (incident) pain. Persistent cancer pain lasts for long periods of time throughout the day. Breakthrough pain is the flare-up of pain that "breaks through" even when the patient is taking pain medications. If you experience breakthrough pain, contact your doctor immediately. He will advise you to take a quick-acting pain medication at the first sign that you are experiencing breakthrough pain. It is important to adjust the frequency and dosage of your pain medications if breakthrough pain occurs often. Always try to do your best to stay ahead of your pain.

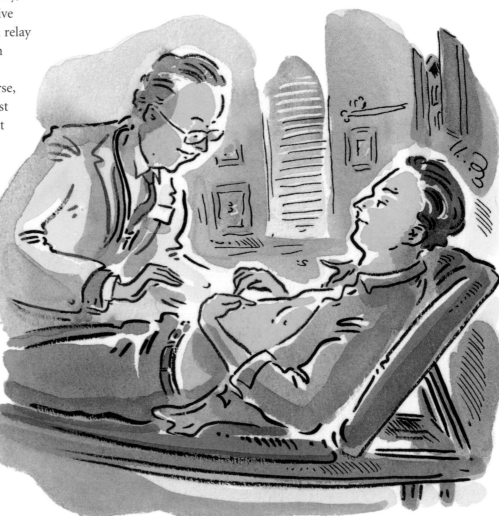

# Pain Diary

It is important to keep an accurate history of your pain, its intensity, and its position for your doctor. For your pain tracking I have provided the following five pages and included a schematic drawing of the human body. When you experience pain, pinpoint it on the body with a pencil so that you can erase your marks and reuse the illustrations at a later date. If the pain is persistent and intensifies after one week, call the doctor.

Date: _____

Pain scale rating: _____

_____

_____

_____

Location of pain: _____

_____

_____

_____

Description of pain _____

_____

_____

_____

Current pain medication: _____

_____

Effectiveness: _____

_____

_____

_____

## SCHEMATIC PAIN MAP

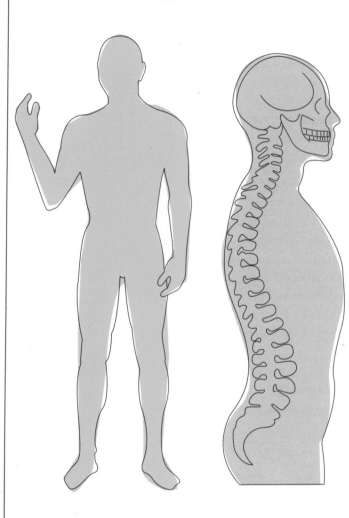

## PAIN RESPONSE BY GENDER

BALTIMORE (Johns Hopkins) – As recently as ten years ago it was believed that people responded more or less the same way to painkillers. Today, medicine knows better.

Recent research has made it increasingly clear that men and women don't always show the same reaction to common pain medications. New work from Australia, for instance, indicates that the anti-inflammatory ibuprofen seems to work better for males than for females. But a common painkiller in the dentist's office, nalbuphine, makes a bigger difference for women.

And it's not just gender. Genes seem to affect even individual responses to pain. "I believe that without a doubt, in the not-so-distant future we'll be able to obtain a genetic profile and determine the most appropriate analgesia for that individual," says Dr. Peter Staatsis, an expert in pain management at Johns Hopkins. But first things first. Researchers can't yet explain why or how gender and genes affect sensitivity to pain and responsiveness to medication. The answers to those riddles will occupy doctors and scientists in the near future.

## *"Simply put, music can heal people."*
– Senator Harry Reid (D-Nevado)

Music is used in hospitals to alleviate pain in conjunction with anesthesia or pain medication; elevate patients' mood and counteract depression; promote movement for physical rehabilitation; calm or sedate, induce sleep; counteract apprehension or fear; and lessen muscle tension for the purpose of relaxation, including the autonomic nervous system. For more information on music therapy, contact:

**American Music Therapy Association, Inc.**
Phone: (301) 589-3300
Online: http://www.musictherapy.org/

Ida Goldman (90-year-old testifying at Senate hearings): "Before I had surgery, they told me I could never walk again. But when I sat and listened to music, I forgot all about the pain," said Goldman, who walked with assistance during the hearing.

REUTERS

Date: _____

Pain scale rating: _____

_____

_____

Location of pain: _____

_____

_____

Description of pain _____

_____

_____

Current pain medication: _____

_____

Effectiveness: _____

_____

_____

_____

### NATIONAL PAIN ORGANIZATIONS

**Addressing Pain, Pain Management, Pain Clinics and Programs, and Pain Specialists**

City of Hope Pain Resource Center (COHPPRC)
National Medical Nursing Research & Education
Duarte, CA 91010
Phone #: (626) 359-8111, extension 3829

**Online: http://prc.coh.org/**

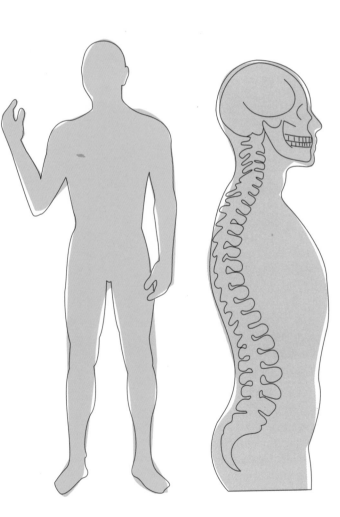

# Pain Diary, cont.

Date: _____

Pain scale rating: _____

_____

_____

_____

Location of pain: _____

_____

_____

_____

Description of pain _____

_____

_____

_____

Current pain medication: _____

_____

Effectiveness: _____

_____

_____

_____

## BRAIN SCAN CONFIRMS ACUPUNCTURE RELIEVES PAIN

### The Medical Tribune

Using a new form of brain imaging, researchers have confirmed that acupuncture does in fact relieve pain. Researchers measured brain activity in 12 subjects using functional magnetic resonance imaging (fMRI). The results showed decreased brain activity in four of the seven subjects (57%) who received manual acupuncture and in all five subjects who received electroacupuncture, compared to the level of brain activity measured during pain stimulation. Scientists led by Dr. Huey-Jen Lee, chief of neuroradiology at the University of Medicine and Dentistry of New Jersey-New Jersey Medical School in Newark found that after acupuncture, the subjects needed stronger stimuli in order to feel pain. "Our study shows that the person actually increases the pain threshold," Lee said. "That's kind of exciting." Despite the results of the study, Lee warned against jumping to general conclusions. "It's still premature," he said. "We'd like to get more data." Lee said that in future research, he and his team would like to see if acupuncture can help relieve chronic pain in cancer patients. He doesn't necessarily expect it to be a cure-all, but he hopes that acupuncture can be used to reduce the dosage needed of pain-relief medications.

*Copyright 1999 The Medical Tribune News Service*

Date: _____

Pain scale rating: _____

_____

_____

Location of pain: _____

_____

_____

Description of pain _____

_____

_____

Current pain medication: _____

_____

Effectiveness: _____

_____

_____

_____

## SOY AND THE PERCEPTION OF PAIN

*February 3, 1999*

BALTIMORE (Johns Hopkins)–- Why can some people bear a great deal of pain and others much less? The latest theories involve biology, genetics, and even diet.

Soybeans, specifically. Working with Israeli researchers, a Johns Hopkins team has found that rats who were fed a diet heavy in soy meal scored far lower on measures of pain sensitivity than rats who dined without soy in their food.

Johns Hopkins neurosurgery professor Dr. James Campbell helped research the study and says that, while the results make a convincing case that diet can affect the perception of pain, it is not yet proven that soy is the magic bullet. So if you hurt, don't start dashing soy sauce over all of your meals.

"We have learned from these studies that diet is important," explains Campbell. "In what ways it's important, do not have practical significance. So this information should in no way affect one's dietary intake at this point." While soy's pain relief benefits remain unproven, it has been shown to help lower cholesterol in people.

# Pain Diary, cont.

Date: _____

Pain scale rating: _____

_____

_____

_____

Location of pain: _____

_____

_____

_____

Description of pain _____

_____

_____

_____

Current pain medication: _____

_____

Effectiveness: _____

_____

_____

_____

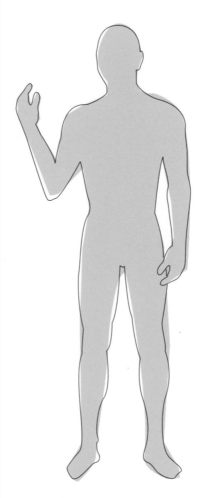
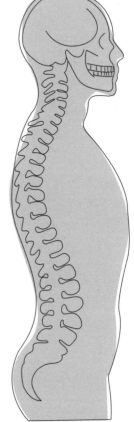

## THE TRAGEDY OF NEEDLESS CANCER PAIN

**You Don't Have to Suffer:** A complete guide to relieving cancer pain for patients and their families explores all the pain-relieving options available in the modern medical arsenal – from drugs and high-tech medical procedures to psychological and cognitive techniques and home nursing tips. Written by Richard B. Patt, MD, one of the country's leading cancer pain experts, and science writer Susan S. Lang.

## PAIN SENSITIVITY IN THE GENES

Researchers at Johns Hopkins University and the National Institute on Drug Abuse (NIDA) have found that much of our sensitivity to pain – and our individual response to opiate pain medications – has a genetic basis. In fact, many of those differences appear to be due to variation in a single key gene. Lead researcher Hopkins/NIDA neuroscientist George R. Uhl, MD, PhD has found that people vary greatly in their sensitivity to pain. A tetanus shot that stings one person may torment another. According to the new research, a particular gene that codes for the body's "mu" opiate receptors is the most likely candidate for both pain sensitivity and responsivity to morphine and morphinelike drugs. "People have long been skeptical that pain has a genetic basis," says Dr. Uhl. "They don't notice that sensitivity can vary because the differences can be subtle and masked by a strong emotional response to pain. Many people assume the way you respond is voluntary. 'Just put up with it' is a common suggestion. But now you can view pain as a genetically regulated problem."

In other words, it's not all in your head – it's in your genes.

Cancer Care provides tips for dealing effectively with your doctor on its website, at "Doctor, Can We Talk?" (http://www.cancercare.org/patients/talking.htm).

• First, remember that you are the consumer. As a patient, it is important for you to realize that you are a consumer of health care. The way to begin making difficult decisions about health care is to educate yourself.
• Bring someone with you. It is always helpful to have support, a second set of ears, and another person to think of questions.
• Write out a list of questions beforehand. When you are discussing something as important as your health, it is easy to become nervous or upset. Make the questions specific and brief, and ask the most important ones first.
• Write down the answers.
• If possible, bring a tape recorder. Taping is helpful because you may find yourself wanting to hear a reassurance or diagnosis again, or share it with friends and family at a later date.
• Make sure you understand exactly what you are saying and hearing.
• When you are talking to your doctor, use "I." The phrase "I don't understand…" is much more effective than "You're being unclear about…"

> Did you call the National Cancer Institute yet? If not, go back to page 35 and do it. The step-by-step instructions make it easy.
> **STOP**

LEAVE YOURSELF AN OUT:
BE CHOOSY ABOUT YOUR HEALTHCARE
TEAM. DON'T SETTLE FOR SECOND BEST.

• Don't be afraid to be assertive. If you don't know what a word means, ask.
• Finally, if something seems confusing to you, try to repeat it back to your doctor. For example, "You mean I should…." If you think you will understand an explanation better with pictures, ask to see X rays, slides, or have the doctor draw a diagram.

## JUST FOR THE FUN OF IT

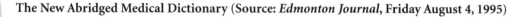

**The New Abridged Medical Dictionary (Source: *Edmonton Journal*, Friday August 4, 1995)**

• Artery: The study of paintings.
• Bacteria: Back door to the cafeteria.
• Barium: What doctors do when patients die.
• Benign: What you be after you be eight.
• Cauterize: Made eye contact with her.
• Coma: A punctuation mark.
• Colic: A sheep dog.
• D&C: Where Bill Clinton lives.
• Dilate: To live longer.
• Enema: Not a friend.

• Fester: Quicker.
• GI Series: World series of military baseball
• Hangnail: Coat hook.
• Impotent: Distinguished, well known.
• Labor Pain: Get hurt at work.
• Medical staff: A doctor's cane.
• Morbid: A higher offer.
• MRI: Who are you?
• Nitrates: Cheaper than day rates.
• Node: Was aware of.
• Outpatient: A patient who fainted.

• Pap smear: A fatherhood test.
• Pelvis: Cousin to Elvis.
• Recovery Room: A place to do upholstery.
• Rectum: Dang near killed 'em.
• Remission: cost of coming BACK into the theater.
• Secretion: Hiding something.
• Terminal illness: Getting sick at the airport.
• Tumor: More than one.
• Ultrasound: The ultimate in music.
• Urine: Opposite of "You're out."

# Scheduling Your Days

This could become a very busy time for you depending on your individual condition. It is conceivable that you might have two diagnostic tests, one doctor's appointment, and a consultation at the hospital all in one day. It would be strenuous under normal circumstances to keep pace with such a schedule, but with the added stress of cancer it is possible to feel overwhelmed and become forgetful. Be smart when you are scheduling your appointments. Make as many for one day as you can handle comfortably and give yourself plenty of time to get from one hospital or doctor's office to another.

I have provided two calendar pages to help you organize your days (you will want to photocopy these pages). Keep your appointments written down so that you do not overlap them or miss one entirely. Use the calendar for hospital stays, treatments, physical therapy, blood tests, diagnostic tests, support groups, and follow-up visits with your doctors.

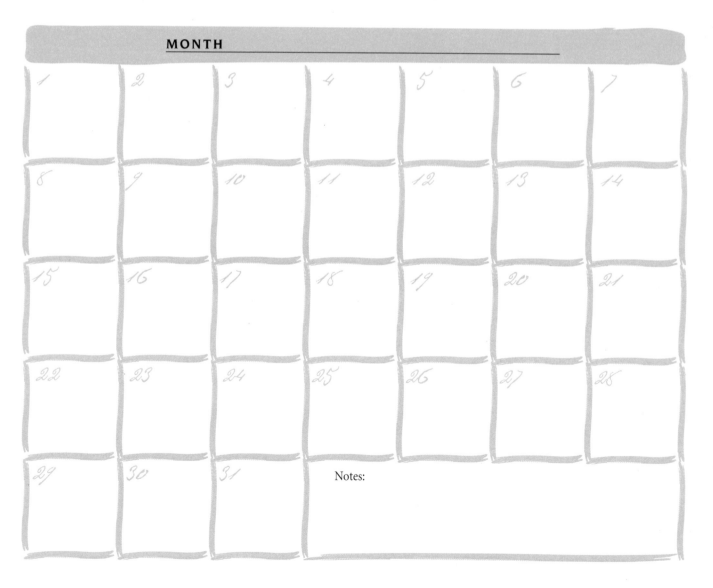

**MONTH**

| 1 | 2 | 3 | 4 | 5 | 6 | 7 |
|---|---|---|---|---|---|---|
| 8 | 9 | 10 | 11 | 12 | 13 | 14 |
| 15 | 16 | 17 | 18 | 19 | 20 | 21 |
| 22 | 23 | 24 | 25 | 26 | 27 | 28 |
| 29 | 30 | 31 | Notes: | | | |

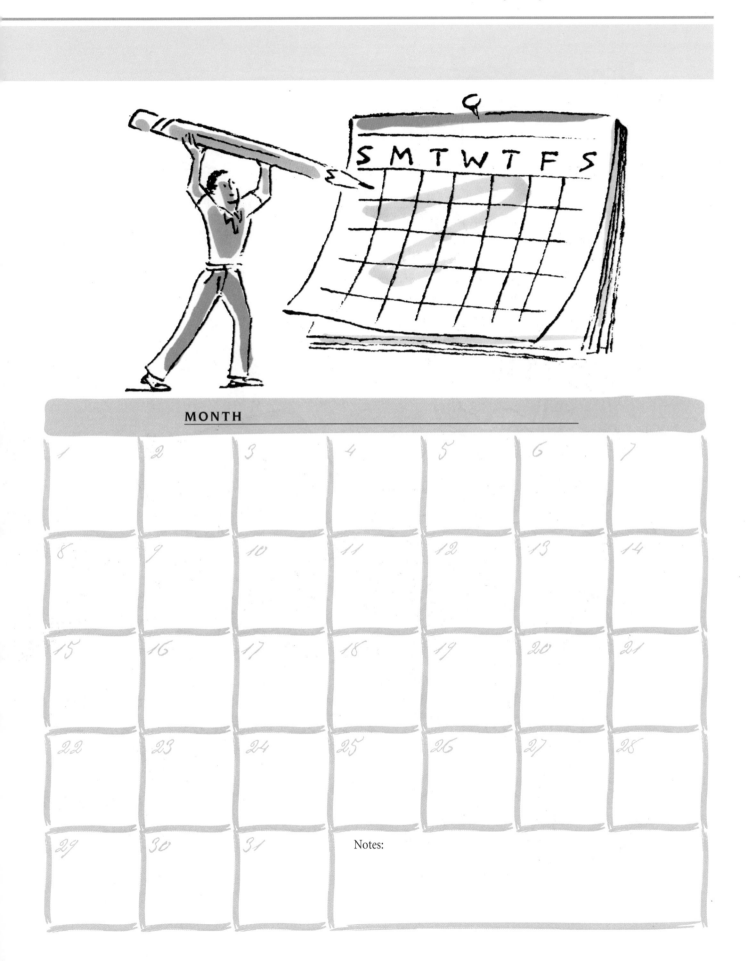

**MONTH**

| 1 | 2 | 3 | 4 | 5 | 6 | 7 |
|---|---|---|---|---|---|---|
| 8 | 9 | 10 | 11 | 12 | 13 | 14 |
| 15 | 16 | 17 | 18 | 19 | 20 | 21 |
| 22 | 23 | 24 | 25 | 26 | 27 | 28 |
| 29 | 30 | 31 | Notes: | | | |

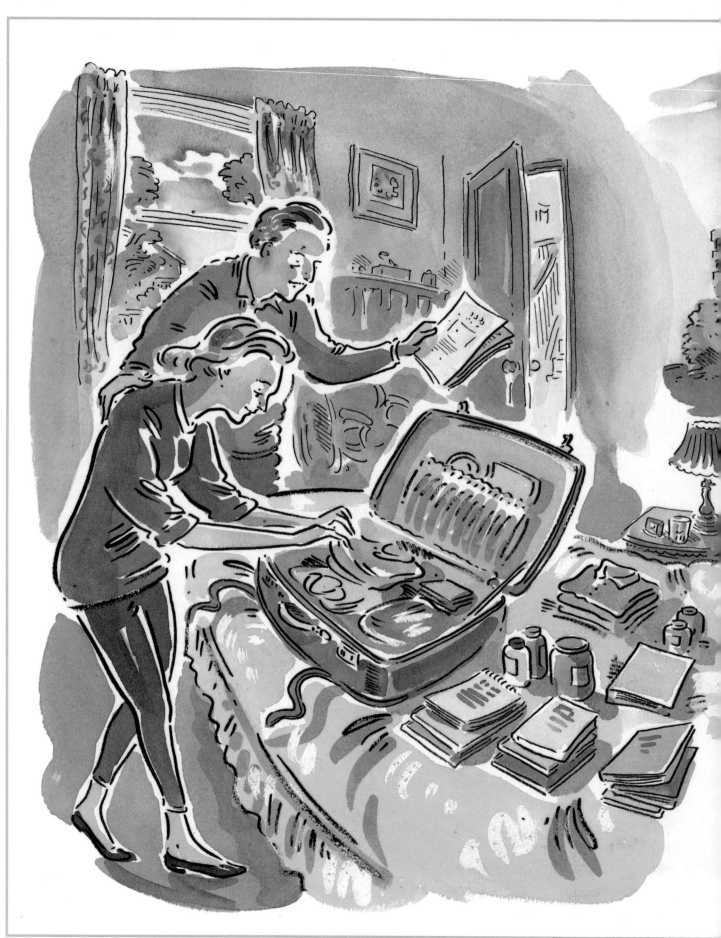

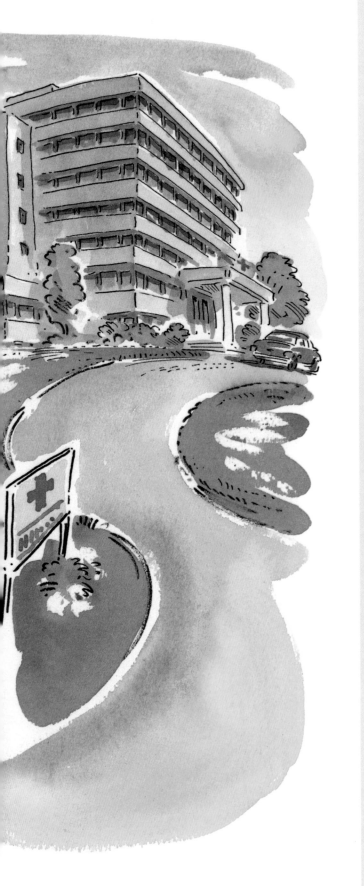

# Your Cancer Plan

## *Chapter 4*

# Be Prepared

Chemotherapy, radiation therapy, and surgery are the primary treatments that doctors use to fight cancer, and they will directly affect your life over the next several months. None of these options to restore you to health are a walk in the park, but there are preparations you can take to help make the time ahead go as smoothly as possible.

First and foremost is your mindset. Maintaining a positive attitude is difficult when you have been given a diagnosis of cancer. You may have feelings of anger, depression, anxiety, and helplessness. Do not suffer with these feelings alone – get help. Talk to your doctor, join a support group, share your concern with your family and friends, or get therapy. It is important to recognize your feelings and deal with them. You have much work and healing to do. Now is not the time to be in conflict with your emotions, it's the time to fight your cancer.

Having made the final decision as to the treatment plan you feel is best for you, now is the time to have a positive attitude and "go with the flow." Cancer patients need to embrace their treatments as much as they possibly can, believe that the therapy will do what it is intended to do, and make every effort to resist going into the fight "kicking and screaming." Take an aggressive stance. Make the doctors, nurses, and technicians your team, and get family members and friends on board to help you do what you are all there to do: fight for your life.

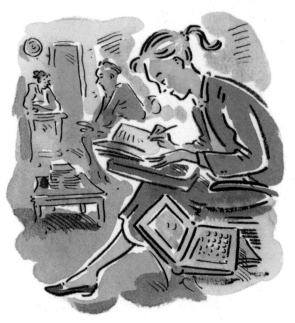

A considerable number of your days will be involved in waiting…waiting in reception areas for doctors, waiting for treatments to start and be completed, waiting for diagnostic tests and their results. The patients that seem to fare the best are the ones who are determined to get through the day making the best of their circumstances. Bringing a loved one, office work, hobbies, or reading material to keep your mind occupied often helps the time go faster.

*It is important to get in control and stay that way in the areas that you can control.*

Do your best to anticipate what you are going to want while in hospitals or treatment centers, and during periods of recuperation. As much as possible, perform responsibilities at home or work before each course of medical care so that you can focus on resting and recovering after your treatment or surgery.

---

The physical and emotional demands placed on you at this time may cause you to feel confused and overwhelmed. Do what you can when you can, keeping focused on only the present. The following pages will help you organize and get through the days ahead. Remember that there is no "right way" to do this, there is only "your way." What you cannot do, ask others to do. What you cannot handle, put off until later. Pamper yourself, rest often, and be mindful not to push past your limitations.

## SPONTANEOUS REMISSION

Simply stated, spontaneous remission is the partial or complete disappearance of a malignant tumor in the absence of any treatment. Oncologists speak of patients whose cancer was believed to be incurable, who had been sent home to live out their lives, and had waltzed back into the doctor's office months later with significantly smaller tumors or no sign of disease at all. This incredible phenomenon has baffled scientists and doctors worldwide. Is it the immune system? If so, what turns it on and why does it now recognize and attack the diseased cells? Does nutrition, prayer, exercise, attitude, vitamins, laughter, or the mind play a part? Those studying spontaneous remissions are trying to unlock the key to understand how to stimulate natural self-healing capacities that exist in everyone to some degree.

# Your Hospital Stay

Surgery is used in about 60 percent of all cancer cases and, when employed solely, has a curative rate of approximately 30 percent. Nearly all people with cancer undergo some form of surgery, whether for a biopsy to stage their disease, determine where and how extensive the malignancy is, or remove the tumor and surrounding tissue (see page 94). Outpatient surgery is now often used for diagnostic surgery or for implanting pumps, catheters, or ports. For more extensive surgery you will be required to stay in the hospital until the doctor finds you well enough to go home. In either case, you should ask plenty of questions and prepare yourself as best you can. See pages 64–65 for questions to ask before and after surgery. Listed below are some items you may want to have with you during your hospital stay.

## TYPES OF SURGERY

- Biopsy: A procedure to remove all or part of a tumor for diagnosis.
- Curative: Complete removal of a tumor.
- Diagnostic: Removal of tissue to test for cancer.
- Elective: Not necessary.
- Emergency: Perfromed to save a person's life, organ, or limb, or to stop bleeding.
- Exploratory: Performed to inspect a suspicious area or organ for cancer.
- Palliative: Used to remove problems or pain.
- Preventative: Removal of a tissue or organ not presently cancerous.
- Staging: Surgery to determine the extent of the disease.
- Treatment: Taking out a tumor or organ to control or cure cancer.

## FACTS ABOUT SURGERY

1. Cancer does not spread because it has been exposed to air during surgery.
2. Biopsies may be done by other doctors, such as radiation oncologists, oncologists, pulmonologists, pathologists, or gastroenterologists.
3. Surgery offers the greatest chance of a cure for many types of cancer.
4. More than one-third of the serious postoperative complications occur 48 hours or more after the procedure.
5. Chemotherapy and radiation therapy are usually more effective after most of the cancer has been removed by surgery.
6. Some insurance companies require a second opinion to approve surgery.

## CHECKLIST OF ITEMS TO TAKE TO THE HOSPITAL

- ☐ Your *Workbook* – write down all questions for your surgeon
- ☐ Health insurance card
- ☐ Address book
- ☐ Playing cards, books, crossword puzzles
- ☐ Stationery, envelopes, and stamps
- ☐ Laptop computer
- ☐ Office-related work
- ☐ Walkman or tape player and favorite tapes
- ☐ Needlepoint, embroidery, or other handicraft projects
- ☐ Dried fruit & healthful snacks
- ☐ Your own pillow if it would make you more comfortable.
- ☐ Comfortable nightclothes, pajamas, or nightgown

- ☐ Bathrobe and slippers
- ☐ Sweater
- ☐ Underwear
- ☐ Socks
- ☐ Comfortable walking shoes
- ☐ Rubber thongs/slaps for the shower
- ☐ Loose-fitting clothing to wear home from the hospital.
- ☐ Medicines and prescriptions
- ☐ Vitamins
- ☐ Shampoo
- ☐ Comb and brush
- ☐ Toothbrush, toothpaste, and floss
- ☐ Lip balm
- ☐ Small towel and washcloth
- ☐ Deodorant
- ☐ Earplugs

- ☐ Hairdryer
- ☐ Hair spray/mousse
- ☐ Extra pair of eyeglasses or contacts
- ☐ Saline solution
- ☐ Makeup
- ☐ Razor and blades
- ☐ Shaving cream
- ☐ Aftershave
- ☐ _____
- ☐ _____
- ☐ _____

Inquire with the hospital if they provide VCRs in the rooms. If so, rent some funny movies to take with you.

# Your Hospital Stay, cont.

## WHY I AM HAVING SURGERY

- ☐ To prevent or lower the risk of developing cancer.
- ☐ To diagnose the disease.
- ☐ To stage the disease.
- ☐ To remove the primary tumor.
- ☐ To relieve painful symptoms.
- ☐ To remove other tumors or affected organs.
- ☐ To reconstruct or rehabilitate.
- ☐ To implant a port, catheter, or pump.
- ☐ To treat complications.

## LIST TO PREPARE FOR SURGERY:

- ☐ Stop smoking.
- ☐ Exercise as much as possible.
- ☐ Gain or lose weight if necessary.
- ☐ Give your own blood if it might be needed during surgery.
- ☐ Pay bills, do errands, get organized.
- ☐ Organize care to start upon your return home.
- ☐ Prepare a living will.
- ☐ If you live alone, arrange to have your home cared for while you are in the hospital.

## THE NIGHT BEFORE SURGERY TO-DO LIST:

- ☐ Pack your bags for the hospital stay.
- ☐ Be certain to include the necessary hospital forms.
- ☐ Enjoy a good balanced dinner.
- ☐ Shower or bathe.
- ☐ Do not drink or eat anything for 12 hours before surgery.
- ☐ Take a laxative if ordered by your doctor.
- ☐ Take a sleeping pill if you have been given one by your doctor. You need a good night's sleep.
- ☐ Make sure you arrive on time in the morning; set your alarm.

## THE DAY OF YOUR SURGERY

- You will be taken to a pre-op room.
- You will dress in a hospital gown.
- An IV will be started to administer drugs.
- You will be given medication that will relax you.
- You may be shaved at the operation site.
- Your skin will be cleaned with an antiseptic.
- Family may be allowed to visit you in pre-op just before your surgery.
- Once in the operating room, anesthesia will be administered and you will go to sleep.

## THE POST-OP RECOVERY ROOM

- You will wake up in a post-op recovery room.
- Your heart rate and breathing will be monitored.
- You will receive IV fluids (painkillers, blood).
- Nurses will supervise and assess you closely.

## WHEN ALL IS SAID AND DONE

- You will be returned to your room.
- The nurses will help you into your bed.
- You will be monitored consistently for pain.
- Family will be allowed to see you.

## TYPES OF ANESTHESIA

Anesthesia is medicine used to make you comfortable during surgery. The medication may be given locally, or through an IV, a face mask, a tube in your nose, or as a shot.

- Epidural anesthesia: A small tube is inserted in the patient's back to numb the area below the waist. Pain medication may also be administered through an epidural after the surgery.
- General anesthesia: Medication used to keep you completely asleep during your surgery. This medication affects the entire body and is most commonly used during surgery.
- Local anesthesia: Medication administered as an injection into the skin where you will have surgery. It is used to dull pain, but you will be awake (but may be sleepy) during the surgery or procedure.

## POSTSURGICAL PAIN

If you feel restless, anxious, sweaty, are unable to move, or cannot walk, talk, or breathe normally, you are experiencing entirely too much pain. Pain after surgery is caused by changes made to your skin, muscles, and nerves during the operation. Most often you will experience pain at the site of the surgery, but you can experience pain in other body locations as well. Keeping your pain level at a minimum will allow your body to heal more quickly. Along with pain medication you may try changing your bed position, having your legs or back rubbed, putting a cool cloth on your face, watching TV, or reading to alleviate pain. Getting up to walk is especially important. Lying in bed allows gas to build up and permits for more intense muscle soreness.

# Ports and Catheters

There are several ways in which chemotherapy drugs can be administered. The most commonly used method is the continuous infusion, which is a tiny plastic catheter inserted into a vein on your hand or forearm on the day of your treatment. The catheter allows the chemotherapy drugs to "drip" into your bloodstream. Generally, the catheter is removed after your treatment, although it may be left in overnight if you are having therapy again the following day.

Another method of drug delivery is the vascular access device (VAD). Doctors will request that you have an implanted VAD device if you are likely to need lengthy treatment or if your veins are small and hard to access. If you have a VAD ask your nurse or doctor for instructions on caring for the device.

## BENEFITS OF VADS

- **You will avoid multiple injections.**
- **Blood can be easily drawn.**
- **There is a smaller chance of chemotherapy leakage from a vein.**
- **It is quickly accessible.**

*There are three major types of VADs:*

**Nontunneled catheters** are placed just beneath the skin near the collarbone and are inserted directly into a vein. This does not require surgery. The catheter is visible and easy to access. It does require cleaning, having the dressing changed, and being flushed with heparin.

**Tunneled catheters** are placed just beneath the skin on the chest and then are tunneled for several inches before being inserted into a vein. Minor surgery is necessary. This has a lower risk of infection. The catheter is visible and requires cleaning and being flushed with heparin.

**Ports** are small devices that are implanted just beneath the skin on the chest and access a vein just below the collarbone. Minor surgery is necessary. Since the port is under the surface of the skin, a needle stick is necessary to access the port. This device requires very little care and only needs to be flushed once a month.

## THE CATHETER VEST

The catheter vest keeps your catheter where you want it. The vest, which comes in styles and sizes that are suitable for children as well as adults, is a soft Lycra/cotton undergarment. By securing one or two central venous catheters inconspicuously, the catheter vest provides easy access to the catheters for nurses and other caregivers, eliminating the need to use tape and thus reducing skin irritation and infection. The catheter vest is durable and machine washable. The cost of the vest may be reimbursed by insurance companies with a prescription written by your doctor. Call (800) 547-6412 or find it online at:

**http://www.cathetervest.com/products.htm**

---

Write the step-by-step cleaning procedure below.

*Step 1.* _____

_____

*Step 2.* _____

_____

*Step 3.* _____

_____

*Step 4.* _____

_____

*Step 5.* _____

_____

Be very aware of redness or soreness around the area of your VAD.

## QUESTIONS ABOUT VADS

**Ask your doctor or nurse for the following information:**

*What kind of VAD would you suggest I have?*

_____

_____

*What are the benefits of this kind of VAD?*

_____

_____

*What are the disadvantages of this VAD?*

_____

_____

_____

## WHAT'S HEPARIN?

It's a drug that prevents blood from clotting and is injected in the tubes of VADs to prevent blockage.

# Chemotherapy

In the last 30 years the use of one or more of the 50 anticancer chemotherapy drugs that are now available has become standard treatment for those diagnosed with cancer. The concept behind this treatment is quite basic: cancer cells divide and multiply rapidly and anticancer drugs interfere with their growth and/or their reproduction. Chemotherapy is administered to the body through the bloodstream, thus treating all tissues and organs. Frequently some cells of a cancerous tumor will have broken off from the original site (metastasis) and spread throughout the body, traveling through the blood and lymph system. Since these cancer cells have yet to form a tumor large enough to be detected by tests, chemotherapy is often used as an adjuvant treatment to eliminate hidden cancer cells.

Great strides have been made in the field of chemotherapy. New chemotherapy agents, antinausea drugs, methods, and timing of administering these drugs have led to larger doses being given while fewer side effects are experienced. The fear that the cure is worse than the disease is shared by many cancer patients, but most would say that the treatment results are well worth the effort.

*Estimates have linked chemotherapy treatment to remission of more than 138,000 cancer cases in the United States each year.*

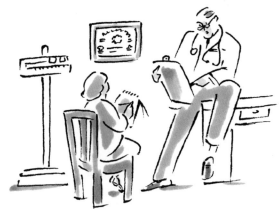

Why will you receive chemotherapy? How will it be administered? What can you expect? Ask your oncologist the questions in pages 54–61 and get a realistic view of what's ahead. It's best to know what to anticipate and this section can help you get organized and prepare you for your chemotherapy treatments. Keep your eyes on the prize.

---

### ADJUVANT TREATMENT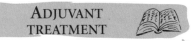

It is a treatment being used "in addition" to the primary form of treatment.

### CHEMOTHERAPY IS BEING USED IN MY CASE TO

**Check all that apply.**

- [ ] Cure my cancer.
- [ ] Stop the spread of cancer.
- [ ] Improve my quality of life.
- [ ] Treat widespread disease.
- [ ] Achieve long-term remission.
- [ ] Control tumor growth.
- [ ] Relieve painful symptoms.
- [ ] Reduce the size of the tumor.
- [ ] Kill cells left behind at the site of surgery.

### HOW WILL CHEMOTHERAPY BE ADMINISTERED TO ME?

- [ ] It will be put on my skin topically.
- [ ] I will swallow it in pill, capsule, or liquid form.
- [ ] It will be given as a shot into the muscle of my arm, thigh, or buttocks.
- [ ] It will be administered intravenously into an artery through an IV or port.
- [ ] It will be delivered directly into the tumor or specific area of my body through a catheter or needle.
- [ ] It will be injected slowly into my body by an ambulatory pump that I wear during my normal activities.

### BEFORE CHEMO TREATMENTS

- Make arrangements to have your dentist clean your teeth and do all necessary dental work.
- It's best to shop and purchase a wig before the loss of your hair.
- Get a short, stylish haircut.
- Receive your yearly flu shot.

### DID YOU KNOW?

**Combining two or more anticancer drugs:**

- Increases the power of the treatments.
- Decreases any single side effect.
- Lowers the chances that cancer cells become "immune" to the drugs given in high doses.

Every cancer and every patient is unique, and it is your doctor's challenge to design a treatment plan tailor-made for your particular case. If you will be receiving chemotherapy as part of your cancer battle plan, then most likely those treatments will be administered to you in an outpatient hospital, doctor's office, or treatment center. Administering the drugs can take from 15 minutes to 8 hours. You may be given one to six weeks off between treatments to rest and recover, and your treatments could last anywhere from a few months to a few years.

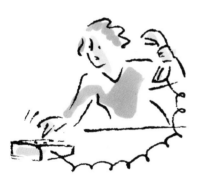

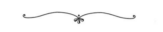

## Yogurt May Be Good For You

Reuters Health reports that a study presented at the Annual Scientific Meeting of the American College of Gastroenterology showed that just two 8-ounce servings of vanilla yogurt a day reduced the rate of antibiotic-associated diarrhea by half in a study of 202 hospitalized patients. Enjoy yogurt for breakfast and lunch. There's more to it than just good taste.

## Record Your Chemotherapy Drugs and the Possible Side Effects

*Drug:*_____

*Side effect:*_____

*Drug:*_____

*Side effect:*_____

*Drug:*_____

*Side effect:*_____

*Drug:*_____

*Side effect:*_____

*Drug:*_____

*Side effect:*_____

## Call Your Doctor Immediately if You Exhibit Any of These Side Effects

- A fever of 100°F or more
- Diarrhea
- A rash
- Bleeding/sudden bruising
- Convulsion or seizure
- Kidney failure
- Violent chills
- Swelling in hands/feet
- Difficulty breathing
- Prolonged vomiting
- Bloody urine
- Pain at injection site

- Symptoms of prostate cancer
- Frequent urination, especially at night
- Trouble starting urine flow
- Blood in the urine
- Interrupted urine flow
- Pain or burning during urination
- Weak urine flow
- Pain in the lower back, pelvis, or upper thighs
- Trouble holding back urine flow

## Complete the Following and Mark Off the Treatments as You Receive Them

Each treatment will take about ____ hours/minutes}

I will have _____ {number} days off between the treatments to rest and recover.

I will receive a total of _____ {number} treatments.

I have already completed the following number of treatments {cross out}

1 2 3 4 5 6 7 8 9 10 11 12 13 14 15 16 17 18 19 20 21 22 23 24

# Before Treatments

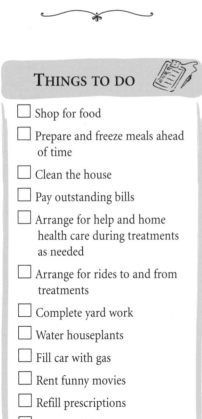

Are fatigue, lethargy, nausea, or other side effects to be expected with your treatment regimen? Coping with chemotherapy is made much easier if you can go home and rest for several days after your treatments. Use the list below as a guideline of chores and tasks that you would like to get accomplished before each chemotherapy session.

*Many patients are able to continue working while being treated for cancer.*

If possible, schedule your therapy right before the weekend so that it interferes with work as little as possible. Pamper yourself. It helps speed your recovery time.

## Things to Do

- [ ] Shop for food
- [ ] Prepare and freeze meals ahead of time
- [ ] Clean the house
- [ ] Pay outstanding bills
- [ ] Arrange for help and home health care during treatments as needed
- [ ] Arrange for rides to and from treatments
- [ ] Complete yard work
- [ ] Water houseplants
- [ ] Fill car with gas
- [ ] Rent funny movies
- [ ] Refill prescriptions
- [ ] Arrange child care

## What to Bring to Chemotherapy Treatments

**Prepare a briefcase, backpack, or carryall with items you may want to have with you while receiving chemotherapy. If possible, leave the case packed and ready for your next treatment.**

- [ ] Your *Cancer Patient's Workbook*; during therapy would be a great time to fill in some pages
- [ ] Laptop computer
- [ ] Office work
- [ ] Sweater or jacket; treatment rooms are cold
- [ ] Walkman and your favorite relaxation tapes
- [ ] Thank-you cards, stationary, envelopes, address book, and stamps
- [ ] Books, crossword puzzles, or needlework
- [ ] Juice and snacks if your treatments are lengthy
- [ ] A friend or family member
- [ ] _____

## What's Your Reaction?

**No one deals with cancer in the same way, but researchers report that most of us do cope rather well. Which best describes you?**

• Denial: A person who goes on without attention to their cancer. Positive avoidance. Doesn't know, doesn't want to know. Proceeds as normal. As long as the patient is getting everything done with regards to the cancer, keeping the disease at a distance serves some people well as a coping technique.

• Fighter: A person who believes completely that he or she can and will affect the outcome of the cancer. Not necessarily an easy patient to get along with but generally ges the best health care. Wants to know every aspect of the cancer. Looks at cancer as a fight to be won.

• Hopeless: A person who believes nothing much will help, that he or she will probably succumb to the disease anyway. Can be a sign of depression. Is also a coping style to handle the impending end of life.

• Stoic: A person with serious and resigned tendencies who accepts his or her "fate." Keeps emotions tightly reigned in. Calm, composed, and impassive.

If you are very tired and weak, or not a fighter by nature, ask a family member or friend to be aggressive and seek answers, and to assist you in making choices.

# Radiation Treatments

Nearly one-half of all people diagnosed with cancer will receive radiation therapy, alone or combined with surgery and/or chemotherapy. Radiation treatments most often consist of high-energy X rays aimed directly at tumors in an effort to shrink or destroy malignant growths. Radiation therapy targets cancer cells that are multiplying rapidly by killing the cell or injuring it so that it cannot divide. Although radiation causes severe damage to cancerous cells, it causes minimal permanent damage to the normal cells surrounding the area and healthy tissue typically recovers with little permanent damage.

## RADIATION'S POSSIBLE SIDE EFFECTS

Side effect: _____

Side effect: _____

**Call your doctor immediately if you exhibit any of these side effects:**

- A fever of 100°F or more
- Diarrhea
- Moist or wet skin areas
- New pain
- Severe appetite or eating problem
- Swelling in hands/feet
- Hoarseness/difficulty swallowing
- Difficulty breathing
- Burned, cracked skin
- Bloody urine

## COMPLETE THE FOLLOWING AND MARK OFF THE WEEKS AS YOU COMPLETE THEM

I will receive a total of _____ (number) treatments.

They will be administered over _____ (how many) weeks.

I have already completed the following number of weeks (cross out).

1    2    3    4    5    6    7    8    9    10

## RADIATION IS BEING USED IN MY CASE TO:

**Check all that apply.**

- ☐ Cure my cancer.
- ☐ Shrink the tumor.
- ☐ Prevent spread.
- ☐ Reduce an inoperable tumor.
- ☐ Reduce pain or pressure, (palliative care).
- ☐ Be used as whole-body radiation for abone marrow transplant.
- ☐ Reduce the size of the tumor before surgery.
- ☐ Kill cells left behind at the site of surgery.

## HOW WILL RADIATION BE ADMINISTERED TO ME?

- ☐ External radiation (a machine directing high-energy rays at the cancer and a small margin of normal tissue surrounding it).
- ☐ Internal radiation: What will be the source of the radiation?
  cesium ____ gold ____ iodine ____
  iridium ____ phosphorus _____
  other _____

What form of internal radiation will be used?

- ☐ Implant placed in tumor and surrounding tissues, later filled with radioactive "seeds"
- ☐ Hollow applicator placed in body space; removed after radiation dose has been delivered

## EXTERNAL RADIATION

The most common type of radiation given during outpatient visits to a treatment center or hospital is external radiation. A machine directs high-energy rays at the tumor and a small margin of tissue surrounding it.

## INTERNAL RADIATION

Brachytherapy is a method of implanting a source of radiation directly into a tumor, body cavity, or "tumor bed" after surgery to wipe up errant cancer cells. The radiation implant may be thin wires, plastic catheters, capsules, or seeds. Internal radiation may be given by injecting a radioactive solution into the bloodstream or a body cavity.

## HUGS AND KISSES

Receiving external radiation therapy does not cause you to become radioactive. You do not need to avoid anyone. Hugging, kissing, or having sexual relations poses no risk to your loved ones.

BECAUSE YOU MAY LOOK NORMAL IT CAN BE VERY FRUSTRATING THAT OTHERS CAN'T BEGIN TO COMPREHEND HOW EXHAUSTED YOU ARE. DON'T LET EXPECTATIONS OF YOU DRIVE YOU BEYOND YOUR LIMITS. LISTEN TO YOURSELF!

# Fatigue

If you receive chemotherapy or radiation therapy, you are likely to encounter fatigue as a side effect. The fatigue may accumulate during the weeks of treatment and may linger for a period of time after the regimen has been completed. Several factors play a part in your weariness. The treatments will suppress your bone marrow's ability to make red blood cells, which can cause you to feel lethargic and may lead to anemia. In addition, your body will be dealing with the expulsion of dead cancerous cells and toxic waste, while using whatever energy you have in reserve in an effort to heal you after each treatment.

Fatigue is the number-one complaint of those receiving treatments. Not only does it affect you physically but fatigue can cause emotional problems as well. Do not make the mistake of confusing this overwhelming exhaustion with the belief that your cancer is growing out

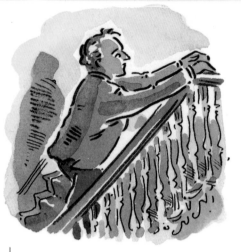

of control. Don't hesitate to speak with your doctor if you are concerned and need reassurance.

## CLOTTING PROBLEMS

Anticancer drugs can affect your platelets, the blood cells that help stop bleeding, by making your blood clot. Let your doctor know if you experience the following:

- Pinkish urine
- Bleeding gums or nose
- Unexpected bruising
- Black or bloody bowel movements
- Small red spots under the skin

### IF YOUR PLATELET COUNT IS LOW:

- Don't drink alcoholic beverages.
- Clean your nose with a soft tissue; do not give a hearty blow.
- Be careful while shaving.
- Do not take vitamin E.
- Do not take aspirin, ibuprofen, acetaminophen, or any other medications without first checking with your doctor.
- Use a very soft toothbrush.
- Do not floss your teeth.
- Avoid sports or other activities that could cause injury.
- Take extra care when using knives, scissors, needles, or tools.
- Do not rub or scratch wounds or cuts.
- Be extremely careful not to burn yourself while you are cooking or ironing.
- Do not use enemas without your doctor's approval.

## SIGNS OF ANEMIA

Some of the signs of anemia closely resemble normal chemotherapy side effects. Do not take chances. Call your physician or nurse if you have several of the symptoms below.

- Weakness, fatigue
- Light-headedness
- Shortness of breath
- Pounding heartbeat rate
- Lining of your lower eyelids looks pale
- Chills

## SIGNS OF FATIGUE

- Anxiety
- Boredom
- Decreased energy
- Impatience / irritability
- Nervousness
- Lack of motivation
- Inability to concentrate
- Sleeplessness
- Tired legs, eyes
- Whole-body exhaustion

## DEALING WITH FATIGUE – THINGS YOU CAN DO

**Rest often, and take short naps.**

- Eat high-energy snacks often.
- Drink at least eight glasses of liquid a day to aid in eliminating waste.
- Do quiet activities, read, watch funny movies.
- Drink protein shakes.
- Go for short walks to build strength.
- Limit visitor time.
- Delegate to family and friends the chores of shopping, housekeeping, yard care, driving, cooking, and childcare.
- Do not let yourself become socially isolated.
- Go to bed early at night.
- Do only those things that are important to you.
- Pace yourself and do not overdo when you are feeling energetic.
- When sitting or lying down, get up slowly to prevent dizziness.
- Eat a well-balanced diet. Make an effort to sustain your weight.

# Nausea

Chemotherapy may make food taste metallic, salty, or bitter. Normal taste sensations will come back after the treatments end. Chemotherapy side effects vary greatly from person to person and from drug to drug. Some people may never feel nauseated, others may experience mild nausea most of the time, and others may be severely nauseated for several days during and after their treatments. Chemotherapy causes nausea because it affects the stomach and the area of the brain that controls vomiting. However, nausea and vomiting may be controlled effectively with the new antinausea medicines that are now available.

During the administration of chemotherapy, you will receive antinausea medication and possibly steroids to prevent queasiness. In addition, your doctor will prescribe medication to keep you comfortable at home.

Determining the right antinausea drugs for you may take a short period of trial and error. Do not give up – work with your doctor. While the side effects are unpleasant, keep in mind that the same drugs that are making you sick are also killing the cancer cells.

## DEALING WITH NAUSEA

- Eat small, frequent meals throughout the day.
- Eat and drink slowly.
- Do not eat past full.
- Start with what "sounds good" and try a large variety of foods.
- Stay away from sweet, fatty, spicy, and fried foods.
- Drink liquids 30 minutes to 60 minutes before or after meals.
- Chew your food well for easier digestion.
- Wear loose-fitting clothes.

- If strong foods bother you, stay away from cooking areas and eat foods cold or at room temperature to prevent strong aromas.
- If nausea is a problem in the morning, eat crackers or dry toast before getting out of bed.
- Rest upright after meals. Don't lie flat for at least 2 hours after eating.
- Get fresh air. Breathe deeply and slowly when you feel nauseated.
- Try relaxation or imagery therapy. Listen to music or watch TV.

## FOODS THAT GO DOWN EASILY

- Ginger snaps, ginger ale without the fizz, ginger capsules, or tea
- Crackers, toast, pretzels, vanilla wafers, dry cereal
- Miso soup, broths
- Clear fruit juices
- Oatmeal
- Mashed potatoes
- Eggs
- Plain noodles
- Jell-O®, pudding
- Popsicles®, sherbet
- Gatorade®
- Ensure®, Boost®, or Carnation® drinks
- Cooked vegetables

## CALL YOUR DOCTOR IMMEDIATELY IF:

- Vomiting occurs more than 3 times per hour for more than 3 hours.
- You think you may have inhaled some vomited material into your lungs.
- There is evidence of blood.
- Your vomit resembles coffee grounds.
- You cannot keep the medications down.
- You are dizzy, very weak, or lose consciousness.
- You are unable to eat or hold down at least 4 cups of fluid over a 2-day period.

## "ANTICIPATORY NAUSEA AND VOMITING"

If you get nauseated just before a radiation or chemotherapy treatment or in anticipation of a doctor's visit, your mind has formed a connection between your medical treatments and nausea or vomiting. Inform your doctor or nurse before your next visit.

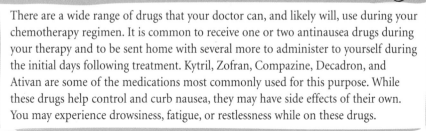

## ANTINAUSEA DRUGS

There are a wide range of drugs that your doctor can, and likely will, use during your chemotherapy regimen. It is common to receive one or two antinausea drugs during your therapy and to be sent home with several more to administer to yourself during the initial days following treatment. Kytril, Zofran, Compazine, Decadron, and Ativan are some of the medications most commonly used for this purpose. While these drugs help control and curb nausea, they may have side effects of their own. You may experience drowsiness, fatigue, or restlessness while on these drugs.

# Fighting Infection

The defense mechanisms of your immune system are the most complicated and miraculous bodily functions you have. Very simply stated, the white blood cells are the soldiers in your body that work hard fighting bacterial, viral, and fungal infections. Chemotherapy wipes out these cells during treatment and affects the bone marrow, decreasing its ability to produce more white blood cells. This compromises your defenses, leaving you vulnerable to infections of the mouth, urinary tract, lungs, skin, rectum, and just about any other part of your body you can name. Don't panic. Your doctor will monitor your white blood count carefully while you are receiving treatment, and there is much you can do on your own to decrease your risk as described below.

## What to watch for

Since chemotherapy plays havoc with all of the cells in your body, both normal and abnormal, damage is done inadvertently to your healthy platelets and red and white blood cells. There are three areas of concern you need to watch for and alert your doctor to that may be associated with depressed blood counts: infection, fatigue, and blood clotting problems. If, during the period following your treatment, your body is having difficulty regenerating your blood back to its more normal standards, your doctor may prescribe something that can artificially stimulate your bone marrow cells to make new red or white blood cells. The drugs Procrit (epoetin alfa), Leukine (sargramostim), and Neupogen (filgrastim) are important additions to the armaments of oncologists. Not only will they quickly get you back to normal, but they also help prevent lapses and breaks in your chemotherapy regimen due to low blood counts. Now that's progress!

Nadir is the condition during the course of treatment when your white blood count is at its lowest. The blood tests that are performed will keep your doctor apprised of your nadir point. You may be given injections to raise your white blood counts. Do everything you can to avoid sources of infection when you are at your nadir and get plenty of rest.

### SIGNS OF INFECTION

- Fever over 100°F.
- Shaking chills
- A sore IV site
- Headache or neck stiffness with fever
- Nausea and vomiting or loose bowels not associated with chemotherapy
- A burning feeling when you urinate
- A severe cough
- A sore throat
- Drenching sweats
- Redness, swelling, or tenderness around a wound or sore
- Unusual vaginal discharge

### STEPS TO TAKE

- Wash your hands often and well, with hot water and soap.
- Stay away from anyone who has a cold, flu, or any other obvious illness. Avoid crowds whenever possible.
- Don't cut or tear the cuticles of your nails.
- Shave with an electric razor instead of a blade.
- Don't eat undercooked meat or poultry.
- Clean your rectal area very carefully after each bowel movement. Avoid constipation since straining can cause a small tear in the anus.
- Do not take enemas and avoid rectal thermometers.
- Don't clean out litter boxes or bird cages. Avoid all contact with animal stools and urine.
- Avoid dental work and cleaning during chemotherapy treatments.
- Use a soft toothbrush and be careful of your gums.
- Don't garden.
- Use gloves doing housework.
- Don't squeeze or scratch pimples.
- Take a bath or shower everyday and pat yourself dry.
- Use lotion to prevent dryness of your skin.
- Do not get any immunization shots without first getting approval from your doctor.

### GENE THERAPY TRIAL ACTIVATES THE ENTIRE HUMAN IMMUNE SYSTEM AGAINST PROSTATE CANCER

John Hopkins researchers reported the successful use of human gene therapy to activate the human immune system against metastatic prostate cancer. The study results were published in the October 15, 1999 issue of *Cancer Research*. This achievement could have implications in the treatment of many kinds of cancer.

# Hair Loss

Not all chemotherapy drugs cause hair loss, but many do, and it can be one of the most devastating side effects of cancer treatment. Ask your doctor whether you should expect no hair loss, just thinning, or total hair loss. Your hair will not fall out right away. It generally takes 2 to 4 weeks after your first treatment and it may come out gradually or in clumps all at once. The first sign will be finding more than the normal amount of hair in your brush or comb and seeing hair on your pillow or clothes. Your scalp may feel tender and have tingling sensations. These sensations disappear in a week or so.

I have lost my hair twice, not just the hair on my head but my eyebrows, eyelashes, facial, arm, leg, pubic, and underarm hair. The association between being attractive and our hair is a powerful one, causing patients who lose their hair to feel uneasy, homely, and unappealing. Hair loss for many patients also means "seeing" that you are really sick with cancer every time you look at yourself in the mirror. It puts physical evidence of your disease in plain view as a constant reminder to you and those around you. But don't forget: As the chemotherapy is killing the fast-growing hair cells, it is doing the same to your cancer cells.

Men have an easier time with hair loss than women and find wearing baseball caps helpful if they don't care for the Telle Savalis look. Wigs, bandanas, and scarves can improve a women's self-image. I highly recommend that cancer patients take extra time with their appearance each morning. Keep in mind that your hair will begin to grow back before or soon after you have finished your treatments, and it will most likely be more lush and exquisite than ever before.

> A hairpiece needed during cancer treatment is a tax-deductible expense and may be partially covered by your health insurance. Cancer Care has great and inexpensive hats and turbans, as well as free wigs. Call (800) 813-HOPE.

## DEALING WITH IT

**Before you lose your hair:**
- Cut your hair short.
- Wash your hair with a mild shampoo.
- Don't pull or tug when combing.
- Use soft hairbrushes.
- If you must use a hairdryer, use the low setting.
- Don't use brush rollers to set your hair.
- Don't use dye or get a permanent.
- Sleep on a satin pillow.

**During and after you lose your hair:**
- If you are buying a wig, you should do it before all your hair is gone.
- Once you begin to bald, cover your head while in the sun.
- If having your hair fall out on a daily basis is difficult for you, you may want to consider having your head shaved.
- Cancer Care provides terry-cloth turbans free of charge to keep your head warm at night.

## ORAL HYGIENE

**Treatments can cause painful mouth sores and/or a dry mouth that occurs 5 to 10 days after therapy. Call your doctor as soon as you notice mouth ulcers. Your doctor may prescribe Magic Mouthwash, in addition to an artificial saliva product that can provide relief.**

- Take special care to maintain good oral hygiene.
- Brush carefully after every meal to prevent infection.
- Rinse your mouth with baking soda and salt diluted in warm water.
- Use a soft toothbrush.
- Ask your dentist for special toothpaste for sensitive gums.
- Use a cotton swab to apply milk of magnesia or Maalox to soothe mouth sores.
- Chew sugarless gum.
- Moisten food with butter, gravy, or sauce.
- Avoid citrus fruits and acidic, salty, or spicy foods.
- Eat foods at room temperature.
- Stop drinking alcoholic beverages.
- Stop smoking.
- Eat soft foods such as ice cream, mashed potatoes. pudding, gelatin, eggs, and milkshakes.
- Suck on ice chips, hard candy, and popsicles.
- Drink plenty of fluids
- Use a straw to avoid liquid coming in contact with problem areas.
- Use lip balm.

# Other Concerns

Remember that not everyone has side effects and that not all side effects are experienced by every patient. Don't make the mistake of reading this chapter and thinking you will never get through the repercussions of treatments. That is simply not true.

One patient may encounter fatigue and mouth sores and another nausea and hair loss. No one person will experience every single side effect. Stay tuned to how your body is feeling and if you have questions don't hesitate to call your doctor.

## CAN'T GO?

Constipation can be one of the most uncomfortable aspects of surgery, radiation therapy, and chemotherapy. The inactivity, drugs, and changes brought about by treatments can alter your daily routine and normal habits and cause problems for you. Give the following a try and if things don't get moving, call your doctor.

**Increase your fiber intake:**
- Fruits
- Vegetables
- Whole grain breads
- Cereals
- Beans
- Nuts & seeds

**Drink plenty of fluids (8 to 10 glasses a day):**
- Prune juice
- Fruit juices
- Lots of water

**Exercise:**
- Walk
- Swim
- Light housework
- Light yard work

**Take a fiber supplement:**
- Metamucil
- Fiberall
- Citrucel

## CAN'T STOP?

Diarrhea is the result of chemotherapy affecting the cells that line the intestines. Call your doctor before taking over-the-counter antidiarrhea medication or if the problem persists for more than 24 hours. Dehydration is serious, so be careful.

**Foods to avoid:**

**High-fiber foods**
- Fruits
- Vegetables
- Whole grain bread
- Cereal
- Beans
- Nuts & seeds

**Other foods**
- Coffee, tea, alcohol, and sweets
- Fried or spicy foods
- Milk products

**Foods to eat:**

**Low-fiber foods**
- White bread
- Rice & noodles
- Eggs
- Pureed vegetables
- Chicken, turkey, or fish

**Potassium-rich foods:**
- Bananas, oranges, potatoes, peaches, and apricots

**Drink plenty of fluids to replace those you have lost.**

## OTHER SIDE EFFECTS OF CHEMOTHERAPY

**Peripheral neuropathy** is a chemotherapy-related condition that causes tingling and burning sensations and/or weakness or numbness in the hands or feet. Other nerve-related symptoms include loss of balance, clumsiness, difficulty picking up objects, walking problems, jaw pain, hearing loss, and stomach pain. Call your doctor if you experience any of these symptoms.

**Fluid retention** can be a side effect of chemotherapy. Avoid table salt and high-sodium foods. Call your doctor if you notice swelling in your hands, face, feet, or abdomen. A diuretic may be prescribed to get rid of excess body fluids.

**Bladder and kidney problems** may arise with some chemotherapy drugs. Drink plenty of fluids to keep your bladder and kidneys flushed out when receiving treatment. Be aware that some anticancer drugs can change the color or smell of your urine. Call your doctor if you experience any of

the following during urination: pain or burning, frequency, "urgency," bloody urine, chills, or fever.

**Skin problems,** including redness, dryness, itching, and peeling, can occur. Apply skin lotion and take quick showers for dry skin. Sprinkle corn starch on areas that itch. Do not use alcohol-based products. Call your doctor right away if you develop a rash or hives. Fingernails may become brittle, darkened, or cracked and could develop vertical lines or bands.

# Working Toward Wellness

Exercising can be difficult for many in the best of circumstances. Add surgery, radiation therapy, and/or chemotherapy, and exercising sounds about as appealing as jumping off the highest mountain. Is exercising worth the effort then? Dr. Kerry S. Courneya of the University of Alberta and Dr. Christine M. Friedenreich of the Alberta Cancer Board in Canada analyzed 24 studies of exercise in cancer patients that had been published between 1980 and 1997 to find out if exercise programs can improve the physical and mental well-being of the nearly 8 million Americans living with cancer today. All of the exercise programs included aerobic activity for at least 20 minutes 3 to 5 days per week. Taken as a group, "the studies have consistently demonstrated that physical exercise following cancer diagnosis has a positive effect on quality of life, including physical, functional, psychological, and emotional well-being," concluded Courneya and Friedenreich. Physical benefits of exercise observed in the studies included lung capacity, muscle strength, flexibility, and increased energy, as well as reduced nausea, fatigue, pain, and diarrhea. Blood markers and the activity of anticancer cells also improved in patients who exercised, the researchers report. Psychological benefits included increased feelings of competence, control, and self-esteem, improvement in

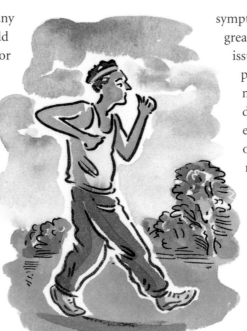

symptoms of depression and anxiety, and greater satisfaction with life. The authors issued two cautions, however. First, they pointed out that some cancer patients may require close medical supervision during exercise, and not all are able to exercise. Second, although the results of these 24 studies are strong, more research needs to be done, using larger groups of patients with a greater variety of cancers and stages. More specific research into the best kinds of activities and programs is also needed. SOURCE: *Annals of Behavioral Medicine*, September, 1999 (Reuters Health).

## NEED IDEAS?

Don't worry, there are many fun ways to get physical exercise. Just pick a few and stick to them.

| | | |
|---|---|---|
| Archery | Dancing | Skating |
| Aerobics | Gardening | Step-climbing |
| Badminton | Golfing | Swimming |
| Bowling | Hiking | Tennis |
| Biking | Jogging | Walking |
| Canoeing | Kayaking | Weights |
| Croquet | Racquetball | Yoga |

## MAKING EXERCISE A HABIT THAT YOU CAN LIVE WITH

**Before you start an exercise program, ask your doctor for advice on how best to proceed.**

- Start right away. Putting it off is only putting it off.
- Begin moderately. Be realistic. Take baby steps at first. Don't push yourself beyond what is comfortable. If you have been bedridden, remember that walking around your house might be all the exercise you can do at first.
- Set goals you are sure to achieve, increasing your exercise in very small increments. If you are really hurting the next day, you have done too much and you need to scale back.

- Do something you LIKE. Don't pick an exercise you are sure to hate because you are setting yourself up for failure.
- Include a friend or family member in your exercise routine. • Ask for company and encouragement.
- Don't skip a day for any reason. Make exercising a priority. If it's a "bad day," do half of your exercise program.

# Working Toward Wellness, cont.

Let the games begin! You have to start someday, so why not today? Get the okay from your doctor, record your goals, and exercise for a few minutes. There is no time like the present.

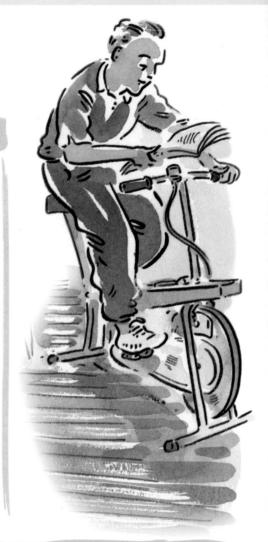

## CALL YOUR DOCTOR OR NURSE TODAY AND HAVE YOUR EXERCISE PLAN APPROVED

**Pick the time you will exercise everyday**

a.m. _____     p.m. _____

**Pick the exercise you are going to start with:**

_____

**If you want an exercise partner, call one today:**

Name: _____

Tel #: _____

• Carefully assess how your body feels before you start. Estimate your strength and endurance and reassess yourself every two months. It will give you great encouragement to look back and see the progress you have made.

• Make your goals attainable. Count extras like housework, shopping, etcetera. An example of the first month might be: walk 10 minutes a day for the first week; 12 minutes the second week; 15 minutes the third week, and so on. Add activities as you gain strength.

• Do not push. "No pain, no gain" should not be a cancer patient's motto.

• Photocopy the daily calendar on the opposite page. Put it in a handy spot (next to your treadmill or equipment) and complete it after each session.

## STRENGTH AND ENDURANCE

| | | |
|---|---|---|
| Date: _____ | Date: _____ | Date: _____ |
| How do I feel physically in regard to strength and endurance? | How do I feel physically in regard to strength and endurance? | How do I feel physically in regard to strength and endurance? |
| **Short-term goal:** | **Mid-term goal:** | **Long-term goal:** |
| First week: _____ | First week: _____ | First week: _____ |
| Second week: _____ | Second week: _____ | Second week: _____ |
| Third week: _____ | Third week: _____ | Third week: _____ |
| Fourth week: _____ | Fourth week: _____ | Fourth week: _____ |
| Fifth week: _____ | Fifth week: _____ | Fifth week: _____ |
| Sixth week: _____ | Sixth week: _____ | Sixth veek: _____ |
| Seventh week: _____ | Seventh week: _____ | Seventh week: _____ |
| Eighth week: _____ | Eighth week: _____ | Eighth week: _____ |

**DIG IT!** Want to stay limber, build muscle, be outdoors, accomplish something, and exercise? Try a moderate-intensity, effective form of resistance training. Gardening is more than just fun. Not only does your body and health benefit as you plant, rake, and mow but you will have the nicest looking yard in the neighborhood. What a bonus!

**MONTH** _____

| | | | | | | |
|---|---|---|---|---|---|---|
| Exercise *1* | Exercise *2* | Exercise *3* | Exercise *4* | Exercise *5* | Exercise *6* | Exercise *7* |
| Distance | Distance | Distance | Distance | Distance | Distance | Distance |
| Time | Time | Time | Time | Time | Time | Time |
| Extras | Extras | Extras | Extras | Extras | Extras | Extras |
| Exercise *8* | Exercise *9* | Exercise *10* | Exercise *11* | Exercise *12* | Exercise *13* | Exercise *14* |
| Distance | Distance | Distance | Distance | Distance | Distance | Distance |
| Time | Time | Time | Time | Time | Time | Time |
| Extras | Extras | Extras | Extras | Extras | Extras | Extras |
| Exercise *15* | Exercise *16* | Exercise *17* | Exercise *18* | Exercise *19* | Exercise *20* | Exercise *21* |
| Distance | Distance | Distance | Distance | Distance | Distance | Distance |
| Time | Time | Time | Time | Time | Time | Time |
| Extras | Extras | Extras | Extras | Extras | Extras | Extras |
| Exercise *22* | Exercise *23* | Exercise *24* | Exercise *25* | Exercise *26* | Exercise *27* | Exercise *28* |
| Distance | Distance | Distance | Distance | Distance | Distance | Distance |
| Time | Time | Time | Time | Time | Time | Time |
| Extras | Extras | Extras | Extras | Extras | Extras | Extras |
| Exercise *29* | Exercise *30* | Exercise *31* | Exercising on the 1st | How I felt starting the month | | |
| Distance | Distance | Distance | Exercising on the 31st | How I feel finishing the month | | |
| Time | Time | Time | Increased time | | | |
| Extras | Extras | Extras | | | | |

# Cancer Support Groups

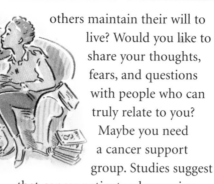

Now that you have been diagnosed with cancer, do you have a desire to talk with a person who has had cancer and the same course of treatments as you? Do you want to know what to expect from someone who has been there? Do you need to lay eyes on people who have gone through the same crisis and survived? Would you like to know how others handle pain and side effects? Do you wonder how others maintain their will to live? Would you like to share your thoughts, fears, and questions with people who can truly relate to you?

Maybe you need a cancer support group. Studies suggest that cancer patients who receive social support in groups experience less anxiety, depression, and stress. Research also shows that the effects of emotional and educational support enhance the immune system and extends longevity. Try it!

## LOCAL GROUPS

Attend several different self-help or cancer support groups in your area until you find one you feel comfortable with. Try to stay focused on getting the help and education you need. Be careful to pick a group with high positive energy and not a group with a "poor me" approach. Don't give up. Every group is different.

Name: _____
Tel #: _____
Address: _____
Meeting time: _____
Fee: _____
What they offer: _____

Name: _____
Tel #: _____
Address: _____
Meeting time: _____
Fee: _____
What they offer: _____

Name: _____
Tel #: _____
Address: _____
Meeting time: _____
Fee: _____
What they offer: _____

Name: _____
Tel #: _____
Address: _____
Meeting time: _____
Fee: _____
What they offer: _____

Name: _____
Tel #: _____
Address: _____
Meeting time: _____
Fee: _____
What they offer: _____

Name: _____
Tel #: _____
Address: _____
Meeting time: _____
Fee: _____
What they offer: _____

## WHAT ARE YOU LOOKING FOR?

Cancer support groups offer different options and preferences from which to choose. Look over the selection below and check those that are important to you. Your local Cancer Care can assist you in finding various cancer support groups that fill your requirements.

- ☐ All male
- ☐ All women
- ☐ Specialized group – for example, breast, prostrate, ostomy, or larynx cancer
- ☐ Children with cancer
- ☐ Led by a professional
- ☐ Led by a lay person
- ☐ Specific culture (African-American, Native American, Hispanic, etcetera)
- ☐ Group open to family members
- ☐ Small group (6 to 12 members)
- ☐ Large group (12 members and up)
- ☐ Provides psychotherapy and/or counseling

## AVOID ANY GROUPS THAT

- Suggest that they are a substitute for medical treatments.
- Get you down, not lift you up.
- Are focused on issues not of interest to you.

In addition, some groups may help certain patients but not be what you want. You might avoid groups that:

- You are not comfortable and honest with.
- Focus on feelings.
- Focus on exchange of information and advice.
- Focus on religion.
- Weekly meetings.
- Monthly meetings.
- Daytime gathering.
- Nighttime gathering.

## THE BURDEN OF ATTITUDE

Can a person's attitude influence cancer survival? Surveys show that the majority of cancer patients certainly do think so. However, despite the importance of attitude to the quality of life, the patient who believes that one's disposition and resolve can and will have total control over the malignancy of the cancer is accepting a tremendous burden. Attitude CANNOT override biology. If a treatment is ineffective and the cancer progresses, many times a patient feels that he or she just wasn't trying hard enough and that the lack of a cure is his or her fault. Nothing could be further from the truth. Biology is biology is biology.

Why then do some studies show that mental well-being, strong social ties, and a solid spiritual connection appear to be factors in long-term survival? It's thought that being isolated and detached during a crisis such as cancer can be a risk factor. In addition, churches, support groups, family, and friends encourage patients to eat right, exercise, demand the best in health care, and struggle heroically for survival. Bottom line is this: you have to have some sort of attitude, positive or negative, so which is it going to be?

---

**STOP**

Have you made the attempt to find a cancer support group that might be a benefit to you?

Read the opposite page and make some calls. You've got nothing to lose.

---

## JUST FOR THE FUN OF IT

**These quotes were collected from essays, exams, and discussions, mostly from fifth- and sixth-graders.**

- One horsepower is the amount of energy it takes to drag one horse 500 feet in one second.
- You can listen to thunder after lightning and tell how close you came.
- The law of gravity says no fair jumping up without coming back down.
- When people run around and around in circles we say they are crazy. When planets do it we say they are orbiting.
- Rainbows are just to look at, not to really understand.
- Someday we may discover how to make magnets that can point in any direction.
- South America has cold summers and hot winters, but somehow they still manage.
- The wind is like the air, only pushier.
- A vibration is a motion that cannot make up its mind which way it wants to go.
- There are 26 vitamins in all, but some of the letters are yet to be discovered. Finding them all means living forever.

- We keep track of the humidity in the air so we won't drown when we breathe.
- Lime is a green-tasting rock.
- Many dead animals in the past changed to fossils, while others preferred to be oil.
- Vacuums are nothings. We only mention them to let them know we know they're there.
- Some oxygen molecules help fires burn while others help make water, so sometimes it's brother against brother.
- Some people can tell what time it is by looking at the sun. But I have never been able to make out the numbers.
- We say the cause of perfume disappearing is evaporation. Evaporation gets blamed for a lot of things people forget to put the top on.
- In looking at a drop of water under a microscope, we find there are twice as many H's as O's.
- Clouds are high-flying fogs.

- I am not sure how clouds get formed. But the clouds know how to do it, and that is the important thing.
- Water vapor gets together in a cloud. When it is big enough to be called a drop, it does.
- Humidity is the experience of looking for air and finding water.
- Rain is often known as soft water, oppositely known as hail.
- Rain is saved up in cloud banks.
- In some rocks you can find the fossil footprints of fishes.
- Cyanide is so poisonous that one drop of it on a dog's tongue will kill the strongest man.
- A monsoon is a French gentleman.
- Thunder is a rich source of loudness.
- Isotherms and isobars are even more important than their names sound.
- It is so hot in some places that the people there have to live in other places.

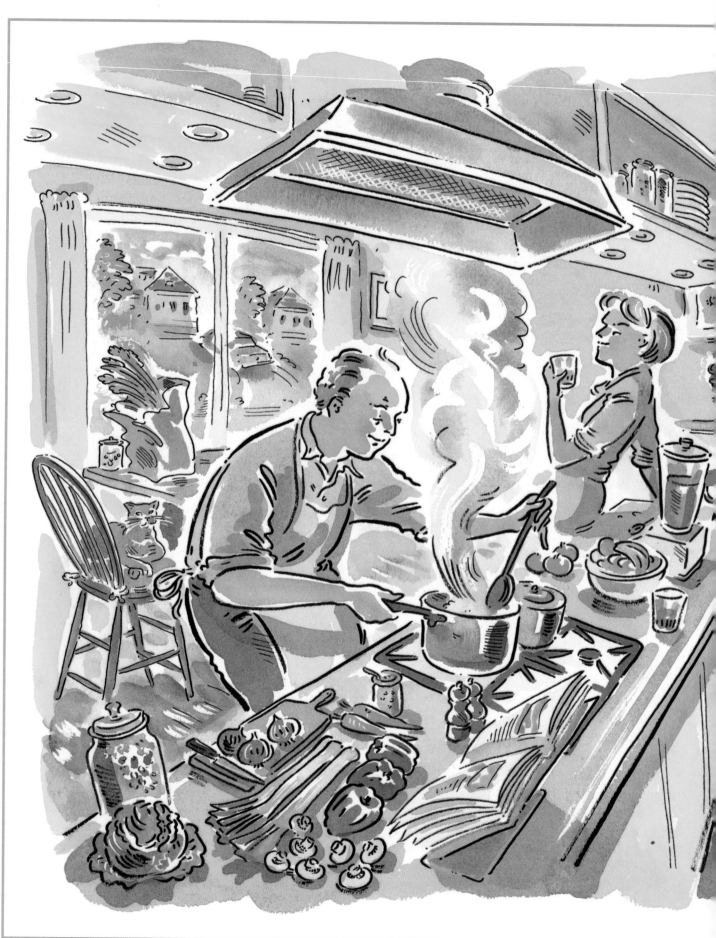

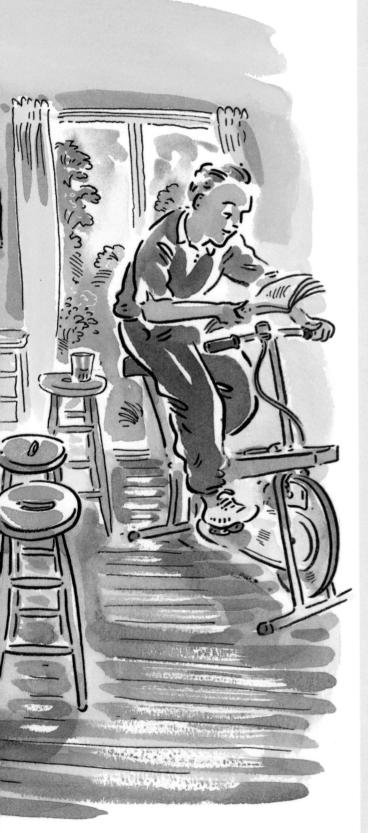

# Nature's Pharmacy
## *Chapter 5*

# Patient, Heal Thyself: The 1% Plan of Action

At this point we will assume that your doctor has decided on your treatment plan and that you have made the decision to bravely march forward to face the chemotherapy, radiation, and/or surgery. You are a fighter and will do whatever the doctor says and whatever it takes. It troubles you, though, that your fate now lies entirely in someone else's hands – or does it?

What if (and I realize this is a big "what if") someone in your cancer support group brings in research about the benefits of tea? Through discussion you come to believe that drinking green or black tea is effective in preventing and fighting cancer. You decide that, even if it only increases your chances by 1 percent, it's worth doing. On the way home from your support group you stop at the supermarket to purchase the tea and you notice a magazine with a headline reading; "Researchers believe frequent laughter increases the number of killer white cells."

You consider that true so, keeping in line with your new 1 percent "it's worth doing" rule, you stop by the video store to rent a funny movie. You arrive home, make a glass of tea, fix a nice little fruit plate (you have no doubt that fruits are high in antioxidants and you believe they fight cancer, giving you another 1 percent boost), turn your funny movie on, begin to chuckle, and the thought occurs: "the tea, the laughter, the fruit…that's 3 points – I'm helping myself, I'm going to beat this disease!"

❦

When I was first diagnosed with cancer, I needed a yardstick by which I could evaluate my own efforts to help myself. I made up the 1 percent plan of action because I could not handle the thought that I had only a 4 percent chance of surviving. I convinced myself that I could increase my chances. My plan was simple. I gave myself one point for those actions I believed were benefiting my immune system. A point for every glass of carrot juice drank, every half-mile walked, every prayer said. I believed that the combination of the doctors' treatments and my efforts would heal me. At night I would get into bed, count my points, and fall asleep

## THE PLACEBO EFFECT

A placebo is a "medication" that is prescribed more for the mental relief of the patient than for its actual effect on a disorder. A patient who has high expectations in a cure or medication often shows improvement even though the treatment or medication did nothing at all. While researchers do not understand the placebo effect, there is some evidence that it may be related to the brain chemicals called endorphins, the body's natural opiates.

buoyed by the thought, "not bad, a 17 percent chance today…."

Research is ongoing to determine the positive health benefits of such things as exercise, relaxation therapy, herbs, laughter, nutrition, positive attitudes, prayer, and massage, to name just a few. Each one has its proponents, both in the medical profession and among cancer patients, as means to augment conventional medical treatment.

The **Cancer Patient's Workbook** has addressed many immune-promoting subjects and you are encouraged to investigate each one more fully. This chapter is devoted to what many consider the most important immune-enhancing weapons of all; nutrition, vitamins, minerals, and herbs. Read it through carefully, determine for yourself what may help you, and then formulate a tailormade plan that you can believe in and live with. I cannot say that my 1 percent plan helped heal me. Nor can I say for sure that it didn't. What I do know is that my method gave me purpose, control, hope, power, and a goal to focus on. No one should tell you what to believe in, but I do suggest that you believe in something.

## DIETICIANS AND NUTRITIONISTS

Registered dietitians (R.D.) have been scientifically trained in the study of diet and its effect on health. They have passed a national exam, are licensed, and are your most accurate and reliable source for information about nutrition.

In most states a nutritionist is not legally licensed and there are no regulations as to the education and training that a nutritionist must have. While many nutritionists are experts in their field and can give profession advice, it is important to remember that anyone can hang a sign over their door and call himself or herself a "nutritionist."

**Watch out for:**
- Fancy private clinics that do not have accredited, licensed health professionals on staff.
- Establishments that sell their own vitamins, herbs, and prepackaged foods at extravagant prices.
- Anyone who claims the ability to cure cancer with unconventional treatments.
- Dietitians who rely more on supplements than foods.

# The Immune System: *Free Radicals & Antioxidants*

Your immune system holds the key to your health; it's as simple as that. Colds and flu, heart disease, arthritis, and cancer are all examples of ailments resulting from an overwhelmed immune system. Scientists now suspect that different nutrients work together in an intricate way to give your immune system the tools it needs to protect you from illnesses. If you understand the immune system and the impact that food and nutrition have on its ability to fight cancer, you may find the incentive to make tough dietary choices that cannot hurt you and might actually augment your medical treatment. Regardless of your cancer situation, a balanced diet high in vegetables, fruits, vitamins, and fiber and low in fats and processed foods will improve your overall health.

The immune system is one of the most complex functions of the human body. It is made up of many different cell types, each one working to protect you from fungal, parasitic, bacterial, and viral infections. Every time we breathe, eat, or drink, free radicals are produced. Free radicals are unstable oxygen atoms. They are normally

## IMMUNE SYSTEM FAST FACTS

- Air pollutants, stress, too much exercise, sunshine, tobacco smoke, toxins, rancid oils and fats, overcooked meats, smog, chemicals, some food preservatives, pesticides, malnourishment, radiation, and chemotherapy all cause free radicals.
- Bioflavonoids – which are found in the white pith of lemons, limes, grapefruits, oranges, and tangerines – not only bolster the immune system but they increase the effectiveness of vitamin C.
- Vegetarians have lower rates of cancer and heart disease, not just because of what they don't eat (meat) but because of what they do eat.
- 28% of Americans have adjusted their eating habits to achieve a healthier lifestyle.
- Some cancers produce a defense system by which they protect themselves and prevent the immune system from attacking them. Getting past this barrier is the focus of much research.

used by a strong immune system to kill bacteria and viruses. As we grow older, however, our bodies do not always have the ready supply of enzymes, hormones, vitamins, and minerals that our immune system counts on to keep extra free radicals under control. If the immune system becomes too weak to destroy the erratic free radicals, they can cause a chain reaction that overpowers our bodies' intricate checks and balances. Some free radical damage is inevitable (as in the aging process), but serious trouble can result when free radicals damage a cell's DNA, attack cell membranes, or turn substances into carcinogens.

The rust on a car, an apple slice turning brown due to air exposure, or a tumor forming in the human body are all examples of free radical damage. Common sense tells you that a good paint job will protect your car and plastic wrap will keep your apple wedge perfect. But what is a human's best defense?

There are literally thousands of chemicals and compounds that occur naturally in our food. Phytochemicals such as allylic sulfides, indoles, quercetin, and lutein, and antioxidants such as vitamins E, A, and C, and beta-carotene and selenium strengthen and stimulate our immune systems. These compounds are the focus of much research in medical and academic laboratories. Is the hope for a cancer vaccine unrealistic? Researchers don't think so. We already have immunizations for illnesses such as the flu, measles, polio, and hepatitis. While scientists are analyzing the chemicals and compounds in our foods, looking for answers on how best to support our immune systems, doesn't it make sense for us to eat those very same foods, even while waiting for the final results of these studies?

We are in the middle of rigorous testing of phytochemicals in foods

## ANTIPERSPIRANTS DON'T CAUSE BREAST CANCER

The new internet e-mail buzz  that's circulating is that antiperspirants prevent perspiration and cause toxins to build up in an woman's underarm, and that eventually leads to breast cancer. Lillie Shockney, R.N., B.S., M.A.S., director of education and outreach for the Johns Hopkins Breast Center, and a seven-year breast cancer survivor, states that there is no valid documentation that antiperspirants cause breast cancer.

that show great promise as anticancer agents," according to Dr. Richard Rivlin of Memorial Sloan-Kettering Cancer Center. "The end product of this research into phytochemicals will be powerful and precise tools for reducing incidence of cancer," Rivlin said.

## RESEARCH FAST FACTS

- Over the past 26 years, the National Cancer Institute has spent over $37 billion in research.
- More than 25% of today's medicines are made from plant sources.
- Some cancers produce a defense system by which they protect and block the immune system from attacking it. Getting past the barrier that cancer utilizes is the focus of much research.

*"Faced with an individual at risk for a specific kind of cancer, we will be able to prescribe specific foods and perhaps supplements that, consumed together, will significantly reduce that risk."*

## MAKING THE COMMITMENT

I, _____, am willing to make lifestyle changes in my eating habits. I comprehend the significant role my diet plays in fighting my cancer. I realize that the only nutrition I will receive is from the foods, vitamins, and minerals that I eat. I understand that no one food is the magic bullet and that I need to eat a variety of good foods featuring fruits and vegetables. I recognize that consuming antioxidants and phytochemicals may have a positive effect on every stage of my cancer. I am convinced that certain foods stimulate my immune system, activate enzymes that neutralize cancer-causing substances, deactivate estrogen, suppress runaway cell reproduction and growth, block enzymes that activate cancer genes, and assist in producing enzymes that destroy cancer cells. From this day forward my focus will be to help my body battle cancer by attending to its nutritional needs. My goal is to prevent further cancer spread, giving my conventional medical treatments time to kill any and all existing cancer cells. I will nutritionally support my body's healing and detoxification process to whatever degree possible. I believe that I have the power to make decisions during my illness that will positively affect my health.

Signed_____ Date_____

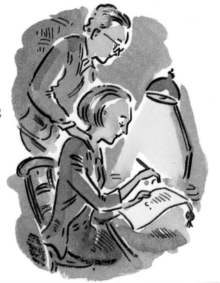

# Medicinal Foods

Would you believe that this year the average American will consume 263 eggs, 27 pounds of cheese, 134 pounds of sugar, 19 pounds of cereal, 116 pounds of beef, 117 pounds of potatoes, 100 pounds of fresh vegetables, 80 pounds of fresh fruit, 22 pounds of tomatoes, out of 1,500 pounds of food, total? You heard right, 1,500 pounds.

Over 80% of adult Americans know that eating more vegetables and fruits decreases cancer risk, and 60% are aware that exercise also lowers the risk. However, the nation's collective girth is expanding at an alarming rate. The incidence for developing some form of cancer in America is now 1 out of every 2 men and 1 out of every 3 women.

*Over 560,000 cases of cancer could be prevented each year by simply eating right, staying physically active, maintaining a healthy weight, and by quitting smoking.*

While the specific roles of naturally occurring substances in individual foods are not yet fully understood, much research has been done in recent years on the compounds found in foods that actually promote freedom from disease. It is crucial that we begin to look at our food as health products, the very foundation of our well-being, responsible for supplying our bodies with the vitamins and minerals that it needs to protect, repair, build, and sustain us as healthy individuals.

We know that diets high in fruits, vegetables, legumes, and whole grains help prevent and fight cancer. One of the most exciting discoveries in recent years has been the phytochemicals (plant chemicals). These substances give plants their odor, color, and flavor, and function as powerful antioxidants. Phytochemicals interfere with cancer at many stages. They prevent carcinogens from damaging cells, suppress runaway cell reproduction and growth, block enzymes that activate cancer genes, deactivate excess estrogen, and assist in producing other enzymes that help destroy cancer cells.

❈

The field of nutrition is new territory for those in the medical profession but it is not far-fetched to believe that one day your doctor may grab his prescription pad and scribble down: "take one serving of each daily for the rest of your life: broccoli, tomatoes, onions, oranges, strawberries, grapefruit" (you get the point). Bear in mind that all fruits and vegetables are disease-fighters and that science has just scratched the surface of only a few.

Do not for a moment think to yourself that it is too late to make lifestyle changes simply because you already have cancer. After all, you are going to put over a thousand pounds of food in your mouth in the next year. Isn't it feasible that if you concentrate on eating the most nutrient-rich food, ounce for ounce, it might give you an edge over this disease? To get an idea of what your diet truly consists of, take the Eating Smart Quiz on pages 116–117.

## TO ENTICE EATING

- Do not fill up on soup, salads, or drinks before your meal.
- Make the plate look appetizing using color.
- Eat small portions throughout the day.
- Allow the aroma of simmering food to fill your home.
- Prepare meals that sound good, even if you eat spaghetti for breakfast and bacon and eggs for supper.
- Eat sitting up.
- Dine as often as you can in a group setting.
- If your appetite is small, make sure you eat the most nutrient-rich food you can.
- When dining out go to buffets.
- Make plans to eat with someone special.
- Play relaxing music or watch your favorite television show while you are eating.

## THE BENEFITS OF WATER

- Replenishes the body's cells and tissues.
- Regulates body temperature.
- Prevents heatstroke.
- Is a major component of blood and lymph.
- Helps digest food by stimulating gastric juices.
- Assists in dissolving and circulating nutrients.
- Lubricates joints.
- Adds much needed bulk to the bowel movements and helps maintain regularity.

In what areas does your diet need to change? Are you willing to make those changes?

# Eating Smart Quiz

The American Cancer Society created the "Eating Smart Quiz" to help you take a realistic look at the food you eat. Don't kid yourself; be honest. If you are not sure what you consume in a day, keep a list of everything you eat for four days before you take the test. If you never eat meat, poultry, or fish, give yourself 2 points for each meat category. Use a pencil so that you can erase your answers and take the test again every 3 months.

## FOOD FAST FACTS

- One-third of adults say they regularly choose foods for medicinal purposes; for example, chicken soup for a cold or cranberry juice for a urinary tract infection.
- The average American throws away almost $250 worth of fruits and vegetables each year.
- Antioxidants in turmeric, one of the herbs in curry powder, prevent DNA damage and block tumor growth.
- Fruits are digested in twenty to thirty minutes.
- Most vegetables are digested within forty-five to sixty minutes.
- Pork takes nine hours.
- One-third of adults and one-fifth of adolescents in the US are overweight.
- Sugar produces faster-growing and more deadly tumors in animal tests.
- Shiitake mushrooms stimulate immune function.

## ACS "EATING SMART" QUIZ

*Points*

**Oils and fats: butter, margarine, shortening, lard, mayonnaise, oil, sour cream, and salad dressing**

| | |
|---|---|
| I always add these to foods in cooking and/or at the table. | 0 |
| I occasionally add these to foods in cooking and/or at the table. | 1 |
| I rarely add these to foods in cooking and/or at the table. | 2 |

| | |
|---|---|
| I eat fried food 3 or more times a week. | 0 |
| I eat fried food 1–2 times a week. | 1 |
| I rarely eat fried food. | 2 |

**Dairy: milk, ice cream, yogurt, cheese, sherbet**

| | |
|---|---|
| I drink whole milk. | 0 |
| I drink 1–2% fat milk. | 1 |
| I seldom eat frozen desserts or ice cream. | 2 |

| | |
|---|---|
| I eat ice cream almost every day. | 0 |
| Instead of ice cream, I eat ice milk, low-fat frozen yogurt, and sherbet. | 1 |
| I eat only fruit ices and seldom eat frozen dairy dessert. | 2 |

| | |
|---|---|
| I eat mostly high-fat cheese (jack, cheddar, Colby, Swiss, cream). | 0 |
| I eat both low and high-fat cheeses. | 1 |
| I eat mostly low-fat cheeses (pot, 2% cottage, skim milk, mozzarella). | 2 |

**Snacks: potato/corn chips, nuts, buttered popcorn, candy**

| | |
|---|---|
| I eat these every day. | 0 |
| I eat some occasionally. | 1 |
| I seldom or never eat these snacks. | 2 |

**Baked goods: pies, cakes, cookies, sweet rolls, donuts**

| | |
|---|---|
| I eat them 5 or more times a week. | 0 |
| I eat them 2–4 times a week. | 1 |
| I seldom eat baked goods or eat only low-fat baked goods. | 2 |

**Poultry and fish: chicken, hens, duck, fish, shellfish**

| | |
|---|---|
| I rarely eat these foods. | 0 |
| I eat them 1–2 times a week. | 1 |
| I eat them 3 or more times a week. | 2 |

**Low-fat meats: extra lean hamburger, round steak, pork loin roast, tenderloin, chuck roast**

| | |
|---|---|
| I rarely eat these foods. | 0 |
| I eat these foods occasionally. | 1 |
| I eat mostly fat-trimmed red meats. | 2 |

**High-fat meats: luncheon meats, bacon, hot dogs, sausage, steak, regular & lean ground beef**

| | |
|---|---|
| I eat these foods every day. | 0 |
| I eat these foods occasionally. | 1 |
| I rarely eat these foods. | 2 |

**Cured and smoked meat & fish: luncheon meats, hot dogs, ham, & other smoked or pickled meats and fish**

| | |
|---|---|
| I eat these foods 4 or more times a week. | 0 |
| I eat some 1–3 times a week. | 1 |
| I seldom eat these foods. | 2 |

**Legumes: kidney, navy, lima, pinto, garbanzo beans, lentils**

| | |
|---|---|
| I eat legumes less that once a week. | 0 |
| I eat these foods 1–2 times a week. | 1 |
| I eat them 3 or more times a week. | 2 |

## ACS "Eating Smart" Quiz, cont.

**Whole grains & cereals: whole grain breads, brown rice, pasta, whole grain cereals**

| | |
|---|---|
| I seldom eat them. | 0 |
| I eat them 3–5 times a week. | 1 |
| I eat them 1–2 times a day. | 2 |

**Vitamin C-rich fruits & vegetables: citrus fruits, juices, green peppers, strawberries, tomatoes**

| | |
|---|---|
| I seldom eat them. | 0 |
| I eat them 3–5 times a week. | 1 |
| I eat them daily. | 2 |

**Dark green & deep yellow fruits & vegetables: broccoli, greens, carrots, peaches, etcetera**

| | |
|---|---|
| I seldom eat them. | 0 |
| I eat them 3–5 times a week. | 1 |
| I eat them daily. | 2 |

**Vegetables of the cabbage family: broccoli, cabbage, Brussels sprouts, cauliflower, etcetera**

| | |
|---|---|
| I seldom eat them. | 0 |
| I eat them 1–2 times a week. | 1 |
| I eat them 3–4 times a week. | 2 |

**Alcohol: beer, wine, hard liquor**

| | |
|---|---|
| I drink more than 2 oz. daily. | 0 |
| I drink alcohol every week but not daily. | 1 |
| I occasionally or never drink alcohol. | 2 |

**Personal weight**

| | |
|---|---|
| I am more than 20 lbs. over my ideal weight. | 0 |
| I am 10–20 lbs. over my ideal weight. | 1 |
| I am within 10 lbs. of my ideal weight. | 2 |

## Scoring yourself

**Add the numbers to get your total score.**

**1–12: Warning signal**

Your diet is too high in fat and too low in fiber-rich foods. It would be wise to assess your eating habits to see where you could make improvements.

**13–17: Not bad!**

You're partway there. You still have a way to go, however.

**18–36: Good for you!**

You're eating smart. You should feel good about yourself. You have been careful to limit your fats and eat a varied diet. Keep up the good habits and continue to look for ways to improve.

## Science says saccharin's safe

A US government report from the National Institute for Environmental Health Sciences removed saccharin as a potential cancer-causing agent because tests that showed it caused tumors in rats did not apply to humans. "Two decades ago, when saccharin was shown to produce bladder tumors in rats, it was a prudent, protective step to consider the sweetener to be a likely human carcinogen," institute director Dr. Kenneth Olden said. He also said humans had used saccharin for decades without increasing rates of cancer.

## Dioxin

This chemical is emitted from garbage incinerators and the paper and pulp industry. Simply put, dioxin gets into our water and air, enters our food chain, and accumulates in the fat of mammals and fish that we eat. Dioxin is linked to several cancers in humans, including lymphomas and lung cancer. The EPA concludes that for those eating a lot of fatty foods the risk could be as high as 1 in 100. Exposure to dioxin occurs over a person's lifetime and is cumulative.

# Fats Can Be Confusing

Some fats are held responsible for illnesses such as cancer, heart disease, arthritis, diabetes, and strokes. Other fats are praised for preventing cancer, heart disease, rheumatoid arthritis, psoriasis, and headaches. It's important that you know your fats and can distinguish between the good, the bad, and the ugly. It is just as important that you consume 30 percent or less of your total daily calories from fat, with 10 percent or less of those calories coming from saturated fat.

| If you eat this number of calories per day: | Total fat per day (grams) | Total saturated fat per day (grams) |
| --- | --- | --- |
| 1,600 | 53 or less | 18 or less |
| 2,000 | 65 or less | 20 or less |
| 2,200 | 73 or less | 24 or less |

## The Good

Fish, olive, canola, sesame, and flaxseed oils are all monounsaturated fats. These compounds prevent free radical damage and detoxify the body. Sesamin, a compound found in sesame oil, inhibited growth of tumors in animal studies. High consumption of olive oil in Mediterranean countries has been linked to lower rates of breast cancer. The antioxidants in these oils are so beneficial that fish oil and flaxseed oil are even sold as supplements in health food stores.

*Use canola, sesame, and extra virgin olive oil for cooking.*

Grapeseed, avocado, and walnut oils are good as well and also belong in this category. Search your kitchen cabinets, and throw out all the other oils that don't fall into the monounsaturated fat category.

## The Bad

Fat from meat, milk, cheese, and butter are all saturated fats. Saturated fats are blamed for heart disease, gout, arthritis, osteoporosis, autoimmune diseases, and strokes. A report in the *International Journal of Cancer* links red meat to prostate, pancreatic, stomach, colon, rectal, bladder, and breast cancers, among others. This fat is bad stuff. It is a major source of cholesterol, which causes enormous free radical damage, putting a terrible strain on the body and the immune system. Eat skinless chicken

---

### MEAT & CANCER

**Question:** According to a study of 11,000 people in the UK published in the *American Journal of Clinical Nutrition*, who had 40% fewer cancer-related deaths?
**Answer:** Non-meat-eaters, of course. Red meat (pork, beef, and lamb) may be a risk factor for cancers of the lung, pancreas, and digestive system. A study at the Harvard School of Public Health in Boston of 88,000 women found that those who ate large quantities of meat may be at a higher risk for non-Hodgkins lymphoma. In addition, the 1996 American Cancer Society Dietary Guidelines states that diets high in fats have been linked with an increase in the risk of cancers of the colon, rectum, prostate, and endometrium (the lining of the uterus).

---

and fish whenever possible. When you do eat red meat, make sure it is lean and eat only small (4-ounce) portions. The best way to remember what belongs in the saturated fat category is to remember that one way or the other all these fats come from animals.

## The Ugly

If you thought saturated fats were bad, there is worse news in store. Polyunsaturated fats and trans fatty acids are the absolute worst of the worst. Polyunsaturated fats are your corn, peanut, sunflower, and safflower oils. These fats mix readily with oxygen (it only takes a minute or two), become rancid, and create total havoc in the body. Once these fats are consumed, they start a chain reaction that causes one cell right after another to become unstable

---

### THE LOWDOWN ON MILK AND CHEESE

Researchers from Harvard found in an ongoing study of 80,000 nurses that women who drink 2 or more glasses of milk a day had a 44% higher chance of getting ovarian cancer and men consuming 2½ servings of diary products daily may be at a slightly higher risk for prostate cancer. Whole milk and whole cheese are high in saturated fats. Stay away from them and whenever possible try these alternatives: low-fat hard cheeses, part-skim ricotta or mozzarella, low-fat cottage, pot, or farmers cheese, parmesan or Romano cheese, and light cream cheese. Also stick with the tub-form light margarine, low-fat sour cream, and skim or 1% milk.

## GRILLING, MARINADES, & CANCER

The American Institute for Cancer Research (AICR) maintains that when meat is grilled, the fat drips onto hot coals and carcinogens called polycyclic aromatic hydrocarbons are formed and deposited onto food by smoke or flame-ups that char or blacken it. What's more, meats cooked at high temperatures have the cancer-causing agents called heterocyclic aromatic amines (HCAs). Take a few precautions:

- Use lean cuts of beef.
- Trim off all fat and remove skin from poultry.
- Marinate meat using a vinegar, lemon, or an orange juice base. This will significantly protect it from the formation of carcinogenic substances.
- Precook the meat in the microwave or oven before grilling.
- Remove any charred material from your food.

and destruct or mutate. If the fats are consumed on a regular basis, this domino effect produces so much damage that the result is often cancer or heart disease.

So, you conclude, making an effort to cook with olive oil and eliminating these vegetable oils should make it easy to stay away from the noxious polyunsaturated fats, right? WRONG! Many of the prepackaged foods on the supermarket shelves are made with polyunsaturated fats. Cakes and cake mixes, cereals, chips, cookies, crackers, donuts, frostings, mayonnaise, muffins, pastries, peanut butter, pizza, puddings, salad dressings, and more. You may not be able to completely eliminate these oils from your diet, but if you make an effort to choose processed food that is fat free, it will help.

Unfortunately, there is more offensive news on the fat front. Trans fatty acids are made from vegetable oils so they have all the ugly traits that polyunsaturates do with an added nasty twist. They have been converted from liquids to semisolid or solid products such as margarine and shortening. When trans fatty acids get into your body their molecules make the membranes of your cells so rigid and inflexible that the cells can barely circulate. Not only can they no longer do their specific jobs, they can't move easily through the arteries either. The slower blood flow to the heart causes heart disease and an increase of the

## YOGURT AND IMMUNITY

Live cultures in yogurt are antibacterial and can help digestion, relieve yeast infections, aid in alleviating urinary tract infections, reduce cholesterol, and suppress upper respiratory infections. Yogurt is high in calcium, riboflavin, vitamin B2, and protein. Apparently, yogurt made with live *L. acidophilus* stimulates the production of gamma interferon, which has been shown to slow tumor growth, provide protection from cancer, and boost the immune system. In-vitro studies show that some lactic acid bacteria can lower levels of enzymes in the colon that are known to be involved in the development of colon cancer. Yogurt assists in the recovery from diarrhea, one of the nasty side effects of antibiotics.

## HENS HATCH GOLDEN NUTRITION

Lucky hens feasting on a diet enriched with vitamin E, lutein, and DHA have produced "designer eggs" for Dr. Peter F. Surai, a biochemist at the Scottish Agricultural College and his research team. Surai's team found that the volunteers who had eaten one fortified egg a day for 8 weeks had higher blood levels of the nutrients. Cholesterol levels did not rise. Vitamin E and lutein are potent antioxidants that fight free radicals, which can cause cancer. DHA is an omega-3 fatty acid, which can reduce blood pressure, help Crohn's disease, relieve arthritis pain, lower triglyceride and cholesterol levels, and slow tumor growth by preventing the nutrients that cancer needs to grow from entering the cells. This is just the beginning. Expect other "designer" foods in the meat, fish, and dairy cases of your supermarket.

cholesterol LDL. The damage doesn't stop there. The entire process serves to suppress the immune system and promote cancer. Here's the bottom line:

### Fat is dangerous to people battling cancer.

By the way, Olestra is a fake fat known to deplete the body of certain vitamins. That is the last thing you need right now, so stay away from products made with it.

# Vegetables

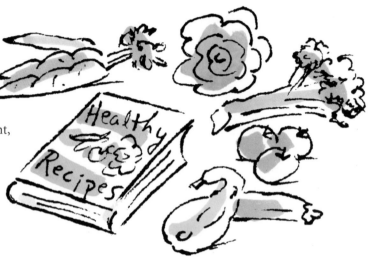

The typical American eats only 1½ servings of vegetables each day. That isn't enough for the average Joe and certainly not for a cancer patient trying to shrink tumors, prevent further spread, and rebuild a body being hammered by treatments. All vegetables are good for you; the following pages highlight a few in which scientists have isolated many chemicals and compounds that help prevent, and possibly even promote cures of cancer of, the breast, colon, stomach, prostrate, esophagus, bladder, pancreas, and lungs, to mention a few.

Make no mistake, the food you eat may possibly interfere with roving cancer cells, give you an edge for a cure, or prolong life after diagnosis. Nothing, however, is good in excess; a balanced diet should always be your goal. Making changes in your diet won't be easy, but it will be worth it. Hippocrates said, "Let food be thy medicine and medicine be thy food."

*Strive for at least five servings of fruits and vegetables a day – nine would be better. Remember, you are what you eat.*

**Broccoli** is the king of kings when it comes to fighting cancer. It is high in the antioxidant beta-carotene, vitamins C and E, rich in iron, calcium, zinc, and folic acid. Broccoli contains the phytochemical sulforaphane, which activates the production of anticancer enzymes and bolsters the body's ability to fight cancer. The indoles found in broccoli stimulate enzymes that make the hormone estrogen less effective, possibly reducing breast cancer risk. Broccoli is also abundant in substances called isothiocyanates – chemicals shown to initiate the body's production of its own cancer-fighting substances. According to findings published in 1999 in *The Journal of Nutrition and Cancer*, scientists at Tokyo's Graduate School of Agriculture have shown that isothiocyanates can block the growth of melanoma skin cancer cells. In addition, scientists at the World Cancer Research Fund reviewed 206 human and 22 animal studies and found convincing evidence that cruciferous vegetables, such as broccoli, cabbage,

---

## Cancer "phyters"

Different phytochemicals are present in different foods. Scientists are beginning to look at these food chemicals as "chemoprevention." Eating an assortment of fruits and vegetables will provide your guarantee that you are getting all the food "phyters" you need to battle your cancer on a nutritional level.

ALLIUM COMPOUNDS are found in onions, garlic, leeks, and chives. These compounds boost natural killer cells, activate enzymes that neutralize cancer-causing substances, and are powerful antibiotics.

CAROTENOIDS are abundant in carrots, spinach, apricots, tomatoes, broccoli, sweet potatoes, and cantaloupe. These compounds (beta-carotene, lutein, lycopene) are potent antioxidants. Their main job: to attack free radicals.

FLAVONOIDS are found in soybeans, tea, yams, berries, citrus, tomatoes, broccoli, carrots, onions, and peppers, to name a few. Flavonoids (of which there are over 600) give fruits and veggies their color and taste. They are powerful antioxidants, preventing and fighting cancer at every level.

GLUCOSINOLATES are present in cruciferous vegetables, such as broccoli, cabbage, and Brussels sprouts. Their two most significant phytochemicals, isothiocyanates and indoles, trigger production of protective enzymes, destroy estrogen, stimulate the immune system, and overpower precancerous cell mutations.

POLYPHENOLS are concentrated in blackberries, raspberries, grapes, strawberries, soybeans, and green tea. They inhibit mutations and prevent the alteration of substances into carcinogens.

## FROZEN FOODS FIND FAVOR FROM THE FDA

"In efforts to evaluate the nutrient content of frozen fruits and vegetables compared to that of raw fruits and vegetables, the agency reviewed both supplemental data from the American Frozen Foods Institute (AFFI) and similar data from the US Department of Agriculture (USDA). The nutrient profiles of selected raw fruits and vegetables and frozen versions of the same fruits and vegetables revealed relatively equivalent nutrient profiles. "In fact, some data showed that the nutrient content level for certain nutrients was higher in the frozen version of the food than in the raw version of the food."

**Bottom line – frozen is just as good as fresh!**

cauliflower, and Brussels sprouts, in general lowered risk for many forms of cancer, including tumors of the stomach, esophagus, lung, oral cavity and pharynx (throat), endometrium (lining of the uterus), pancreas, and colon. Dr. Paul Talalay and his research team at Johns Hopkins University in Baltimore discovered the power of broccoli sprouts. According to Fahey, "we determined that three-day old broccoli sprouts were between 20 and 50 times richer in sulforaphane than mature broccoli. In our research, sulforaphane-fed rats developed fewer cancerous tumors and their tumors developed at a slower rate."

---

**Cabbage** is in the same cruciferous family as broccoli and contains many of the same properties. It is rich in vitamins B, C, and E, beta-carotene, folic acid, and potassium. Cabbage juice is commonly used to cure ulcers, and studies suggest that cabbage lowers the rate of stomach, bladder, colon, lung, and skin cancers. Like broccoli, it contains indoles and isothiocyanates, which prevent the formation of carcinogens in the body, and sulforaphane, which increases the body's production of phase-two enzymes that help inactivate and eliminate carcinogens. A study at Johns Hopkins University found that only 26 percent of the rats injected with a chemical known to cause mammary cancer developed tumors when they were injected with sulfora-phane, compared to 69 percent injected with solely the cancer-causing chemical. A study of 47,909 men, published in the *Journal of the National Cancer Institute,* found the higher the intake of cruciferous vegetables, particularly cabbage and broccoli, the lower the risk for bladder cancer.

## WHAT IS A SERVING?

**A serving of fruit can be a:**
- ¾ cup of fruit juice
- a medium-size piece of fruit (apple, banana, etcetera)
- ½ cup of canned fruit
- ¼ cup of dried fruit
- 1 cup cut up fresh fruit

**A serving of vegetables can be:**
- ½ cup of chopped raw vegetables
- ¾ cup vegetable juice
- ½ cup of cooked or canned vegetables
- 1 cup of raw leafy vegetables
- ½ cup of beans/peas

### HOW TO GET 5 A DAY

- Drink a glass of 100% fruit or vegetable juice.
- Slice bananas or strawberries on your cereal.
- Eat a cup of fruit yogurt once a day.
- Eat an apple or banana for midmorning snack.
- Buy and keep on hand precut raw baby carrots, broccoli spears, cherry tomatoes, celery, grapes, strawberries, and other finger fruits and vegetables.
- Keep boxes of raisins and prepackaged snacks of dried dates, apricots, figs, and prunes handy.
- Order your pizza with veggies on it.
- Eat a salad for lunch.
- Put lettuce & tomato on your sandwich.
- For more information on the "5 a day" plan go to:

**http://www.5aday.com**

**Carrots** are a good source of vitamins C and E and potassium. A medium-size carrot has enough beta-carotene to provide over 200 percent of the daily vitamin A requirement. Beta-carotene is believed to block the formation of tumors and boost the immune system. The American Cancer Society maintains that lower risk of cancers of the larynx, esophagus, and lung are associated with a high carotene intake. The National Cancer Institute is sponsoring cancer prevention studies testing beta-carotene; several of these studies are specifically geared toward lung cancer. Researchers at John Hopkins University found that people with low levels of beta-carotene were four times more likely to develop lung cancer.

# Vegetables, cont.

Further research has shown that beta-carotene lowers the risk of breast, stomach, colon, and mouth cancer and may help reverse cancers of the uterus and cervix. The American Society of Clinical Oncology presented research that foods rich in beta-carotene could help men ward off prostate cancer. WARNING: Taking beta-carotene supplements does not have the same benefits. One study was stopped two years early when the group of smokers that were taking beta-carotene supplements actually showed a higher rate of lung cancer.

**Cauliflower** is a cruciferous vegetable that has many of the same attributes as broccoli, thus making it one of nature's powerful panaceas. Cauliflower contains sulforaphane, considered the most powerful anticancer compound found to date, as well as other phytochemicals, including dithiolthiones. Indoles, found in cruciferous vegetables, may help inhibit breast cancer. These compounds work by triggering enzymes that may act to block carcinogenic damage to your cells'

DNA. Other cruciferous vegetables include kale, Brussels sprouts, collards, mustard, and turnip greens.

**Garlic** stands alone in its power as a natural healer. Widely accepted as beneficial for afflictions such as asthma, heart disease, ulcers, tuberculosis, infections, rheumatism, high cholesterol, bronchitis, and cancer, garlic's curative capabilities have been the subject of hundreds of studies. Garlic's main claim to fame is the phytochemical allicin, a very active antioxidant. A study of 41,837 women in Iowa found that those who ate garlic at least once a week had a 35-percent lower risk of colon cancer, and epidemiologic studies in China show that eating a lot of garlic can protect against stomach cancer. Researchers believe that garlic is a promising ally against prostate cancer. Test-tube experiments show that compounds present in garlic also inhibit the growth of existing cancerous tumors of the skin, prostate, colon, rectum,

esophagus, and breast. It is difficult to get enough of garlic's medicinal compounds through a daily diet, so taking a supplement is important (see page 137).

IMPORTANT: crush fresh garlic 10 minutes before cooking so that the beneficial chemicals are released and not lost due to heating.

Katharine Milton, a professor of environmental science, policy, and management at the University of California at Berkeley, reported in the publication *Nutrition* that a 15-pound wild monkey consumes 600 milligrams of vitamin C a day (10 times more than the recommended daily allowance or RDA for a 150-pound human being), 4,571 milligrams of calcium (our RDA is 800) and 6,419 milligrams of potassium (our RDA is 2,000). Monkeys' food sources are excellent. Their fruits have higher levels of calcium, potassium, and iron than the cultivated varieties that we buy. Milton also reported that monkeys ate a high content of alpha linolenic acid, a nutrient found in Brussels sprouts, cabbage, and kale. "Throughout our history, humans have suffered from all sorts of diet-related disease," said Milton. Maybe now we know why.

The average American eats more than 10 pounds of chocolate a year and that may be a good thing. Tests show that chocolate has high levels of the powerful antioxidants catechins and phenolics. In a study published by the British medical journal *Lancet*, Dutch researchers found that dark chocolates had the highest levels of catechins – 53.5 mg per 100 grams – and that milk chocolate had 15.9 mg per 100 grams. Andrew Waterhouse of the University of California at Davis found that a 1.5-ounce chocolate bar had 205 mg of phenolics. Phenolics suppress cell-damaging chemicals and boost immune function. In addition, chocolate makes us happy (it contains phenylethylalanine and anandamide, naturally occurring mood-altering chemicals). So delight in your favorites, just don't overdo.

**Greens** abound – there are over one hundred different types, including iceberg, endive, Boston, romaine, chard, kale, and escarole. They are high in lutein, folic acid, iron, vitamins A, C, and E, as well as potassium. Just one serving of leafy greens is estimated to contain over 100 different phytochemicals. According to nutritionist Melanie Polk, R.D., Director of Nutrition Education at the American Institute for Cancer Research (AICR), "over the last few years, our understanding of how greens protect our health has greatly expanded. We now know that they are powerful arsenals in the fight against cancer." Greens are abundant in indoles and isothiocyanates, both potent cancer-prevention agents. Indoles, which are nitrogen compounds, may fight hormone-dependant cancers. Isothiocyanates may suppress tumor growth and block cancer-causing substances from reaching their targets. Studies have linked eating greens with the reduction of stomach cancer and a 20-percent lower risk of colon cancer.

**Onions** contain allicin, allylic sulfides, and various sulfur-containing compounds. Onions have several B vitamins, niacin, and potassium, and are good for preventing blood clots, combating infections, controlling cholesterol levels, relieving congestion, and healing wounds. Red and yellow onions are higher in these compounds than white. Onions possess a high level of the flavonoid quercetin, an anticancer, antiviral,

antibacterial, and antifungal antioxidant. A report in the *Journal of the National Cancer Institute* found that the effect of onions was particularly strong against squamous cell carcinoma lung cancer and a Dutch study found that eating half an onion a day reduced the risk of stomach cancer by 50 percent. Dr. Leonard M. Pike, research leader at the Vegetable Improvement Center, located in the Texas A&M Research Park at College Station, has this to say about onions: "there are several sulfur compounds that will actually inhibit cancer cell division. So when we consume these in our diet, they play a major role in inhibiting cancer of the esophagus and cancer of the colon, for example."

**Soybeans**, soy protein, and other soy products are being studied around the world for their ability to inhibit hormone-dependent cancers and reduce the development of blood vessels that nourish tumors. Soy has more than its share of wonderful attributes. It's rich in fiber, calcium, folic acid, potassium, iron, lecithin, vitamin E, zinc, and omega-3 trans fatty acid, and is a significant source of protein. The high level of soy in the Japanese and Chinese diet is credited with the low incidences of breast, prostate, and colon cancers in those populations. Soy also contains phytoestrogen hormones called isoflavones, one of which is genistein. Japanese researchers reported in the *International Journal of Cancer* that genistein decreased lymphatic vessel invasion and metastasis of intestinal adenocarcinomas in rats. It did not

## COFFEE, CAFFEINE, & CANCER

Researchers report that coffee beans may contain multiple anticancer agents and studies show that roasting does not destroy the anticancer activity associated with the beans. Dr. Edward Miller of the Baylor College of Dentistry in Dallas, Texas, and colleagues there and at the Biotechnology Research Institute in Montreal, Canada, say that roasted coffee beans appear to contain "cancer chemopreventive agents." Studies have shown that drinking coffee is associated with a significant reduction in colon cancer. This may be due to coffee's ability to speed up the waste process, inhibiting carcinogenic absorption through the intestinal wall, or possibly due to coffee's many polyphenols, which are potent anticancer agents.

## COMBATING ANEMIA NATURALLY

Chemotherapy can wipe out your red blood cells. The blood tests that your doctor regularly gives you during treatment will indicate whether or not you have become anemic. If this occurs, you will likely receive shots and/or iron supplements. What can you do to help your body recover? PLENTY.

Concentrate on eating the following foods: Raisins, beans, blackstrap molasses, beets, almonds, shellfish, dried apricots, lean red meat, dark green leafy vegetables, oily fish, prunes, tofu, whole wheat bread, and iron-fortified products such as pasta, rice, and cereal. Increase your vitamin C as it helps with iron absorption.

# Vegetables, cont.

however, affect the growth of the primary cancer. Other studies on the impact of genistein on breast and prostate cancer are being conducted by Dr. Stephen Barnes at the University of Alabama at Birmingham. Dr. Barnes postulates that soybeans and the drug tamoxifen are similar in the way they prevent breast cancer. Soy apparently mimics the body's estrogen but without its detrimental effects. As if that weren't enough, soy also contains other chemicals, such as protease inhibitors, phytosterols, phytates, and saponin, which are known to block and stop cancer cells from developing. You can find soy products such as soy flour, tofu, tempeh, miso, soy milk, soy nuts, soybean oil, soy yogurt, and meat substitute products like soy "veggie burgers" and bacon at your local supermarket. I recommend getting a soy cookbook if soy isn't already part of your diet.

IMPORTANT: An article in the *Journal of the National Cancer Institute* stated that genistein seems to modify the metabolism of cancer cells by weakening their defenses against chemotherapy and radiation treatments. Cancer cells have developed a system by which they become resistant to treatment, making it difficult for chemotherapy drugs and radiation to be effective. It looks as if genistein is capable of interfering with the production of cancer's protective proteins, giving chemotherapy and radiation therapy a better shot at killing tumors. It's possible that eating a soy-rich diet during your cancer treatments could make an impact on the outcome of your disease.

———※———

**Spinach** was Popeye's favorite food with good reason. It is loaded with beta-carotene, potassium, fiber, selenium, magnesium, zinc, calcium, lutein, folic acid, iron, and vitamins C, E, A, B6, and B12. Whew! This vegetable decreases the risk of cataracts, lowers blood cholesterol, and helps with anemia. Spinach has three times as much beta-carotene as carrots and is abundant in alpha-carotene as well. As a result, spinach is one of the most powerful anticancer foods you are going to find. Foods high in carotene help prevent lung, stomach, prostate, bladder, colon, esophageal, cervical, and skin cancers. In the *Journal of the National Cancer Institute*, Michiaki Murakoshi, Ph.D., reported that alpha-carotene suppressed the growth of pancreatic and gastric cancer, neuroblastomas, and glioblastomas. In addition, Italian scientists have found in test-tube studies that spinach blocked the formation of nitrosamines, a very powerful carcinogen.

**Squash**, pumpkins, and sweet potatoes are extremely high in polyphenol compounds, beta-carotene, and protease inhibitors (compounds that prevent cancer formation). They are good sources of vitamin E and C, fiber, potassium, and zinc, and they lower blood cholesterol, reduce the incidence of stroke, cataracts, and heart disease. Countless studies have found that the elements in these veggies combat cancer and offer protection against cancer of the esophagus, and gastrointestinal, prostate, colon, bladder, breast, cervical, skin, larynx, and most notably, lung.

———※———

**Tomatoes** contain potassium, iron, vitamins C and E, and quercetin, a flavonoid known for its antioxidant powers. Quercetin helps prevent

## VEGETABLES HAVE DIFFERENT GROWING SEASONS

Below is a list of what you'll get fresh and when.

| Cool-season crops | Warm-season crops |
|---|---|
| Cabbage, Onions, Peas, Carrots, Lettuce, Potatoes, Beets, Radishes | Eggplant, Corn, Squash, Tomatoes, Cucumbers, Melons, Peppers |

## THE BENEFITS OF ONE "ALL-RAW" MEAL A DAY

- Your body will not have to work as hard to digest the food.
- A diet heavy in raw fruits, vegetables, and nuts provides the best food "phyters" you can get.
- Cooking depletes vitamins, damages proteins and fats, and destroys the enzymes.
- Raw foods have more flavor.
- Cooking can create free radicals.
- Raw foods take little time to prepare.
- Clean-up is easy.
- Raw foods are loaded with water.
- Eating raw foods helps keep you "regular."
- Enjoying a meal of raw foods will give you energy.

## MOMENTOUS FISH TALE

Researchers found that eating fish two or more times a week reduces cancers of the stomach, colon, breast, esophagus, ovaries, larynx, rectum, and pancreas by 30 to 50%. Fish and its omega-3 oils reduce heart disease, blood clots, strokes, migraines, and asthma, and benefits ulcerated colitis, psoriasis, Crohn's disease, rheumatoid arthritis, depression, and brain function. Scientists believe that eating fish accounts for low breast cancer rates in Japanese women. An American Institute for Cancer Research study shows that omega-3 fatty acids help cancer patients increase the effectiveness of chemotherapy and reduce the destructive side effects.

**Fish abundant in omega-3 oil: anchovy, bluefish, herring, mackerel, tuna, salmon, and swordfish.**

## IS IT WRONG TO USE YOUR WOK?

Stir-frying is the rage and all those healthy vegetables and herbs that go into the wok are without question good for you. However, a study published in the *Journal of Epidemiology* reports that researchers from Canada and China found that stir-frying increased the risk of lung cancer in a group of nonsmoking women living in Shanghai, China. The study suggests that Chinese–style wok cooking may increase the risk of lung cancer by releasing potentially toxic fumes from cooking oils. While using your wok, watch for smokiness in the kitchen, work in a well-ventilated space, and turn down the wok temperature when you notice the cooking oil getting really hot.

cancer by blocking the growth of cancer cells and is the focus of several test-tube studies. A study at the Harvard Medical School involving 48,000 men found that those who ate tomato-based foods four to seven times a week cut their risk of prostate cancer by 22 percent and those who ate tomatoes more than ten times a week cut their risk by 35 percent.

Tomatoes are also rich in the phytochemical lycopene, a potent antioxidant. According to the *Journal of the National Cancer Institute,* the intake of lycopene from foods such as tomato sauce and pizza may reduce prostate cancer risk and there is now enough data to show convincingly

high consumption of tomatoes and tomato products substantially lessens the risk of many cancers, although probably not all. Dr. Edward Giovannucci of Harvard Medical School reported that 57 of 72 studies linked tomato consumption with a reduced risk of cancers. The studies were most compelling for cancers of the lung, stomach, and prostate. The findings also suggested links between tomatoes and lower levels of several other cancers, including pancreatic, colorectal, esophageal, oral, breast, and cervical cancers. Johns Hopkins researchers have linked pancreatic cancer to low blood levels of lycopene. It is

not destroyed by heat. The highest sources are ketchup, spaghetti sauce, and tomato sauce, followed by fresh tomatoes, tomato juice, tomato soup, and canned tomatoes. Tomato products cooked with a bit of oil have two or three times the absorption of lycopene.

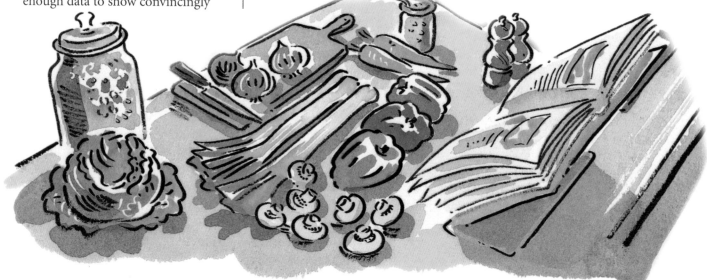

# Fruits

As a cancer patient you have special needs that require special attention. Your body suddenly has the formable task of dealing with cancer and the fallout from your treatments. It needs all the help it can get. Given the chance, fruit can play an enormous role in supporting the immune system and assisting the body's detoxification process.

This is what happens to you during cancer treatments: Typically, billions of cancer and normal cells are killed off when you receive chemo and/or radiation therapy. At that point your body faces the major challenge of eliminating the overload of toxic by-products (dead cells). In addition, the chemicals and radiation beams themselves have produced errant free radicals that your immune system must work overtime to deal with. Fatigue is the outcome of your body's efforts. With each passing treatment the body becomes slower to respond, making fatigue more and more pronounced.

This is where fruit comes in. The chemicals and compounds in fruits are known to assist the kidneys, bowels, lungs, and skin in the natural elimination process. They filter the lymph nodes, work on the adrenal glands, purify the blood system, act as a natural diuretic, and aid in the removal of toxins from the liver, testes, bladder, prostate, and kidneys. Obviously you can't afford to be like the average American, eating only ½ serving of fruit a day. Three servings a day are the minimum.

## CAN THIS BE?

Dietary choices are linked to 70% of all diseases affecting Americans. However, only 30 of the 125 medical schools in the US require doctors to take a course in nutrition. The average doctor gets only about 2.5 hours of nutritional training in four years of school. To date, well over 4,500 studies on the link between diet and cancer have been completed. The connection between what we eat and our health is overwhelming. The National Cancer Institute believes that one-third of all cancers are caused by dietary factors and the American Cancer Society recommends a daily diet of five fruits and vegetables to lower cancer risk. Many Americans searching for better health and longer lives are willing to make major lifestyle changes. Are you?

**Don't forget: Research shows that a varied diet rich in fruits, vegetables, and whole grains is beneficial to a cancer patient.**

One other thing. You do the majority of healing while you are completely at rest or asleep.

*Sleeping more than usual is simply another tool with which you can provide your body with the time to recuperate and rebuild. Never, ever overdo.*

❦

**Apples** lower blood cholesterol and blood pressure, help with diarrhea, boost the immune system, clear the lungs, combat viruses, stabilize blood sugar, assist in relieving constipation, prevent ulcers, and provide arthritis relief. Apples are high in fiber and contain potassium, boron, vitamins A and C, and they are loaded with the antioxidant flavonoid, quercetin. According to a study done by Finland's National Public Health Institute, people who consumed the most flavonoid-rich foods were about 46 percent less likely to develop lung cancer. The *Journal of the National Cancer Institute* reported that a study done at the Cancer Research Center of Hawaii, University of Hawaii, Honolulu showed significantly lower incidence of lung cancer in test subjects who had a high level of quercetin from eating apples. At the University of Kansas, Dr. Jill Pelling found that apigenin, a flavonoid in apples, induces the same protein as the tumor-suppressor gene p53. The protein p53 programs your body to stop out-of-control cell growth and in many cancer patients the p53 is damaged and cancerous cells spread undaunted.

❦

**Berries** are to the fruit empire what broccoli is to the vegetable empire – the kings in fighting cancer. There are blackberries, blueberries, bilberries, cranberries, and straw-berries, to mention just a few. In general, they contain fiber, C, E, and B vitamins, potassium, folic acid, and iron. They fight herpes, urinary tract infections, viruses, and diarrhea; prevent stroke and memory loss; and aid in motor coor-dination, eyesight problems, and damage to the circulatory system. The ellagic acid found in berries slows tumor growth by blocking production of enzymes used by cancer cells and may prevent new free radical damage as well. In addition, blueberries and strawberries registered ounce for ounce the highest in antioxidant activity among 40 different foods that were tested. They are high in salicylates, anthocyanosides, tannins, and oligomeric tannins, and

## GETTING NUTS ABOUT NUTS

In general, nuts are high in selenium, iron, zinc, vitamin E, and some B vitamins, folic acid, calcium, manganese, magnesium, fiber, polyphenols, phytochemicals, and protease inhibitors. Nuts protect the heart and lower cholesterol. Brazil nuts are plentiful in selenium, walnuts are abundant in ellagic acid, and almonds are exceptionally high in vitamin E, all recognized as powerful antioxidants that boost immunity and fight cancer. Peanuts have the same health benefits as nuts but they are technically legumes. Many cancer books suggest eating two brazil nuts, 10 almonds, and a few walnuts each day. Laetrile, found in the kernels of almonds, peaches and apricots, were found by the NCI not to be effective against cancer.

## GREEN & BLACK TEA CHALLENGE CANCER

Green and black tea contain polyphenols, catechins, and other flavonoids that prevent initial cancer development. A study by Dr. Roderick Dashwood of Oregon State University uncovered new evidence that tea stops the promotion, progression, and metastasis of cancer. Said Dr. Dashwood, "This indicates that more than one anticancer mechanism is at work." One of green tea's polyphenols, EGCG, a powerful antioxidant, is 20 times stronger than vitamin E. Japanese tea drinkers who consumed 4 to 6 cups a day had lower incidence of breast, liver, lung, and skin cancer. Green tea relieves allergies, headaches, asthma, colds, hepatitis, coughs, hangovers, diarrhea, congestion, and migraines.
You can order it online at: **www.harney.com**

oligomeric proanthocyanidins, often known as OPCs. These chemicals help protect DNA from free radicals such as radiation and chemicals, and slow down the mutation of cancer. Also, the numerous phenols found in berries shut off the formation of carcinogens, suppress cancer promotion, and increase the body's detoxification defenses. In a study done at the University of Western Ontario, Canadian researchers found that mice fed with dehydrated cranberries and then injected with human breast cancer cells were 50 percent less likely to develop cancer than the mice who did not receive cranberries. In addition, the mice who had cranberries showed a reduction in the spread of tumors to the lungs and lymph nodes. According to researchers with the US Department of Agriculture (USDA), strawberries have as much ability to counteract damaging oxygen-free radicals in the body as a large dose of vitamin C. In one study reported by Ronald L. Prior of the USDA's Human Nutrition Research Center on Aging at Tufts University in Boston, eight elderly women were given special drinks made from strawberry extract. The drinks were the equivalent of about 8 to 10 ounces of the fruit (about one pint of strawberries). The drinks boosted each lady's antioxidant capacity by 20 percent. That's as much as taking 1,250 milligrams of vitamin C.

**Cherries** contain vitamin C, potassium, and fiber and are known to relieve gout, hamper headaches, and prevent tooth decay. According to the American Institute for Cancer Research (AICR), cherries contain substances that fight cancer. The chemical perillyl alcohol binds to protein molecules to inhibit the growth signals that stimulate tumor development. In laboratory studies this phytochemical has caused pancreatic tumors to regress and has shown the potential to help prevent cancers of the breast, lung, liver, and skin. Cherries also contain anthocyanins, potent antioxidants that cut off harmful by-products of the metabolism and rid them from the body. A test at Michigan State University showed that carcinogens from grilled hamburgers could be reduced by 90 percent if ground cherries were mixed into the raw hamburger meat prior to grilling. Use 1 part cherries to 9 parts hamburger.

**Grapefruit** contains vitamin C, potassium, folic acid, calcium, and pectin. Pink grapefruit gets its color from carotenoids and contains over fifty times the amount of carotene as white grapefruit. Grapefruit contains limonene, which increases the production of enzymes that may break down carcinogens and stimulate cancer-killing immune cells. Limonene is contained in the peels of citrus fruits and studies have shown that it blocks the development of breast, colon, liver, and lung tumors in addition to causing existing tumors to shrink in laboratory animals. The phytochemical lycopene, found in red grapefruit, is actually twice as powerful as beta-carotene at eliminating free radicals and is linked to the reduction of cancers such as prostate, esophageal, oral,

# Fruits, cont.

colorectal, pancreatic, breast, cervical, and stomach. Recent studies at the Institute of Bioscience and Technology in Houston have shown that lycopene helps patients with prostate cancer by slowing down cancer cells and stabilizing normal cell growth. Grapefruit also contains chemicals known as monoterpenes, which are believed to rid the body of carcinogens, thus preventing cancer. According to the *Journal of the National Cancer Institute*, high consumption of white grapefruit is associated with significantly less lung cancer.

WARNING: If you are taking medication of any kind, ask your doctor if it is safe to eat grapefruit or drink grapefruit juice while taking the drugs. Grapefruit juice amplifies some drugs and inhibits the body's absorption of other drugs. Therefore, do not drink grapefruit juice on the days when you will be receiving chemotherapy, especially if you are receiving vinblastine.

**Grapes** help prevent coronary artery disease, strokes, and blood clots. They lower cholesterol, fight viruses, prevent tooth decay, cleanse the body of toxins, and contain many cancer-fighting compounds such as quercetin, polyphenols, and tannins. Dark purple grapes contain more antioxidants than do green grapes, with the majority of the antioxidants found in the seeds and skin. Red wine contains catechins, a very powerful antioxidant, but you shouldn't use that as an excuse to drink bottles of the stuff. Purple grape juice is almost as high in catechins, so drink purple grape juice if you're a teetotaler. According to a report in the journal *Science*, reservatrol, detected in the skin of grapes, has been found to block three major mechanisms of cancer-cell development.

**Melons** are high in beta-carotene, potassium, and vitamins A and C. Cantaloupe assists with high blood pressure, lessens risk of heart attack and strokes, thins the blood, and boosts the immune system. The high concentrations of beta-carotene in cantaloupe is believed to lower the risk of lung cancer. Studies show that people with high levels of beta-carotene in their blood are half as likely to develop cancers of the breast, stomach, larynx, throat, mouth, and bladder. Beta-carotene keeps cancer cells from multiplying. Watermelon also contains high concentrations of iron. Ounce for ounce, watermelon has the highest concentration of lycopene, the most powerful antioxidant discovered to date. In a study conducted by Harvard University, researchers found lycopene lowered the risk of developing certain cancers, especially prostate cancer.

**Oranges** and citrus fruits are abundant in vitamin C, calcium, fiber, folic acid, and potassium. A study testing the anticancer power of flavonoids in tangerine and orange juice found that tumor incidence was inhibited by 50 percent. These citrus juices

## FROM THE STORE SHELVES: 100% JUICE

If your not inclined to make your own juices than try to buy the 100% fruit juices. Some of the top picks in the *Environmental Nutritional Newsletter* comparison study were as follows:

- V8 100% Juice
- Dole Pineapple Juice
- Sunsweet Prune Juice
- Mott's 100% Apple Juice
- Ocean Spray Pink Grapefruit Juice
- Lakewood Organic Mango Juice
- Hollywood 100% Pure Carrot Juice
- Tropicana Pure Premium Orange Juice Double Vitamin C

## FRUIT FAST FACTS

- From Tufts University: Prunes are number 1 in antioxidant activity of 50 fruits and vegetables measured.
- From the University of Hawaii: lung cancer patients who eat the most fruits and vegetables, especially broccoli, survive a year and a half longer than those who skimped on produce.
- Half a cantaloupe contains 100% of the RDA of vitamins A and C.
- From the University of Maryland: Zeaxanthin, an antioxidant new to the cancer-prevention scene, is "one of the best" in stimulating enzymes that detoxify carcinogens. It's available in squash, oranges, peaches, and apricots.

obstructed cell reproduction in melanomas and lung, stomach, prostate, and colon cancer. Tangeretin from tangerine juice was the most active of the 22 flavonoids studied. Another compound found in citrus fruit, limonoids, is the focus of studies led by Dr. Takuji Tanaka of Kanazawa Medical University in Uchinada, Japan. His team has found that limonoids may protect against colon cancer In another study Dr. Luke K.T. Lam and others at LKT Laboratories, Inc. in St. Paul, Minnesota, and the USDA's Western Regional Research Center in Albany, California, found that fewer liver or lung cancer tumors were formed in those mice that had been given limonoids than those in the control group. In addition, the American Cancer Society believes that orange juice, when it is included as part of a healthy diet, helps in the fight against cancer.

**Pineapples** contain vitamins A and C, potassium, manganese, and chlorine. They are antiviral and antibacterial, help prevent blood clots and osteoporosis, soothe sore throats, and help relieve the symptoms of the common cold. Pineapples' big claim to fame is that they contains the enzyme bromelain. Bromelain is a very effective enzyme that is popular for providing relief from indigestion, one of chemotherapy's common side effects. Eating fresh pineapple or drinking 6–8 ounces of pineapple juice before each meal can make eating more pleasant on the days of treatment and for several days thereafter. There are also bromelain enzymes in tablet form in health food

stores, and while they don't have all the elements that fresh pineapple does, they are still effective. In a test-tube study, bromelain was found to have anti-tumor effects. In-vitro studies showed that bromelain fought leukemia by normalizing blood cells and that it helped prevent lung cancer metastasis.

---

### FUN IS FUN, BUT ENOUGH IS ENOUGH

Two or more alcoholic drinks a day can increase your risk for cancers of the mouth, throat, esophagus, and liver. Add tobacco to the mix and you are 15 times more likely to enhance your risk for cancer of the head and neck region. Studies show alcohol increases the risk of breast cancer in women as well. It isn't clear whether alcohol directly causes cancer or promotes tumor growth by other cancer-causing substances. Alcohol can inhibit the body's ability to handle stress and may indirectly lead to cancer by causing nutrient deficiencies. The American Institute for Cancer Research suggests the following:

• Eat before you drink and while you drink.

• Order diluted drinks like white-wine spritzers.

• Never guzzle alcohol when you're thirsty.

### PANICKY ABOUT PESTICIDES?

Pesticide residues found on foods are well below the EPA limits for children and adults. However, even a minimal amount can cause free radicals.

A cancer patient should take special care to eliminate free radical damage whenever possible. What do you do?

• Buy organic produce when you can.

• Avoid buying produce that has mold, bruising, cuts, insect holes, or decay.

• Remove the outer leaves of lettuce, cabbage, and other leafy vegetables before washing.

• Wash fresh produce very well in freshwater or with soap made specifically for cleaning produce, whether you plan to eat it raw or cook it.

**For more information call (703) 305-5017 and order your free Pesticides on Food pamphlet.**

# Fiber

Fiber is the part of food that does not get fully digested. There are two types of fiber: Water-soluble fiber is found primarily in fruits, vegetables, nuts, oats, legumes (dried beans and peas), and whole grains. Insoluble fiber is found in unrefined cereal grains such as wheat bran. High-fiber diets protect against heart disease (in one study it cut a woman's risk nearly in half), diverticulosis, and obesity, reduces blood cholesterol, lowers blood pressure, helps steady blood sugar levels, and lowers the risk of ulcers. Fiber intake is believed to have a positive impact on the risk of rectal, stomach, thyroid, and mouth cancers, and studies have found that fiber lowered estrogen levels, which can promote cancers of the breast and prostate.

The evidence regarding fiber and colon cancer remains confusing. Some studies discovered that diets high in fiber reduced the growth of polyps and colon cancer. Other studies have found that there is no link between the two. Many scientists feel that the jury is still out on this one because it takes up to 15 years for colon cancer to develop and most trials were done over a three-year period. In the bowel, fiber bulk pushes fat and toxins through the colon quickly, giving them less time to damage the body. This is especially important for the cancer patient, who needs to detoxify as soon after treatments as possible. Drinking plenty of water while consuming fiber actually helps this process along and can help relieve constipation, which is a common side effect of chemotherapy. Legumes are one of the best sources of fiber that you can get. They are rich in protein and contain zinc, potassium, B vitamins, calcium, magnesium, and iron. Strive for at least one serving of beans a day between treatments. Your intake of fiber should be 25 to 35 grams daily. To make sure that you get enough fiber in your diet, increase your intake of wholewheat bread, beans, whole-grain pastas, and brown rice.

*Don't forget fruits and vegetables are a great source of fiber, as well.*

Avoid highly refined foods such as white bread, pastries, pies, cakes, noodles, and white rice. Most of these items have little in the way of nutritional value, some are high in fat content, and all are merely fillers you can learn to do without.

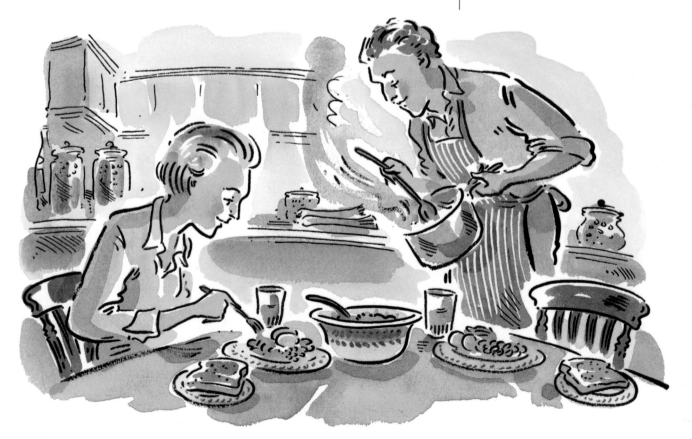

# Juicing

Juicing fresh fruits and vegetables takes organization, time, and energy, all of which you may feel you have precious little at this point in your life. The fatigue that many people experience during treatments prevents them from being able to juice at the time when fresh juices would help them the most. Think hard. Do you have a neighbor or family member who loves to cook and spend time in the kitchen? Could you explain the importance of fresh juices and ask him or her to make a few glasses a day until you feel able to do it yourself? The benefits of fresh fruit and vegetable juice far outweigh the time and mess involved.

Vegetables that are thought to be potent cancer fighters and are good for juicing are: kale, parsley, broccoli, carrots, cabbage, and beets. Incidentally, to relieve an upset stomach, juice 2 apples and 4 slices of pineapple. Pineapple is loaded with bromelain, an enzyme that assists digestion.

## Why you would want to juice

- When you juice you receive the highest concentration, ounce for ounce, of nutrition and phytochemicals that fruits and vegetables have to offer. This is especially important while you're in therapy or during periods of recuperation when you have little or no appetite.

- Fresh juice is a concentrated source of chlorophyll, enzymes, proteins, vitamins, minerals, carbohydrates, refined water, phytochemicals, and antioxidants.

- Juicing will add much-needed liquids to your daily intake. Be sure to drink plenty of water too.

- When you drink fresh juice your body will have less digestive work to do than if you were to eat a snack or a full meal.

- Nutrients are absorbed quickly into your body when you drink fresh juice because your body does not have to extract the liquid from the fiber.

- Fresh juice can oftentimes give you a boost of energy when you are feeling tired or weak.

- Fresh fruit and vegetable juices have no added preservatives or refined sugars.

- Fruit juices are the energizers and cleansers of the body, while vegetable juices are the body builders.

Drink up!

## JUICING HELPFUL HINTS

- You will need a cutting board, a sharp knife, Ziploc® bags, a salad spinner (if you are going to juice kale, parsley, or other greens), a vegetable brush, and a good vegetable juicer. A blender won't work for this purpose.

- Don't buy more produce than you can use in one week. Try to buy organic produce if you can.

- Have a friend or family member clean all your fruit and veggies for you when you bring them home from the store.

- Store your fresh produce in large Ziploc® bags.

- Do not juice the rind or skin.

- Remove pits from the fruit.

- Include stems and leaves along with the fruit and vegetables, making sure all pieces are small enough to fit easily into the juicer.

- Drink the juices immediately. They do not keep and they will lose their nutrients quickly.

- Remember that variety of fruits and vegetables are key. Try different combinations. If you have fruits or vegetables that are too ripe to eat but are still good, toss them in the juicer.

- Clean your juicer immediately after juicing; otherwise, you will have a messy job on your hands.

- Remember that these drinks are concentrated. In the beginning start with 4-ounce glasses of juice, working your way up to 6 or 8 ounces.

- Try to drink a minimum of one fruit and two vegetable drinks a day. Go light on green leafy veggies.

- Fruit and vegetable juices do not mix, with the exception of juicing carrots and apples together.

### Joanie's Favorite
1 beet
4 carrots
3 broccoli flowerets with the stems
small handfull of parsley
¼ head of cabbage

### The Prize Fighter
½ green pepper
3 broccoli flowerets with the stems
5 carrots
2 stalks of celery
small handful of spinach

### The Champion
½ orange or tangerine
3 slices of pineapple (lengthwise)
1 apple
5 or 6 large strawberries
½ banana

### The Eliminator
12 green or red grapes
½ cup raspberries (frozen is fine)
2 slices of pineapple (lengthwise)
½ cup blackberries (frozen is fine)

# The ORAC *of Fruits & Vegetables*

What is ORAC? Oxygen Radical Absorbence Capacity per serving. The USDA Agricultural Research Service uses a test that measures the total antioxidant power of foods and other chemical substances called the oxygen radical absorbence capacity (ORAC). The higher the level of ORACs in a food, the more beneficial it is to the body. Think of it in terms of war. The territory (cells of the body) come under attack every ten seconds. The troops (antioxidant enzymes) are part of the armed forces (the immune system), whose soldiers are constantly on patrol looking for the enemy (free radicals). The strength and number of troops depends entirely on the supply lines (the foods you eat). If the soldiers are well equipped (high-ORAC foods), they will locate the position of the enemy (free radicals), surround them, and then neutralize them so that they can not declare war on other cells. The more soldiers you have, the fewer successful invasions

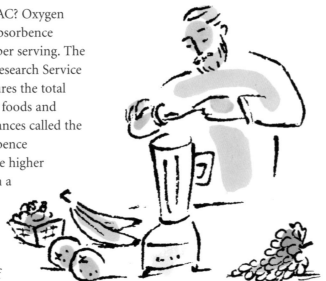

from free radicals. Studies published in the *Journal of Nutrition* and the *American Journal of Clinical Nutrition* show that eating high-ORAC fruits and vegetables raises the antioxidant power of the blood between 13 and 25 percent.

*Remember: don't fill up the supply trucks (your body) with shoddy ammunition (junk food). Your troops have a hard battle ahead.*

## QUICK AND EASY
**Immune-boosting Smoothie**

In your blender add approximately 1/2 cup of each:
Frozen Blueberries
Frozen Strawberries
Frozen Blackberries
Frozen Raspberries

Pour in enough Orange Juice (about 1 1/2 cups) to make the mixture blend easily but still maintain a milkshake-like consistency. When the ingredients are blended well and while the blender is still on, add Soy or protein powder. Continue to blend for approximately 30 seconds.

Note: you may substitute fresh fruit and ice cubes instead of frozen fruit. You may also substitute your favorite fruit drink for the orange juice.

Are You Curious? The total amount of ORAC per Immune-boosting Smoothy is about 6,930. Beat that!

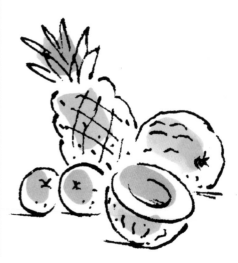

| Antioxidant Power of Veggies | |
|---|---|
| **Vegetables** | **ORAC** |
| Kale (1 cup) | 1,186 |
| Beets (1/2 cup) | 571 |
| Red bell peppers (1/2 cup) | 533 |
| Brussels sprouts (1/2 cup) | 431 |
| Corn (1/2 cup) | 420 |
| Spinach (1 cup) | 378 |
| Onions (1/2 cup) | 360 |
| Broccoli florets (1/2 cup) | 320 |
| Eggplant (1 cup) | 320 |
| Alfalfa sprouts (1/2 cup) | 149 |

| Antioxidant Power of Fruit: | |
|---|---|
| **Fruits** | **ORAC** |
| Prunes (4) | 1,939 |
| Blueberries (1/2 cup) | 1,740 |
| Blackberries (1/2 cup) | 1,466 |
| Strawberries (1/2 cup) | 1,170 |
| Raisins (1/4 cup) | 1,026 |
| Raspberries (1/2 cup) | 756 |
| Oranges (1/2 cup) | 675 |
| Plums (1) | 626 |
| Red grapes (1/2 cup) | 591 |
| Cherries (1/2 cup pitted) | 516 |

# What Did You Learn *about* Nutrition?

**W**hy is it significant that we grasp the fine points of how nutrition impacts our health? In most aspects of our lives what we believe dictates our behavior. It follows then that having a clear and concise understanding of the immune system and its connection to our diet is terribly important to our health.

*Remember: knowledge is power!*

**SCORING YOURSELF**

The answers to these questions on nutrition can be found on page 146. If you missed more than two or three questions, go back and read pages 112–132.

## TRUE OR FALSE

1. A nutritionist is always licensed and is the best source for information on what food and vitamins you should consume.

2. Cancer is most often the result of a weak or overwhelmed immune system.

3. Meat and some fats produce free radicals, creating work for the immune system.

4. Rust on a car, cancer, and an apple turning brown are examples of antioxidants.

5. The average American eats 1½ servings of vegetables and ½ serving of fruit each day, which is sufficient to maintain one's health.

6. Phytochemicals can not deter cancer once it's large enough to be diagnosed.

7. "Phyto" means antioxidant.

8. Free radicals attack the body's cells every ten seconds.

9. As we age the levels of vitamins, minerals, enzymes, and hormones diminish, leaving us more vulnerable to more ailments.

10. Over ½ million cancers a year could be prevented by healthier living.

11. Scientists are calling phytochemicals "chemoprevention" and believe them to hold promise in the war against cancer.

12. Fruits and vegetables that have been frozen lose much of their nutritional value.

13. Fruits help the body eliminate dead cancer cells and boost the immune system.

14. The omega-3 fat in fish causes free radicals and heart damage.

15. The juice of fresh fruits and vegetables gives you concentrated amounts of nutrients.

16. ORAC denotes the amount of antioxidant power a food has against free radicals.

17. Vegetables are the energizers and cleansers of the body while fruit juices are the body builders.

18. The worst fat you can consume comes in the form of margarine and shortenings.

19. Most medical schools provide doctors with ample education in nutrition.

20. Grilled meats create cancer-causing carcinogens so you need to take precautions.

# Vitamins, Minerals, & Herbs

Having cancer means having billions of out-of-control mutated cells creating havoc in your body. Whatever you ate and whatever supplements you took before your diagnosis were not enough to prevent you from getting cancer. It follows then that you need to concentrate at this point on providing your immune system with the support it needs to play "catch up" to destroy cells already malignant and to stop metastasis.

You can not substitute good nutrition with a vitamin capsule. However, researchers are starting to confirm the benefits that nutritional supplements have in reversing established cancers. For the first time medicine is looking not only at chemotherapy, surgery, and radiation as cancer treatments but at chemoprevention (the use of nutritional supplements to halt or suppress the carcinogenic process), as well.

❧

Decide for yourself if you want to fight your illness combining the best that medicine has to offer with your own individual arsenal of vitamins and minerals. In general, an antioxidant multivitamin is the very least you should take, although you should consult your doctor if you are on chemotherapy.

I believe passionately that supplements fight cancer. I've kept many personal convictions out of these pages but this is the one area where I can't stay silent. Every cancer patient I have ever spoken with has wanted to know to what I attribute my survival. I'll tell you: I think it's because I have strong

## CHEMO, RADIATION, AND VITAMINS

If you doubt the power of vitamins, minerals and herbs, you only need to look at the scientific research that has come out in recent years regarding cancer therapy and supplementation. As a cancer patient you need to know what to take and when. Some vitamins have been proven to enhance cancer therapy while others may hinder treatments. Let's take a look at what is what.

Dr. David Golde, physician-in-chief at Memorial Sloan-Kettering Cancer Center, reported to the ACS that taking mega doses of vitamin C during treatments may actually insulate and protect the tumor from radiation and chemotherapy.

Drs. Elaine Hardman and Ivan Cameron, researchers at the University of Texas Health Science Center, who are funded by the American Institute for Cancer Research, discovered that polyunsaturated fatty acids found in fish oil may increase the effectiveness of chemotherapy while protecting the patient against side effects such as fatigue, dry mouth, nausea, vomiting, and weight loss. Omega-3 fatty acids are also known to slow or prevent the growth of tumors. According to Dr. Hardman, the study's principal investigator. "Studies suggest that the more types of these fatty acids the cancer cells incorporate, the more sensitive they become to damage by certain chemotherapeutic drugs."

A combination of vitamins A, C, and E may protect cancer patients from the side effects of radioimmunotherapy, a treatment that uses the immune systems' antibodies to carry cancer-killing radioactive agents directly to tumor cells. This would allow increased doses of radiation to be given without harming surrounding tissues.

## THE OPTIMIST VERSUS THE PESSIMIST

A set of twins were being evaluated because one was always happy and the other always sad. The psychiatrist put the sad little boy in a room full of toys and the happy little boy in a room full of horse manure. Returning an hour later he found the sad little boy crying because he had realized the toys were not his to keep. Checking in on the happy little boy, the doctor found tunnels dug throughout the manure. Finally locating the boy in one of the tunnels, he asked "what are you doing?" The boy replied " With all this horse manure I just know there has to be a horse in here somewhere."

Findings at the Mayo Clinic suggest that optimists tend to live longer and enjoy better health then pessimists, indicating that the mind can strongly influence the body. While no one expects you to have a positive outlook all the time, it might just benefit your health occasionally to look for horses in the manure.

faith in God and medical science; I've picked aggressive doctors who have given me aggressive treatments; I get diagnostic tests regularly; I eat and juice tons of fruits and vegetables; and I consume large doses of vitamins, herbs, and supplements.

I take about 60 supplements a day, and while that may seem a bit extreme, keep in mind that many supplements are just concentrated foods that have been put into various capsules or gel caps. I believe the supplements I take boost my immune system, fight cancer, detoxify my body, cleanse my lymph glands, purify my blood, and protect my heart.

**Beta-carotene & vitamin A:** Vitamin A plays an important role in immune system function, is key to preventing infections, assists new cell growth, and works in combination with vitamins C and E. Since vitamin A is fat-soluble it is safer to take beta-carotene, the precursor to vitamin A. As a precursor, beta-carotene is stored in the liver where it is converted to vitamin A every time the body needs it.

*Beta-carotene increases the number and activity of white blood cells enhancing cancer fighting immune functions.*

Research found that beta-carotene supplements boosted immunity in people with colon cancer. Waun Ki Hong, MD, and his colleagues at M.D. Anderson Cancer Center have made significant advances in the use of chemopreventive agents related to vitamin A against epithelial cancers of the head and neck, lung, and esophagus cancers. Studies of former smokers who take beta-carotene supplements (30 mg daily) show a "dramatic" reduction in the risk of oral cancer, according to researcher Harinder Garewal of the University of Arizona, and beta-carotene reverses growth of precancers of the mouth in up to 70 percent of patients. Beta-carotene and vitamin A are the focus of many on-going cancer clinical trials. In one study, patients given large doses of beta-carotene responded well to chemotherapy and had less progression of cancer. Beta-carotene is water-soluble and very safe; however, if you continue to smoke, do not take beta-carotene. Two studies have found that beta-carotene may slightly accelerate lung cancer in smokers.

❋

**Vitamin C** has tremendous benefits to those who have cancer. Not only does vitamin C help protect the heart during treatments but it also elevates interferon levels, which stimulates the immune system and enhances the activity of specific immune cells. Researchers detected a 37-percent lower risk of death from cancer in men taking at least 138 mg of vitamin C and 5.3 mg of beta-carotene a day. Dr. Gladys Block, M.D., from the National Cancer Institute, found that vitamin C has a protective effect in a number of cancers. In nearly 90 studies involving thousands of people, vitamin C exhibited positive effects in cancer-prevention for cancers of the pancreas, oral cavity, stomach, esophagus, cervix, rectum, breast, and lung. Research shows that vitamin C not only slows tumor growth and prolongs life, but in some cases causes tumor regression as well. Supplementation with vitamin C has been shown to inhibit nerve, lung, kidney, and skin cancers. Studies show that vitamin C is capable of inhibiting tumor cell growth and carcinogen-induced DNA damage.

❋

**Vitamin E** is one of nature's most important antioxidants, and when teamed up with the antioxidant vitamins A and C, there is a significant improvement in the number of immune cells that protect against and fight cancer. Vitamin E helps preserve oxygen, protects against harmful free radicals, helps prevent heart attacks, improves circulation, and increases energy and stamina. One study showed that people who had the lowest blood levels of vitamin E were at the highest risk for all types of cancer. Other research found that vitamin E inhibits cancer cell proliferation and causes cancer cell death. A study published in the *Journal of the National Cancer Institute* reported

## THE FDA "CONSPIRACY THEORY"

No one feels more anger than I that there is no cure for cancer. Nonetheless, common sense and personal experiences tells me the following "theory" that some people believe is pure bunk. Here it is: "The good news is that a cure for all cancers has been discovered and it's a common, natural substance making it very inexpensive. The bad news is that the FDA , the ACS, and the NCI are all in cahoots with the pharmaceutical companies in concealing the treatment. Hundreds of scientists, biologists, administrators, doctors, and pharmaceutical employees are keeping quiet due to the vast amounts of money involved. None of the conspirators has lost a loved one to cancer, thus the secret is secure. The various clinical trials being conducted on food compounds, vitamins, minerals, plants, herbs, and trees is simply a ruse by the government to make us think they looking for a natural cure." Does anyone really buy all that?!

# Vitamins, Minerals, & Herbs, cont.

that the risk of prostate cancer was reduced by one-third and the death rate by 41 percent in men taking vitamin E compared to those taking a placebo. Vitamin E decreases DNA damage (important for cancer patients receiving chemo or radiation therapy) and inhibits malignant transformations. In the Iowa Women's Health Study, researchers found that women who developed colon cancer consumed the smallest amount of vitamin E. British researchers found that women with the highest blood levels of vitamin E had only one-fifth the risk of breast cancer compared with women with the lowest blood levels. It's nearly impossible to get enough vitamin E from foods, so I strongly suggest a supplement of natural vitamin E. Selenium increases the beneficial effects of vitamin E, so you should always take them together.

**Selenium** supplements have been found to reduce overall cancer incidence by 42 percent in studies done by Dr. Larry Clark of the University of Arizona. They also appeared to reduce the risk of dying from cancer in treated patients, reported Dr. Clark. Selenium assists the body in the production of glutathione, a critical antioxidant enzyme. Glutathione helps detoxify cellular fats that lower immunity, foster cancer cells, and destroy arteries. Selenium stimulates the immune system by increasing the activity and number of white blood cells, promotes the formation of natural killer cells, and retards the growth and replication of cancer cells in test-tube studies. Researchers found that

taking 100 mcg of selenium a day improved certain factors of immune functions by 79 percent. According to research reported in the *Journal of the American Medical Association*, patients who took daily doses of selenium had 63 percent fewer cases of prostate cancer, 58 percent fewer colon or rectal cancers, and 45 percent fewer lung cancers. Selenium has been effective against esophageal and liver cancer as well, and research is underway to see if selenium might help those who already have prostate cancer. If you would rather get your daily dose of selenium by eating four Brazil nuts a day, eat them when you take your vitamin E supplements.

**Coenzyme Q10 (CoQ10)** functions as a super antioxidant, maintains the vitality of the heart, the gums, and the immune system, and is an extremely important nutrient needed by every cell in your body in order to produce energy. As we grow older, our ready supply of CoQ10 is depleted, and while we can obtain small amounts from our foods, it isn't nearly enough for a cancer patient.

The effects of chemotherapy on the heart and gums make this nutrient especially important in protecting the patient during treatments. Adriamycin (doxorubicin), an effective chemotherapeutic drug used for many different cancers, including breast cancer, carries the serious risk of cardiac toxicity and a significant number of patients experience serious complications of cardiomyopathy. Studies have shown that patients taking CoQ10 during treatments did not develope cardiac

## Buyer beware!

- Aloe Vera has many healing properties. However, in recent years several cancer patients have died as a direct result of getting T-UP (concentrated aloe) injections. There is no evidence that aloe cures cancer.
- The National Cancer Institute (NCI) evaluated Cancell and found that it had no effect on cancer cells. An injunction prohibits the distribution of Cancell but it's being sold under various names as a dietary supplement in some health food stores.
- Laetrile is a toxic drug. According to research at seven different institutions and a NCI clinical trial, laetrile had no benefit in the treatment of cancer.
- DMSO, an industrial solvent, is given orally, by injection, or by enema as a cancer treatment. DMSO may cause damage to the liver, kidneys, and central nervous system. There's no proof that it cures cancer.

toxicity. Furthermore, CoQ10 did not interfere with the therapeutic effects of Adriamycin.

Many chemotherapeutic drugs are known to cause periodontal and gum problems. CoQ10 effectively protects cancer patients against deterioration of the gums, inflamed gum tissue, and tooth loss.

Several studies assessing the effects of CoQ10 on breast and prostate cancer patients found some regressions of tumors and remarkable survival times for both. CoQ10 requires four to eight weeks to build up to peak concentration in the body and has no known adverse side effects even at extremely large doses.

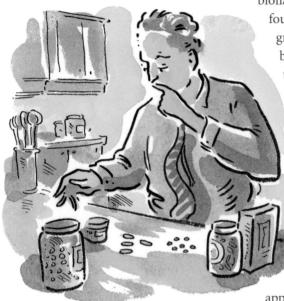

**EPA Fish Oil** (omega-3 fatty acids and linolenic acid) is the focus of several ongoing clinical animal studies that show omega-3 fatty acids may delay tumor development and decrease rate of growth, size, and the number of tumors. In humans, researchers have found reduced tumor metastasis in women when there were high levels of alpha-linolenic acid in breast fat tissue, while low alpha-linolenic acid in breast tissue near the site of cancer were associated with increased risk of lymph node involvement and the spread of cancer. EPA supplements reduce chemotherapy side effects such as fatigue, nausea, vomiting, and malnutrition. EPA supplements are safe and nontoxic and should be taken while receiving treatments. For more information, see page 118.

**Pycnogenol and grapeseed extract,** which are also known as OPCs or proanthocyanidins, are a class of nutrients that belong to the bioflavonoid family. OPCs are found in pine bark and grapeseed extract and have been shown to have 20 times the antioxidant potency of vitamin C and 50 times the potency of vitamin E. In addition to being powerful antioxidants, they boost immune function, strengthen capillaries, prevent varicose veins, significantly reduce heart attacks and strokes, repair connective tissue, assist with allergy control, and appear to have antimutagenic activity. Since they are one of the few supplements that crosses the blood-brain barrier, they may be important in the prevention of cancer metastasis to the brain. Proanthocyanidins and flavonoids, in general, are free of side effects since they are water-soluble nutrients and any excess intake is simply excreted in the urine. Take this supplement with vitamins C and E because it may preserve the body's stores of vitamin C and strengthen the antioxidant effects of vitamin E.

**Garlic** is high in the anticancer phytochemical allicin, and sulfur compounds, which inhibit the growth of different types of cancer, especially breast and skin tumors. For those who like the flavor of garlic, Kyolic™ or Kwai™ are garlic extracts that come in pill form. In laboratory studies, the potent anticancer compounds allyl sulfides were found to intensify in the presence of selenium and vitamin A. The garlic compound, diallyl sulfide, was given to mice prior to exposure to a colon

## DESIGNER FOODS AND NUTRACEUTICALS

As a result of recent scientific developments in the field of nutrition, consumers are beginning to realize the important role that functional foods (those containing positive druglike benefits) have in providing optimum health. Food manufactures interested in enticing consumers into buying their products are adding vitamins, minerals, and antioxidants to their merchandise, creating "designer foods." Nutriceucticals, most often referring to food compounds that have been processed and/or concentrated into a pill, capsule, or powder, is now a $17 billion dollar industry in the US alone. Within the next ten years, as new food chemicals and compounds are discovered, the nutraceuticals market is expected to skyrocket to $80 billion. Fish oil gel caps and garlic capsules are examples.

## VITAMIN FAST FACTS

• It's estimated that 66% of cancer patients use alternative therapy and herbal medicine but usually only divulge they are doing so when directly questioned by their doctors.

• Mayo Clinic radiologists and biochemists at the University of Minnesota have developed a new way to image cancerous tumors using vitamin B12.

• The National Center for Complementary and Alternative Medicine, along with the NCI, are enrolling pancreatic cancer patients in a study involving pancreatic enzymes, coffee enemas, 160 vitamins a day, and a mostly vegetarian diet. The testing process is scheduled to be completed in three years, but so far the results are good.

# Vitamins, Minerals, & Herbs, cont.

cancer-inducing agent. The treated animals got 75 percent fewer tumors than control animals not given garlic. In other research, garlic against esophageal cancer. Garlic protects the heart, a bonus for cancer patients receiving chemotherapy, and enables the liver to detoxify cancer-causing chemicals before they can do damage. In one study, people who ate 2–3 cloves of garlic a day for 3 weeks showed significantly more activity in special white blood cells that fight tumors. In the test tube, these white blood cells killed more than twice as many tumor cells as white blood cells taken from people who didn't eat garlic. It is difficult to get enough of garlic's medicinal compounds through a daily diet, so taking a supplement is important. For more information on garlic, see page 122.

## HEY HONEY!

Bee pollen contains lipids, amino acids, carbohydrates, calcium, manganese, phosphorous, iron, sodium, potassium, aluminum, magnesium, copper, and vitamins B1, B2, B3, B6, C, D, and E, enzymes, pigments, beta-carotene and sterols. Bee pollen also has five times more protein than beef and is known for increasing stamina & strength. It is said to be nature's most perfect food. Bee pollen combats depression, allergies, colds, flu and colon disorders. Cancer patients experiencing fatigue may find that bee pollen gives them energy. Honey is used for treating wounds, ulcers, burns, sores, and skin lesions. It is an antimicrobial agent, inhibiting certain bacteria and healing skin wounds even when infected with antibiotic resistant germs. It's excellent in helping heal surgery incisions.

**Soy isoflavones** protect the heart, help prevent osteoporosis, and relieve menopausal symptoms. More importantly, soy isoflavones, genistein, and daidzein are the focus of many cancer research studies and are believed to be of benefit to people with skin, breast, colon, prostrate, endometrium, and ovarian cancers. Genistein has produced significant inhibition of adenocarcinoma cell maturation and differentiation, and was found to decrease lymphatic vessel invasion and intestinal adenocarcinoma in rats. In other studies, genistein has shown antiangiogenesis effects. Angiogenesis (new blood vessel growth) is a key factor in tumor growth, invasion, and metastasis. It is believed that cancer patients who carry a mutated form of the tumor suppressor p53 have increased benefits from soy supplementation. It's nearly impossible to get enough soy isoflavones through our diet, though, so for those of us with cancer, taking a soy supplement becomes especially important. See pages 123–124 for more information on soy.

IMPORTANT: Cancer patients should not take soy supplements if they are receiving radiation until their treatments are discontinued.

❦

**Red clover** is commonly used as a cough suppressant, an antibiotic, to heal skin problems, and for kidney problems, liver disease, and inflammation of the intestines. Although the isoflavone compounds found in red clover are being studied in experimental treatments for

## COMFORT FOR CHEMO

An Indian herbal formula called Amrit significantly reduces the instances of nausea, vomiting, diarrhea, insomnia, and anorexia in patients during chemotherapy and has improved their overall well-being by boosting energy levels. Amrit is an antioxidant containing 44 herbs and minerals, including large amounts of vitamins C, E, and beta-carotene. It is sold by Maharishi Aayurveda Products. Call (800) 255-8332 or go online at www.mapi.com. In addition, Researchers at the University of California, San Francisco, have begun several studies of traditional Chinese and Tibetan herbal therapies which they believe show promise in patients with breast cancer. The studies will test the Chinese herbs' ability to reduce chemotherapy side effects such as nausea, vomiting and fatigue and they will research whether or not the herbs enhance patients' immune systems.

different cancers, the important benefit to cancer patients who have had cancer treatments is that red clover is excellent at cleansing toxins from the body. It is best known as a blood purifier, expelling poisons from the bloodstream, and for cleansing, detoxifying, and improving the overall health of the liver and kidneys. Red clover increases the production of mucus and urine flow that helps relieve irritation and inflammation of the urinary tract and stimulates the production of digestive fluids and bile. It also relieves constipation and helps soothe inflammation of the bowel, stomach, and intestines is of utmost importance to cancer patients.

IMPORTANT: Do not use red clover if you have a history of stroke or heart disease, or if you are taking blood thinning agents.

✻

**Blue-green algae** (spirulina) provides the highest known nutrition from any single plant source known to man. It contains minerals, trace minerals, enzymes, vitamins, amino acids, proteins, iron, the rare essential fatty acid GLA, and beta-carotene, and is also one of the richest sources of chlorophyll that you can obtain. As one of the oldest living plants on the planet, spirulina has been used as a food source in some cultures for centuries.

Blue-green alga benefits cancer patients in releasing toxins from the body, providing energy to treatment-fatigued patients (it contains twice the vitamin B12 found in liver), and it is believed to enhance brain function. Since it is the best plant source of protein, the World Health Organization (WHO) has used it in its feeding programs for malnourished children in India. An article published in the *Journal of the American Nutraceutical Association* reported that researchers found that *Aph. flos-aquae* (blue-green algae) helped natural killer immune cells better perform their surveillance function. Natural killer cells are key players in the body's defense system patrolling the body, looking for transformed or infected cells. The National Cancer Institute has identified compounds in blue-green algae that are active against

HIV, the virus that causes AIDS. In addition, Massachusetts General Hospital, Harvard Medical School, McGill University, and The Royal Victoria Hospital are some of the institutions studying *Aph. flos-aquae*. Algae isn't entirely new to the American diet. The seaweed in sushi, for instance, is really just a macro-algae.

✻

**Zinc** is an important trace mineral second only to iron in its natural concentration in the body. It is required for the enzyme activities necessary for cell division, cell growth, and wound healing, and is probably involved in more bodily functions than any other mineral. As zinc becomes depleted in our soils, a dietary deficiency in zinc has become more common.

Zinc contributes more to a cancer patient than just its role in the immune system. In several studies, zinc taken before and after surgery reduced the incidence of postoperative complications and hastened the recovery time, cutting the patient's hospital stay. Zinc supplements are also known to reduce the incidence of pneumonia and diarrhea, detoxify chemicals and metabolic irritants from the body in general and the liver most importantly, prevent infections, reduce fatigue, and help with muscle weakness, all of which are major concerns for a cancer patient. Cancer patients become depleted in zinc due to stress, surgery, alcohol use, and weight loss. Zinc supplements are nontoxic. The therapeutic dose is 30–60 mg a day.

## WHAT'S YOUR DOCTOR GOING TO SAY?

...when you tell him you're taking 60 vitamins, minerals, herbs, and food concentrates a day? Most likely he'll ask why? Be prepared. Explain that you believe they will: 1. help protect your heart; 2. increase your immune system; 3. battle your cancer on a nutritional level; 4. help rid your body of toxins; and 5. assist with fatigue and other side effects. Hopefully, your doctor will: 1. encourage you; 2. tell you not to take megadoses of vitamins A, D, E and K; 3. ask you not to take supplements the day before, the day of, and the day after treatments; and 4. suggest other supplements that might help you. If your doctor panics it may be because he has had experience with snake oil salesmen peddling miracle cures and he is afraid that you will stop conventional treatments to take laetrile and shark cartilage. Reassure him!

## "CHEMO-BRAIN"

For years, cancer patients have complained about the lingering effects that chemotherapy had on their memories and ability to focus and concentrate. For years, doctors have dismissed this subtle problem by reassuring patients that the condition would soon "go away." In a study conducted at Dartmouth Medical School, doctors found that people who get standard chemotherapy appear to be twice as likely as other cancer patients to score poorly on various intelligence tests even 10 years after their treatment. This is no surprise to cancer survivors who can't remember yesterday, need to read a page twice to absorb what they've read, and use calculators to do simple math. While this is not good news, cancer patients are relieved that their doctors are finally taking seriously a complaint they have had all along.

# Vitamins, Minerals, & Herbs, cont.

**Astragalus** contains flavonoids, polysaccharides, trace minerals, and amino acids. It is a member of the legume, or bean, family and is used in China for symptoms such as wasting, diarrhea, fatigue, lack of appetite, colds, flu, arthritis, asthma, autoimmune diseases, and upper respiratory infections. In addition, Chinese hospitals use astragalus to help cancer patients recover from the immune system wipeout caused by chemotherapy. A study done at the University of Texas Medical Center in Houston showed that damaged immune cells from cancer patients were restored with astragalus extracts. Polysaccharides in astragalus help reestablish the white blood count in patients receiving chemotherapy and radiation. Astragalus has antiviral activity and is known to stimulate the body's natural production of interferon, increasing its activity and stimulating the immune system.

In test-tube studies astragalus enhanced the power of interleukin-2. In Chinese cancer patients, a formula containing astragalus made chemotherapy agents more potent but helped protect patients from their toxic side effects. A study at M.D. Anderson Cancer Center found that compounds taken from the astragalus root increased the function of T-cells, key fighters in the body's immune system. However, astragalus by itself is not a cancer cure. IMPORTANT: Do not take this herb prior to surgery, or with warfarin, diabetes drugs, phenobarbital, beta-blockers, or decongestants.

※

**Green tea extract** in capsule form is being studied on cancer patients by researchers at M.D. Anderson Cancer Center. According to Dr. Waun Ki Hong, chairman of the Department of Thoracic/Head and Neck Medical Oncology, "There is tremendous interest right now in using natural substances to treat and prevent disease. Green tea

has been shown to inhibit many kinds of cancer in laboratory and population-based studies in Japan, and since it appears to have very few side effects, it has tremendous potential for widespread use." Dr. Pisters, the principle investigator of the study, explained that the "dose-escalation" study will examine the safety of taking the equivalent of up to 10 cups or more of green tea a day. Another study conducted by Dorothy Morre and D. James Morre, researchers at Purdue University, found that EGCg, a compound in green tea, inhibits an enzyme required for cancer cell growth and

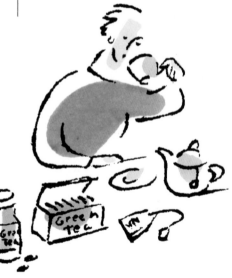

## Herbal fast facts

- Rosemary, ginger, sage, nutmeg, thyme, cumin, basil, cilantro, and black pepper boost the immune system, and have antioxidant and anticancer activity.
- The *Journal of the National Cancer Institute* reported that Italian researchers found that eating rosemary, basil, and parsley may reduce lung cancer risk.
- Feeding basil leaves and cumin seeds blocked liver cancer in animals.
- Researchers at Rutgers University, applying rosemary to the skin of mice, reduced the number of skin tumors by 64%.

## The starflower

Studies found that a substance called gamma linolenic acid (GLA) found in the starflower, or borage as it is more commonly known, can kill brain and prostate tumor cells. In addition, GLA also restricts blood vessel growth, thereby inhibiting the spread of malignant tumors and preventing cancer metastasis. In a study published in the *International Journal of Cancer*, women with breast cancer who were given 8 capsules of GLA a day along with the drug tamoxifen showed a faster clinical response to treatment. GLA has other benefits as well. It relieves inflammation, swelling, pressure in the joints, rheumatoid arthritis, water retention, and gout. It helps nerve transmission, reflexes, chronic fatigue syndrome, and increases the survival rates for patients with acute respiratory distress syndrome. GLA is very safe.

can kill cultured cancer cells with no ill effect on healthy cells. "Our research shows that green tea leaves are rich in this anticancer compound, with concentrations high enough to induce anticancer effects in the body," says Dorothy Morre. This is the first scientific evidence that explains exactly how green tea compounds work within a cell to ward off cancer. Studies show that even cigarette smokers who consumed green tea had a 45-percent lower risk of cancer than nontea drinkers. Green tea contains carotenoids, chlorophyll, polysaccharides, vitamins C and E, manganese, potassium, zinc, and polyphenols (see page 120), and is nontoxic.

**Milk thistle** is well known for its ability to protect the liver from chemical toxins and alcohol and is believed to assist the liver in the cleansing process, important for cancer patients undergoing treatments. In addition, milk thistle contains silymarin, a combination of chemicals called flavonolignans that seem to have a membrane-stabilizing activity preventing toxins from getting into the cells. Silybin has been tested in animals for its ability to protect the kidneys from damage due to chemotherapy drugs. Approximately two weeks after your last round of chemotherapy and/or radiation treatments, you may discontinue the use of milk thistle. It is assumed that the benefits of milk thistle in the detoxification process of the body will, by that time, be accomplished.

**Burdock** is a carrotlike root grown in China, Europe, and the United States and consumed as a vegetable in Japan. Burdock has been used for centuries as a remedy for throat infections, pneumonia, arthritis, and to prevent formation of gall and kidney stones. It is recommended to cancer patients by herbalists as nature's best "blood purifier" and is used to rid the body of dangerous toxins. It clears congestion in the respiratory, lymphatic, urinary, and circulatory systems. Burdock root promotes the flow of bile and eliminates excess fluid in the body. In addition, it stimulates elimination of toxic wastes in body tissues, relieves liver malfunctions, and improves digestion. Burdock is an effective diuretic and is considered a very safe herb and food product.

## PROSTATE HELP

A study conducted by Dr. Eric Small of the University of California, San Francisco Cancer Center, found that a regimen of PC-SPES, a combination of eight herbal supplements, significantly decreased the PSA levels in men who had prostate cancer. In Small's study, patients took nine capsules of the herbal supplement daily. All had a major drop in their PSA level, and in 80% the levels became undetectable. In patients with advanced prostate cancer, the results were not as dramatic, yet over half had a 50% drop in their PSA levels. Some patients had side effects, but, said Small, "by and large they're pretty mild." About 4% had blood clots, constipation, diarrhea, leg cramps, or fatigue. Other patients who complained of pain and other symptoms at the trial's start reported improvement. To learn more or to order, go online at:

**http://www.pc-spes.com**

## WHAT DO HIMALAYAN TREES AND SEA MOSS HAVE IN COMMON?

Scientist looking 6,000 feet high in the Himalayas and hundreds of feet deep in the oceans are finding chemicals that may allow them to make potent anticancer drugs. A marine organism extract called briostatin is now being combined with traditional chemotherapy drugs, resulting in additional anticancer activity. Moreover, the bark and leaves from rare trees with names like resount, herar, and texus baccata are being used and/or studied for their potential in becoming powerful cancer drugs.

## CALCIUM

Calcium supplements were found by researchers at Dartmouth-Hitchcock Medical Center to reduce the risk of recurrent colorectal polyps, the benign tumors that can lead to colon cancer, by 17%.

Researchers at Harvard University found that an excess of calcium may increase the risk of prostate cancer because it may reduce the levels of vitamin D. Vitamin D is known to protect the prostate.

# What Did You Learn *about* Supplements?

There is much to remember when you are deciding which vitamins you want to take, when, and why. I have on occasion added other supplements to my daily regimen, but the ones on the preceding pages I feel are most important. Take the test below.

Remember, knowledge is power! The supplements I have taken for years and now recommend to you are for the most part extremely safe for everyone except where I've indicated. ***There are 13 different vitamins essential to your health.***

### SCORING YOURSELF

The answers to these questions on supplements are on page 146. If you missed more than two or three of these questions, perhaps you should reread pages 134–141.

## TRUE OR FALSE

1. It is best not to take vitamins A, C, and E on the day before, the day of, and the day after treatments.

2. You should take vitamin A and beta-carotene every day.

3. Reputable news agencies discovered our government has concealed proven cancer cures and have dubbed the scandal the FDA "conspiracy theory."

4. You should take the antioxidant vitamin E because it's hard to get enough in your diet.

5. Whether you take a selenium supplement or eat 4 Brazil nuts a day, you should always take it with vitamin E.

6. Nutraceuticals are food products with vitamins, minerals, and antioxidants added.

7. You should take Co Q10 everyday but especially when receiving chemotherapy because it is known to protect the heart.

8. EPA oil, amrit, and astragalus help patient's handle chemotherapy's side effects.

9. Your memory and ability to focus and concentrate will come back immediately after chemotherapy stops.

10. Grapeseed extract has 20 times the antioxidant potency of vitamin C and 50 times the potency of vitamin E.

11. Bee pollen fights fatigue and putting honey on surgery incisions speeds healing.

12. Taking soy isoflavones supplements benefits cancer patients during radiation.

13. *Aph. flos-aquae* (blue-green algae) is the focus of much research in hospitals and universities and is considered rich in nutrients.

14. Zinc, taken before and after surgery, reduces the incidence of postoperative complications and speeds the recovery time.

15. GLA capsules should only be taken under doctor's orders.

16. If you take green tea extract in capsules you don't need to drink green tea.

17. You can stop taking milk thistle a few weeks after your treatments are completed.

18. If you decide to take a multivitamin instead of separate supplements, make certain that you get one that has the Recommended Daily Allowance.

# Getting Organized

One class of vitamins is known as water-soluble: vitamin C and the family of B vitamins. These are not stored in your body and must be replaced every day, either in your diet or as supplements. The fat-soluble vitamins, A, E, D, and K, are stored in your fatty tissues and liver. You should never take megadoses of fat-soluble vitamins since they could build up in your body and cause problems.

Watching the food you eat and making sure that you are consuming the healthiest ones possible should be part of your cancer-fighting regimen. In fact, you can get nearly everything you need if you consume nine servings of fruits and vegetables per day. Taking supplements, especially in large quantities, can get quite costly ($100–$300 per month) and, unfortunately, this cost is not covered by medical insurance. You should not feel guilty or anxious if you cannot or do not want to make this kind of investment. I would suggest at least a multivitamin high in antioxidants; however, you should discuss with your oncologist whether it should be taken when you are receiving chemotherapy.

## THE DIXIE CUP METHOD

For the last 6 years I have taken approximately 20 supplements with my meals to replenish my body with nutrients throughout the day. To make taking supplements convenient, I spend about a half an hour every two weeks organizing my 3 daily doses of supplements. Here's how I do it:

- Have your supplement chart and supplements handy.
- Take 42 dixie cups and place them 14 in a row (two weeks' worth), 3 cups deep (for breakfast, lunch, and dinner).
- Take the first supplement on your chart. If that supplement is checked for breakfast and dinner, place one supplement in all 14 breakfast cups. Then place one supplement in all 14 dinner cups.
- Continue through the list placing the appropriate supplement in the breakfast, lunch, and dinner cups.
- Make stacks of three, with the dinner cup on the bottom, lunch cup in the middle, and breakfast cup on top. Put the stacked cups in a safe, dry cabinet in your kitchen.
- Each day take one stack of breakfast, lunch, and dinner cups and put them in a location where you will remember to take them with each one of your meals.
- Repeat the process every two weeks.

**If you have numerous medications to take with meals every day, you may want to consider the dixie cup method with those as well.**

For a great vitamin sales catalog call Puritan's Pride (800) 645-1039 or
**ONLINE GO TO www.puritanspride.com**

---

I take Green Source Multi Vitamin & Minerals with Whole Food Concentrates from Puritan's Pride. One daily dose is three tablets, so I take one at breakfast, lunch, and dinner. Look for this form of vitamin in your health food store.

- Vitamin A 15,000 I.U.
- Vitamin C 1,000 mg
- Vitamin D 400 I.U.
- Vitamin E 250 I.U.
- Thiamine (B1) 25 mg
- Riboflavin (B2) 25 mg
- Niacin 25 mg
- Vitamin B6 25 mg
- Folic Acid 400 mcg
- Vitamin B12 25 mcg
- Biotin 50 mcg
- Pantothenic acid 25 mg
- Calcium 250 mg
- Iodine 150 mcg
- Magnesium 125 mg
- Zinc 15 mg

- Selenium 25 mcg
- Copper 0.5 mg
- Manganese 4 mg
- Chromium 100 mcg
- Molybdenum 50 mcg
- Potassium 50 mg
- Boron 1 mg
- Choline bitartrate 50mg
- Inositol 25 mg
- PABA 25 mg
- Citrus bioflavonoids complex (prange) 100 mg
- Quercetin 25 mg
- Rutin 25 mg
- Hesperidin 10 mg
- Bromelain (pineapple 2000 GDU/gm) 20 mg

- Betaine hydrochloride (beets) 20 mg
- Papain (papaya) 20 mg
- Amylase 5 mg
- Lipase 5 mg
- Protease 1.0 mg
- Cellulase 2.5 mg
- Proprietary lactobacillus blend 25 mg
- Oat bran 25 mg
- Pectin (apple) 25 mg
- RNA 35 mg
- DNA 10 mg
- Carotenoids 10 mg
- Chlorophyll 4 mg
- Vegetable oil (borage and sunflower) 100 mg

- L-Glutathione 5 mg
- Spirulina 1,000 mg
- Wheat grass juice (dry) 100 mg
- Sprouted barley juice (dry) 100 mg
- Flaxseed oil (dry) 100 mg
- Chlorella 100 mg
- Bee pollen 100 mg
- Siberian ginseng 50 mg
- Dehydrated garlic 10 mg
- Proprietary herbal blend 60 mg
- Echinacea
- Milk thistle goldenseal ginger
- Ginkgo biloba extract cayenne pepper

# Your Daily Supplements Chart

| SUPPLEMENTS | BREAKFAST | LUNCH | DINNER |
|---|:---:|:---:|:---:|
| **Multivitamin:** (a daily dose is three tablets a day) | ☐ | ☐ | ☐ |
| **Beta-carotene:** 15 mg. (25,000 I.U.) soft gels | ☐ | ☐ | ☐ |
| **Vitamin C:** 500 mg | ☐ | ☐ | ☐ |
| **Vitamin E:** emulsified, 200 I.U.; take with selenium | ☐ | ☐ | ☐ |
| **Selenium:** 50 mcg | ☐ | ☐ | ☐ |
| **Co Q10:** 50–100 mg | ☐ | ☐ | ☐ |
| **EPA fish oil concentrate:** 1,000 mg soft gels | ☐ | ☐ | ☐ |
| **Grapeseed or pycnogenol:** 50–100 mg | ☐ | ☐ | ☐ |
| **Garlic:** 1,000–5,000 mg | ☐ | ☐ | ☐ |
| **Soy isoflavones:** 750 mg capsules | ☐ | ☐ | ☐ |
| **Red clover** | ☐ | ☐ | ☐ |
| **Blue-green algae:** 1,500 mg (1 dose is 3 capsules) | ☐ | ☐ | ☐ |
| **Zinc:** 15 mg | ☐ | ☐ | ☐ |
| **Astragalus:** 1,000 mg | ☐ | ☐ | ☐ |
| **Green tea extract:** 1,000 mg | ☐ | ☐ | ☐ |
| **Milk thistle (silymarin):** 1,000 mg soft gels | ☐ | ☐ | ☐ |
| **Burdock root:** 425 mg capsules | ☐ | ☐ | ☐ |

# Shopping List for Supplements

One of our largest expenses has been my vitamins and supplements bill. I was spending about twice what I do now when I first started but with experience and some research, I have found good-quality supplements at affordable prices. Do some investigating on your own. Check your phone book for discount vitamin stores, search your newspaper for sales at your health food stores, or look into the discount vitamin sites online (see Chapter 7, page 205). Keep track of where you buy each supplement, the product number, and price below. When you find a great sale, stock up!

| SUPPLEMENTS | STORE | PRODUCT # | COST |
|---|---|---|---|
| High antioxidant: | | | |
| Multivitamin: | | | |
| Beta-carotene: 15 mg (25,000 I.U.) soft gels | | | |
| Vitamin C: 500 mg | | | |
| Vitamin E: emulsified, 200 I.U. | | | |
| Selenium: 50 mcg | | | |
| Co Q10: 50–100 mg | | | |
| EPA fish oil concentrate: 1,000 mg soft gels | | | |
| Grapeseed or pycnogenol: 50–100 mg | | | |
| Garlic: 1,000 –5,000 mg | | | |
| Soy isoflavones: 750 mg capsules | | | |
| Red clover | | | |
| Blue-green algae: 1,500 mg | | | |
| Zinc: 15 mg | | | |
| Astragalus: 1,000 mg | | | |
| Green tea extract: 1,000 mg | | | |
| Milk thistle (silymarin): 1,000 mg soft gels | | | |
| Burdock root: 425 mg capsules | | | |
| Other: | | | |
| Other: | | | |
| Other: | | | |
| Other: | | | |
| Other: | | | |

# The Importance of Hope

In June, 1998 five brave breast cancer survivors and seven young healthy women joined forces in an expedition to climb Alaska's Mt. McKinley in an expedition known as the Climb Against the Odds. The goal; to raise funds for research, education, and support and to promote the awareness of women's 1 in 8 odds of getting breast cancer. In June of 1998, I faced, if such things are measurable, the most despondent moment of my treatments. I thought of my dear friend MaryAnn Castemore, a breast cancer survivor, a mountain climber, one of the 12 women struggling against the odds. I and countless other cancer patients can think of

*Recognizing the determination and courage that these brave women possessed strengthened me that day and gave me hope.*

no greater gift than the one these women have offered. A beautiful and inspiring one-hour documentary on the climb has been produced by the Breast Cancer Fund and Michelson–Carlson Productions.

Climb Against the Odds has appeared on public television stations throughout the country, at film festivals, and significant fun raisers. Major label artists have donated their songs for an accompanying benefit soundtrack. The CD is extraordinary. You may order the home video and CD at:

**www.breastcancerfund.org/climb.html.**

*All proceeds go to
The Breast Cancer Fund.*

## ANSWERS TO NUTRITION TEST, P. 133

1. False: A nutritionist is not generally licensed.
2. True
3. True
4. False: It is an example of free radical damage.
5. False: A minimum of five (preferably nine) servings a day are recommended.
6. False: Compounds found in phytochemicals actually inhibit cancer cell division.
7. False: "phyto"= plant
8. True
9. True
10. True
11. True
12. False: Sometimes they have more nutrients.
13. True
14. False: Omega-3 oil reduces some cancers by 50 percent and protects against heart disease.
15. True
16. True
17. False: Fruits are the energizes and cleansers, and vegetables are the body builders.
18. True
19. False: Doctors receive only an average of 2.5 hours.
20. True

## ANSWERS TO SUPPLEMENTS TEST, P. 142

1. True
2. False: beta-carotene is all you need to take.
3. False: There is no evidence the government is aware of a cancer cure and is keeping it secret.
4. True
5. True
6. False: Nutraceuticals are food compounds that have been processed and/or concentrated into a pill, capsule, or powder.
7. True
8. True
9. False, the problem may last for years.
10. True
11. True
12. False: large amounts of isoflavones in cancer cells may protect them against radiation.
13. True
14. True.
15. False: it is completely safe to take.
16. False: Supplements are never a replacement for a fresh food source. You should take both.
17. True
18. False: If you got this question wrong, go back and read the entire chapter.

## JUST FOR THE FUN OF IT

- A can of SPAM is opened every 4 seconds.
- Cranberry Jell-0 is the only kind that contains real fruit.
- Lemons contain more sugar than strawberries.
- The largest pumpkin weighed 377 lbs.
- Because of Animal Crackers, many kids until they reach the age of ten, believe a bear is as tall as a giraffe.
- Milk is heavier than cream.
- The left leg of a chicken is more tender than the right one.
- There are more than 15,000 different kind of rice.
- A-1 Steak Sauce contains both orange peels and raisins.
- There are more 25,000 McDonald's restaurants in over 115 countries.
- Apples are more effective at keeping people awake in the morning than caffeine
- Cabbage is 91 percent water.
- The McDonalds at the SkyDome in Toronto, Ontario is the only one in the world that sells hot dogs.
- Japan is the largest exporter of frog's legs.

- Every time you lick a stamp you consume $\frac{1}{10}$ of a calorie.
- George Washington Carver invented peanut butter.
- There are professional tea tasters as well as wine tasters.
- After eating too much, your hearing is less sharp.
- If you ate too many carrots you would turn orange.
- America's best selling ice-cream flavor is vanilla.
- As many as 50 gallons of maple sap are needed to make a single gallon of maple sugar.
- The avocado has the most calories of any fruit.
- A hard-boiled egg will spin. An uncooked or soft-boiled egg will not.
- The state of California raises the most turkeys out of all of the states.
- The largest cabbage weighed 144 lbs.
- Burger King uses approximately $\frac{1}{2}$ million pounds of bacon every month in its restaurants.

- The most common noncontagious disease in the world is tooth decay.
- The first Lifesaver flavor was peppermint.
- Chocolate contains the same chemical, phenylethylamine, that your brain produces when you fall in love.
- One-tenth of the 7 million tons of rice grown in the US each year goes into the making of beer.
- The green stuff on the occasional freak potato chip is chlorophyll.
- A person swallows approximately 295 times while eating dinner.
- Americans eat 18 billion hot dogs a year.
- In a normal lifetime an average American will eat 10,000 pounds of meat and 200 pounds of peanuts.
- Five Jell-O flavors that flopped: celery, coffee, cola, apple, and chocolate.
- Broccoli is a vegetable with a nervous system. Primitive though it may be, it CAN feel pain.
- Cranberries are sorted for ripeness by bouncing them; a fully ripened cranberry can be dribbled like a basketball.

If you haven't already done so, take the test on pages 116–117 to see in what areas you can make changes to your diet. Also, take the tests on pages 133 and 142 to see how much you have learned.

**STOP**

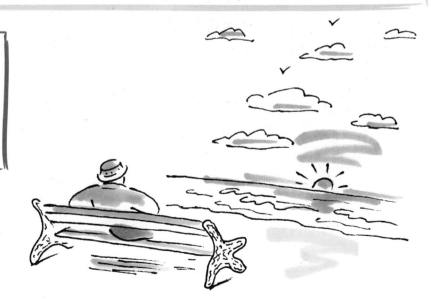

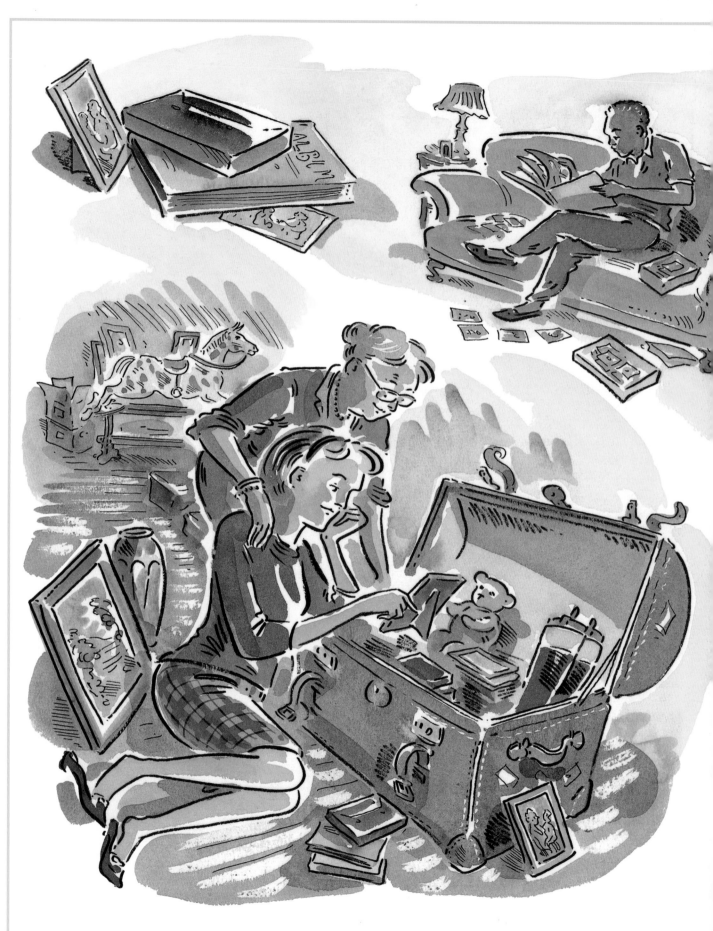

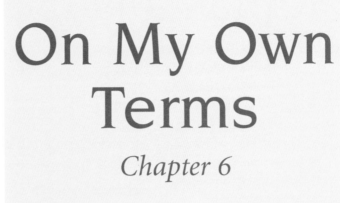

# On My Own Terms

*Chapter 6*

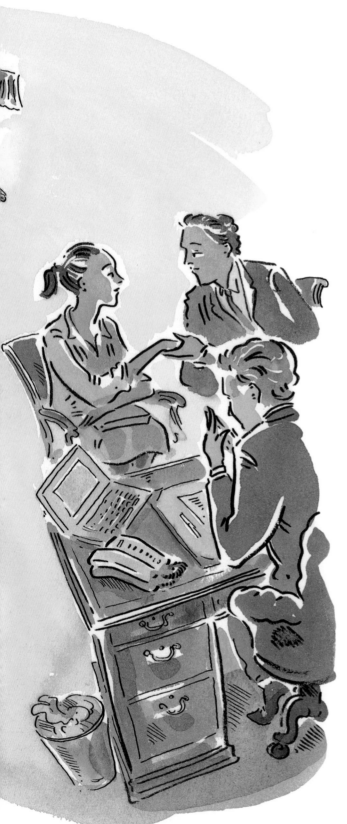

# Preplanning Is Not Giving Up

It is no small wonder that I have procrastinated in writing this chapter. I have found death is a difficult topic to broach with almost anyone, especially a cancer patient. I've faced the prospect of dying twice, and as painful as that may be, it is part and parcel of this disease. Everyone, regardless of one's health, should have all final plans in order. Having cancer merely underscores the importance of preplanning all of your arrangements. I believe that there is a need in each of us to play a role in every aspect of our lives, including the end of it. Designing our funeral service can be the most special gift to our family and friends, whenever that day may come.

## *Someone has survived every type of cancer, at every stage.*

The majority of people who get cancer will not die from it. Over 60 percent of patients diagnosed with cancer are cured and the percentage increases yearly. However, the day you hear "You have cancer" will be the same day you think: "Am I going to die?" Regardless of the prognosis, whether it is excellent, good, fair, or poor, those of us with cancer will forevermore live in a fragile kingdom of speculation concerning our health. We long for answers to such questions as "Is a lasting cure possible?"..."What are my chances?"... "How much time do I have left?" The burden of this disease compels us to look to doctors for solutions that they do not always have, and the uncertainty of our future leaves us feeling vulnerable and exposed.

*While there is no up side to cancer, all of the cancer survivors that I have spoken with have said how precious their life has become since they have had to confront the aspect of their own death.*

Mortality is a reality for all of us, those with and without cancer. It is my hope that you recognize that by reading and completing this chapter you are not closing the door on fighting and living, but rather that you are putting to rest some of the apprehension concerning the details of death. I personally have no intention of giving up my struggle and letting go. However, when it's my time to die, I want my ceremony to be a reflection of who I am, to impart a message to those I love. In addition, I do not want my family to be burdened by hard decisions at a time when they are dealing with their grief.

The objective of your memorial service is to bequeath to your family and friends a genuine insight of your life, the many people you touched and treasured, your beliefs, your values, and what you would want your legacy to be. You should not hesitate to request specific poetry, scripture, music, and speakers for your service. There are many distinct styles and special messages. What is it you want? You may find it helpful to discuss your plans with a loved one and/or spouse.

IMPORTANT: THIS CHAPTER WILL CONTAIN VERY PERSONAL INFORMATION ABOUT YOUR RECORDS, YOUR WISHES, AND THE LOCATION OF IMPORTANT DOCUMENTS. ON COMPLETING THIS SECTION, YOU MIGHT WANT TO REMOVE THE PAGES FROM THE WORKBOOK FOR SAFEKEEPING, OR PHOTOCOPY AN EXTRA SET.

## COMPLETE THIS CHAPTER

- As promptly as you feasibly can.
- When you're feeling fairly good physically.
- On a day when you are thinking positively about your future.

**Keep in mind:**
- The objective is to provide organized information for your family.
- Everyone, yourself included, should preplan his or her funeral needs regardless of health.
- Completing this chapter has nothing to do with the outcome of your disease.
- You are not "giving up" by preplanning.

**When you have finished:**
- Remove the pages from the workbook or photocopy an extra set.
- Place in an envelope marked "In the event of my death."
- Put the issue of your funeral service, "whenever that day comes," to rest.

Use this chapter to guide and assist you in the basic decisions. This workbook is not meant to be a substitute for your local funeral home, nor are the documents in this chapter meant to replace legal documents. The funeral home of your choice can help you with all of your preplanning. Most offer funeral ceremonies from simple to elaborate and, needless to say, the prices reflect that. There is a flat fee for cremation or the preparation of the body for burial, filing the death certificates, and putting the obituaries in the newspapers. The funeral costs vary depending on the merchandise and services requested.

I outlined and experimented with this chapter as a trial run before I went to M.D. Anderson for my lung resection. I cannot tell you the tranquility I experienced knowing my last wishes would be carried out in the event of my death. The details of what I desired and how I wanted my funeral service to be performed were of upmost importance to me. Recording my wishes did not mean I no longer thought about dying, it was just that I thought of it less. Completing this section will alleviate some of the unknowns and help you find a measure of peace.

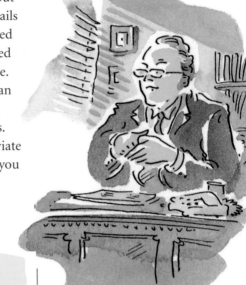

## PREARRANGING AND PREFUNDING A FUNERAL CAN GO HAND-IN-HAND

**Funeral homes are flexible in both prearranging and prefunding.**

### What you want in a funeral home

- Make certain that the company is well established.
- Phone several funeral homes and request their price list for services and merchandise and compare before choosing a funeral home.
- If visiting a funeral home will make you uncomfortable, find a company that sends a representative to your home.
- Investigate the different payment options that are offered.

### Questions about prefunding

- Do I get my money back if the funeral home goes out of business?
- Is my prepayment transferred if the funeral home is sold?
- In the event that I move is the prefunding plan transferable?
- If I decide that I do not want the funeral home's services, may I get a refund in part or in full?
- Is there interest on my prepaid account?
- Who pays the taxes on that interest?

*"It ain't over 'til it's over."*

*– Yogi Berra*

### Services of funeral directors

- Meet with you and your family to discuss arrangement options.
- Help you choose the place, type, and time for the visitation, service, and other details.
- Help you select a casket, outer burial container, urn, memorial stone, marker, and/or other items.
- Assist in decisions about pallbearers, flowers, pictures/easels, and music.
- Provide acknowledgment cards and memorial record book.
- Transport the deceased person's body to the funeral home.

- Prepare, embalm, and cosmetically restore the deceased.
- Obtain information for the death certificate.
- File and get necessary copies of the death certificate.
- Assist with the necessary paperwork, including obituary notices and a variety of government benefit claim forms.
- Help you notify the deceased person's employer, attorney, insurance companies, and banks.
- Arrange for limousines.
- Arrange for gravesite services.

## MEMORIAL DOVES

Memorial dove releases are an inspirational, peaceful tribute to our departed loved one as well as a beautiful gift to family and friends that want a special way of expressing their good-byes. This ceremony can be performed at the end of a church service or at the location of the deceased's final resting place during internment. This is popular in many areas and your funeral director will know of companies in your region that offer this service. Significant prayers, music, or poems can precede the dove release, making it a unique memory for all those present.

# In the Event of My Death

After completing the following pages, you may prefer to remove them from this workbook entirely. Otherwise, photocopy them, put the copy in an envelope marked "In the event of my death," and give the envelope to your personal representative for safe-keeping. Your personal representative is the person or persons (if more than one) that you have chosen to oversee the details of your services.

**After careful consideration I have chosen:**

_____

and/or_____

_____

as my personal representative to oversee the details of my funeral services. If he/she is unable to perform these duties at this time, my alternate representative is

_____

_____

Date: _____

Dearest _____

I am leaving the following instructions for you so that you will know my final wishes.

_____

_____

_____

_____

_____

_____

_____

_____

_____

_____

_____

_____

_____

_____

**In the event of my death please contact:**

Doctor: _____

Phone #: _____

Funeral director: _____

Phone #: _____

Pastor: _____

Phone #: _____

Please ask when the clergy person's schedule would permit the service to be held. Hold the service when the greatest number of my family members and friends can be present. Keep in mind that you will need to allow sufficient time for family and friends to arrive from out of town.

Please call my immediate family members first – parents, grandparents, children, and siblings. In addition, please notify the following friends, my attorney, and the executor of my estate.

**Immediate family and relatives:**

Name: _____

Phone #: _____

Name: _____

Phone #: _____

Name: _____

Phone #: _____

Name: _____

Phone #: _____

Name: _____

Phone #: _____

Name: _____

Phone #: _____

Name: _____

Phone #: _____

**Also notify these following people:**

Attorney: _____

Phone #: _____

Address: _____

Executor of my estate: _____

Phone #: _____

Address: _____

## LOCATION OF ALL IMPORTANT DOCUMENTS

**Record the location of all your important documents:**

- Birth certificate: _____
- Marriage certificate: _____
- Citizenship papers: _____
- Divorce/separation papers: _____
- Adoption papers: _____
- Social Security number/card: _____
- Passport: _____
- Driver's license: _____
- Military records: _____
- Medicare numbers: _____
- Medicaid numbers: _____
- Living will: _____
- Power-of-attorney: _____
- Bank accounts: _____
- IRAs/Roths/Keoghs: _____
- Stocks & bonds: _____
- Life insurance policies: _____
- Deeds: _____
- Car titles: _____
- Boat titles: _____
- Retirement & pension information: _____
- IOUs: _____
- Mortgages: _____
- Credit card numbers: _____
- Debts: _____
- Will: _____
- Organ donor card: _____
- Tax records: _____
- Other: _____
_____
_____
_____

## ESTATE DETAILS

Getting organized can give you a sense of control and a feeling of accomplishment. Most of us have important papers tucked away in every corner of our home. Now is the perfect time to locate all your documents and put them in one central location or note where they are. Take advantage of a "down time" and Just Do It!

*Safety deposit box:*    *yes* ☐    *no* ☐

*Name of bank:* _____

*Number:* _____

*Location of key:* _____

## VIDEO PHOTO ALBUM

Memorial videos are a beautiful keepsake and are being used frequently in funeral services to highlight a loved one's life. Using state-of-the-art software, the photographs you have selected are scanned into a computer. Then they are retouched, fixing color, spots, and creases. Music, graphics, and transitions are added to the photographic montage, creating a flowing, powerful presentation. Many companies provide this service, at an approximate cost of $200 to $400. You can find these companies either by searching the internet using the key words "Memorial Video" or by looking in your local yellow pages for "Video Production Services"; make sure the company you choose specializes in keepsake videos.

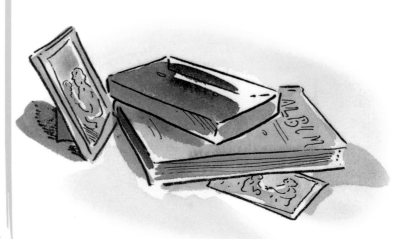

# Obituary Information

## NOTIFY THE FOLLOWING NEWSPAPERS

**For my obituary:**

Newspaper: _____

Phone #: _____

Address: _____

_____

Newspaper: _____

Phone #: _____

Address: _____

_____

Newspaper: _____

Phone #: _____

Address: _____

_____

### A FAMILY AFFAIR

Donating your body to medical science is a decision that needs to be discussed with the whole family. If anyone in your family is not comfortable with it, then don't consider the option. If it is something you want to do, discuss it with your doctor. Medical schools, research facilities, and other agencies need to study bodies to gain knowledge of how the disease of cancer functions. The research does much toward saving and improving lives. Regardless of your decision, your family will still be asked to sign a consent form for the arrangements to be finalized.

- ☐ I DO NOT want to donate my body.
- ☐ I DO want to donate my body.

**Special instructions:**

_____

_____

*"People are like stained-glass windows. They sparkle and shine when the sun is out, but when the darkness sets in, their true beauty is revealed only if there is light is from within."*

*– Elizabeth Kubler Ross*

## PERSONAL INFORMATION

**For obituary and memorial folder**

First: _____ Middle _____

Last: _____ Nickname _____

Maiden name: _____

Place of marriage: _____

Date of birth: _____

Place of birth: _____

Present residency: _____

Marital status: _____

Spouse's name: _____

Date of marriage: _____ Years married: _____

Mother's name: _____

Living? _____ Place of birth: _____

Present residency: _____

Father's name: _____

Living? _____ Place of birth: _____

Present residency: _____

Name of sibling: _____

Place of birth: _____

Name of sibling: _____

Place of birth: _____

Other relatives: _____

_____

_____

_____

_____

_____

_____

_____

_____

_____

_____

_____

_____

_____

_____

_____

_____

_____

_____

Number of children:_____

Name of child:_____

Present residency: _____

_____

Name of child:_____

Present residency: _____

_____

Name of child:_____

Present residency: _____

_____

Name of child:_____

Present residency: _____

_____

Name of child:_____

Present residency: _____

_____

Number of grandchildren:_____

Name of grandchild:_____ Age:_____

Name of grandchild:_____ Age:_____

Name of grandchild:_____ Age:_____

Name of grandchild:_____ Age:_____

Social, religious, community, and private institutions to which you now belong or have belonged in the past.

_____

_____

_____

_____

_____

Employment:_____

_____

Years employed: _____

Names and addresses of present and former employers:

_____

_____

_____

_____

Education:
High school:_____

College: _____

Degrees or honors received:

_____

_____

_____

Were you ever in the Armed Forces?   Yes ☐       No ☐

Branch of service:_____

Date and place of enlistment:_____

Rank:_____

Commendations received: _____

Date of military discharge: _____

Flag desired to drape casket?        Yes ☐       No ☐

Additional information to be included in the obituary:

_____

_____

_____

_____

_____

_____

_____

_____

_____

# Memorial Service

The funeral home will be able to provide as many copies of the death certificate as are requested for a small fee. Make certain your family, attorney, or executor has enough certificates for all the insurance companies, income tax records, investment companies, and pension funds.

My estate/family will need _____ copies of my death certificate.

*"What lies behind us and lies before us are small matters compared to what lies within us."*

*– Ralph Waldo Emerson*

## GIFTS FOR OTHERS TO TREASURE

- Make voice tapes to bequeath to those you love.
- Sign milestone birthday, anniversary, graduation cards etcetera for celebrations in upcoming years.
- Write letters to your grandchildren (born & unborn).
- Make a photo album for each member of the family.
- Record what you know about your family history.
- Purchase gifts to be given to your loved ones for special future occasions: an engraved watch, a locket with a picture in it, a monogrammed briefcase, your portrait. Have foresight and make the gift very personal.
- Make a video of yourself speaking to your family.
- Create a scrapbook centered around yourself.
- Write an autobiography.

## MEMORIAL INSTRUCTIONS

Name of funeral home: _____

Phone #: _____

Funeral director: _____

Phone #: _____

Name and location of cemetery: _____

Phone #: _____

Cemetery representative: _____

Plot/niche number: _____

Deed or title #: _____

Marker/headstone:   Yes ☐   No ☐

To be inscribed:

Name: _____

Dates: _____

Inscription:

_____

_____

_____

_____

_____

_____

**Type of service desired:** Body burial Yes ☐   No ☐

Type of casket:

Wood casket

Pine ☐   Pecan ☐   Mahogany ☐   Oak ☐

Maple ☐   Cherry ☐   Poplar ☐   Walnut ☐

Metal casket

Bronze ☐   Copper ☐   Steel ☐

It would honor me if the following persons would consider being my pallbearers:

_____

_____

_____

| | Yes | No |
|---|---|---|
| I prefer cremation: | ☐ | ☐ |
| I have selected my casket/urn: | ☐ | ☐ |
| Cremation burial: | ☐ | ☐ |
| Vault preferred: | ☐ | ☐ |
| I have selected a vault: | ☐ | ☐ |
| I would like a graveside service or a service of committal of the ashes after my funeral service | ☐ | ☐ |

Family's choice: _____

## THE FUNERAL SERVICE

**My funeral services are to be held at:**

Funeral home: _____

Address: _____

_____

Place of worship: _____

Address: _____

_____

Clergyperson or person to officiate: _____

I would like viewing/visitation
of the body.          Yes ☐        No ☐

I would like my urn
displayed at my service.   Yes ☐        No ☐

My wishes are that the body is to
remain in the church overnight,
with opportunity for friends and
family to keep a vigil.     Yes ☐        No ☐

It would honor me if _____ would preach at my ceremony.

I would also be honored to have these people participate in my service, either by delivering eulogies, reading lessons, or playing particular music selections:

_____

_____

_____

_____

_____

_____

_____

_____

_____

_____

*Do not stand at my grave and weep;*
*I am not there, I do not sleep.*
*I am a thousand winds that blow.*
*I am the diamond glints on snow.*
*I am the sunlight on ripened grain.*
*I am the gentle autumn rain.*
*When you awaken in*
*the morning's hush*
*I am the swift uplifting rush*
*Of quiet birds in circled flight.*
*I am the soft stars that shine at night.*
*Do not stand at my grave and cry;*
*I am not there, I did not die.*

*Anonymous*

## IN LIEU OF FLOWERS

In lieu of flowers, I have chosen this foundation to receive gifts in my name and memory.

Name of charity: _____

Phone #: _____

NEARLY ALL OF US FIND COMFORT KNOWING THERE IS A DESIGNATED SANCTUARY TO CALL UPON WHEN THERE IS A NEED BY FAMILY MEMBERS TO REMEMBER AND EXPERIENCE INTIMACY WITH THE PERSON THEY HAVE LOST. CONSULT YOUR FAMILY TO CHOOSE ONE THAT WILL BEST FIT THEIR EMOTIONAL NEEDS. THE FUNERAL DIRECTOR WILL SUGGEST MANY OPTIONS FOR YOU TO CONSIDER.

# Scriptures & Other Sayings

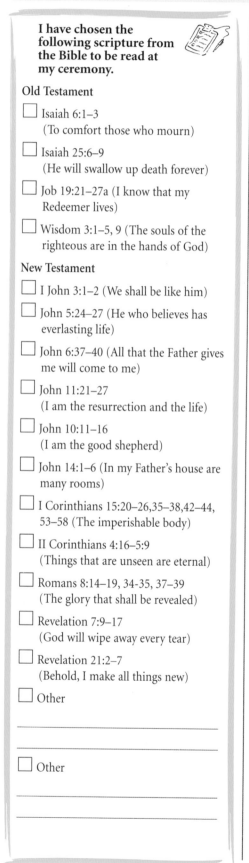

**I have chosen the following scripture from the Bible to be read at my ceremony.**

## Old Testament

☐ Isaiah 6:1–3
  (To comfort those who mourn)

☐ Isaiah 25:6–9
  (He will swallow up death forever)

☐ Job 19:21–27a (I know that my Redeemer lives)

☐ Wisdom 3:1–5, 9 (The souls of the righteous are in the hands of God)

## New Testament

☐ I John 3:1–2 (We shall be like him)

☐ John 5:24–27 (He who believes has everlasting life)

☐ John 6:37–40 (All that the Father gives me will come to me)

☐ John 11:21–27
  (I am the resurrection and the life)

☐ John 10:11–16
  (I am the good shepherd)

☐ John 14:1–6 (In my Father's house are many rooms)

☐ I Corinthians 15:20–26,35–38,42–44, 53–58 (The imperishable body)

☐ II Corinthians 4:16–5:9
  (Things that are unseen are eternal)

☐ Romans 8:14–19, 34-35, 37–39
  (The glory that shall be revealed)

☐ Revelation 7:9–17
  (God will wipe away every tear)

☐ Revelation 21:2–7
  (Behold, I make all things new)

☐ Other

_____

_____

☐ Other

_____

_____

## The Mourner's Kaddish

Let the Glory of God be exalted, let God's great name be hallowed in the world whose creation God willed. May God's rule soon prevail, in our own day, our own lives, and the life of all Israel, and let us say: Amen

Let God's great name be blessed for ever and ever.

Let the name of the Holy One, blessed is God, be glorified, exalted, and honored, though God is beyond all the praises, songs and adorations that are uttered in this world, and let us say: Amen.

May there be abundant peace from heaven, and life for us and all Israel, and let us say: Amen.

May the one who makes peace in the high heavens, make peace descend on us and upon all Israel, and let us say: Amen.

## Job 19:25–27a (I know that my Redeemer lives)

I know that my Redeemer lives, and that in the end he will stand upon the earth And after my skin has been destroyed, yet in my flesh I will see God; I myself will see him with my own eyes – I, and not another. How my heart yearns within me!

## Revelation 21:2–7 (Behold, I make all things new)

I saw the Holy City, the new Jerusalem, coming down out of heaven from God, prepared as a bride beautifully dressed for her husband. And I heard a loud voice from the throne saying, "Now the dwelling of God is with men, and he will live with them. They will be his people, and God himself will be with them and be their God. He will wipe every tear from their eyes. There will be no more death or mourning or crying or pain, for the old order of things has passed away." He who was seated on the throne said, "I am making everything new!" Then he said, "Write this down, for these words are trustworthy and true." He said to me: "It is done. I am the Alpha and the Omega, the Beginning and the End. To him who is thirsty I will give to drink without cost from the spring of the water of life. He who overcomes will inherit all this, and I will be his God and he will be my son."

## II Corinthians 4:16–18 (Things that are unseen are eternal)

Therefore we do not lose heart. Though outwardly we are wasting away, yet inwardly we are being renewed day by day. For our light and momentary troubles are achieving for us an eternal glory that far outweighs them all. So we fix our eyes not on what is seen, but on what is unseen. For what is seen is temporary, but what is unseen is eternal.

Life is a stage in time and death is a stage in time, like, for example, winter and spring. We do not suppose that winter becomes spring, or say that spring becomes summer.

He who knows not and knows that he knows is a fool. Shun him. He who knows not and knows that he knows not is ignorant. Teach him. He who knows and knows not that he knows is asleep. Wake him. He who knows and knows that he knows is a wise man. Seek him.

Anonymous

The lotus has its roots in the mud,
Grows up through the deep water,
And rises to the surface.
It blooms into perfect beauty and purity in the sunlight.
It is like the mind unfolding to perfect joy and wisdom.

### John 5:24–27 (He who believes has everlasting life)

"I tell you the truth, whoever hears my word and believes him who sent me has eternal life and will not be condemned; he has crossed over from death to life. I tell you the truth, a time is coming and has now come when the dead will hear the voice of the Son of God and those who hear will live. For as the Father has life in himself, so he has granted the Son to have life in himself. And he has given him authority to judge because he is the Son of Man."

Follow the coherence in your heart, beware of anything towards which it feels despondent, and disregard what it declines to concur with.
`Abdullah bin Mas`oud

It ended...
With his body changed to light,
A star that burns forever in that sky.
Aztec

**Treat the earth well:**

it was not given to you by your parents,
it was loaned to you by your children.
We do not inherit the Earth from our Ancestors, we borrow it from our Children.

Hatred never ceases by hatred;
But love alone is healed.
This is an ancient and eternal law.

You have noticed that everything that an Indian does is in a circle, and that is because the Power of the World always works in circles, and everything tries to be round....The Sky is round, and I have heard that the earth is round like a ball, and so are all the stars. The wind, in its greatest power, whirls. Birds make their nest in circles, for theirs is the same religion as ours....Even the seasons form a great circle in their changing, and always come back again to where they were. The life of a man is a circle from childhood to childhood, and so it is in everything where power moves.

Black Elk – Oglala

# Music

## HYMNS/MUSIC
### THAT HAVE MEANING FOR ME

**I would appreciate it if they could be incorporated at my service.**

_____
_____
_____
_____

**Special instruction to the choirmaster or worship leader:**

_____
_____
_____
_____
_____
_____

Ave Maria

Because He Lives

Coming Home

Every Hour

Face To Face

God Bless America

God Will Take Care of You

Great Is Thy Faithfulness

He Touched Me

Hero

How Great Thou Art

Holy, Holy, Holy

In the Garden

In the Sweet By and By

I Surrender All

Let There Be Peace On Earth

My Heart Will Go On

Nearer My God to Thee

On Eagle's Wings

O God, Our Help in Ages Past

O, How I Love Jesus

Rock of Ages

Rise Again

Shall We Gather at the River

Softly and Tenderly

Some Where

Stairway to Heaven

There Is a Balm in Gilead

The Lord Is My Shepherd

The Lord's Prayer

The Old Rugged Cross

There's Something About That Name

Turn Your Eyes Upon Jesus

Through It All

Until Then

What a Friend We Have in Jesus

Wind Beneath My Wings

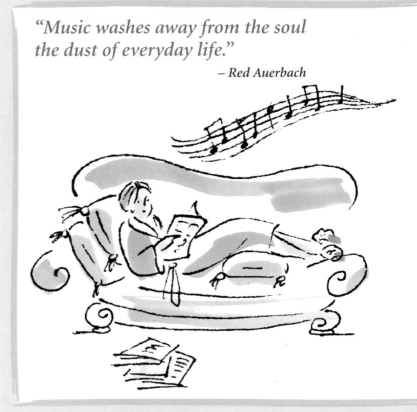

_"Music washes away from the soul the dust of everyday life."_

– Red Auerbach

**Danny Boy**

Oh Danny boy, the pipes, the pipes are calling
From glen to glen, and down the mountain side
The summer's gone, and all the flowers are dying
'Tis you, 'tis you must go and I must bide.
But come ye back when summer's in the meadow
Or when the valley's hushed and white with snow
'Tis I'll be here in sunshine or in shadow
Oh Danny boy, oh Danny boy, I love you so.

**I'll Fly Away**

Some glad morning when this life is o'er, I'll fly away;
To a home on God's celestial shore, I'll fly away.
I'll fly away, O glory, I'll fly away;
When I die, Hallelujah, by and by, I'll fly away.
When the shadows of this life is gone, I'll fly away;
Like a bird from prison bars have flown, I'll fly away.
I'll fly away, O glory, I'll fly away;
When I die, Hallelujah, by and by, I'll fly away.

### Open My Eyes that I May See

Open my eyes, that I may see
glimpses of truth thou hast for me;
place in my hands the wonderful key
that shall unclasp and set me free.
Silently now I wait for thee,
ready, my God, thy will to see.
Open my eyes, illumine me, Spirit divine!

### Morning Has Broken

Morning has broken like the first morning
Blackbird has spoken like the first bird
Praise for the singing Praise for the morning
Praise for them springing fresh from the world
Sweet the rain's new fall
Sunlit from heaven
Like the first dew fall on the first glass
Praise for the sweetness of the wet garden
Sprung in completeness where His feet pass
Mine in the sunlight Mine is the morning
Born of the one light Eden saw play
Praise with elation Praise every morning
God's recreation of the new day

### Just a Closer Walk with Thee

I am weak, but Thou art strong;
Jesus, keep me from all wrong;
I'll be satisfied as long
As I walk, let me walk close to Thee.
Refrain
Just a closer walk with Thee,
Grant it, Jesus, is my plea,
Daily walking close to Thee,
Let it be, dear Lord, let it be.

### Will the Circle Be Unbroken?

I was standing by my window on a cold and cloudy day
When I saw the hearse come rolling for to carry my mother away
Will the circle be unbroken by and by, Lord, by and by?

There's a better home a-waiting in the sky, Lord, in the sky
Lord, I told that undertaker "Undertaker, please drive slow
For this body you're a-hauling, Lord, I hate to see her go."
Will the circle be unbroken by and by, Lord, by and by?

There's a better home a-waiting in the sky, Lord, in the sky
I followed close behind her, tried to hold up and be brave
But I could not hide my sorrow when they laid her in the grave
Will the circle be unbroken by and by, Lord, by and by?

There's a better home a-waiting in the sky, Lord, in the sky
Went back home, Lord, my home was lonesome,
'cause my mother, she was gone
All my brothers, sisters cryin', what a home, so sad and lone
Will the circle be unbroken by and by, Lord, by and by?

There's a better home a-waiting in the sky, Lord, in the sky
One by one the seats were emptied, one by one, they went away
Now that family, they are parted; will they meet again someday?
Will the circle be unbroken by and by, Lord, by and by?

There's a better home a-waiting in the sky, Lord, in the sky
I was singing with my sisters, I was singing with my friends
And we all can sing together, 'cause the circle never ends
Will the circle be unbroken by and by, Lord, by and by?

There's a better home a-waiting in the sky, Lord, in the sky
I was born down in the valley where the sun refused to shine
But I'm climbing up to the highland, gonna make that mountain mine!

### It Is Well with My Soul

When peace, like a river, attendeth my way,
When sorrows like sea billows roll;
Whatever my lot, Thou has taught me to say,
It is well, it is well, with my soul.

### Amazing Grace

Amazing Grace
how sweet the sound
that saved a wretch like me
I once was lost but now am found,
was blind but now I see

### Precious Lord, Take my Hand

Precious Lord, take my hand.
Lead me on, let me stand.
I am tired, I am weak, and worn.
Through the storm, through the night,
Lead me on to the light.
Take my hand, precious Lord,
Lead me home.

# Memorial Folders

**M**emorial folders may be used as a remembrance of the deceased and may be the only keepsake that some friends will have to treasure. The folders are handed out to the family and friends at the time of the service and/or visitation. Not only do the folders serve the purpose of celebrating the life of the departed love one, they can also include information about the remaining family members, the service itself, and the final resting place of the deceased.

Many people want to design their own memorial folders, while others would prefer their families to take care of it when it is necessary. It is completely up to you; there is no right or wrong way. Regardless of who designs the folder, keep in mind that its primary purpose is to honor and represent the deceased.

## MEMORIAL RECORD BOOKS

Memorial record books are displayed at your service to register guests attending the service. They also record personal information about the departed love one and archive details about the funeral service.

### PRAYER CARDS

Prayer cards may be made available at the time of the service as a memento of the deceased. On one side of the card is the name, dates, and picture of the deceased as well as a prayer or poem. On the reverse side is a religious, nature, or secular image.

### BOOKMARKS

These are similar to the prayer cards and are generally laminated.

Memorial folders can come in all sizes and styles. Some are very simple while others are quite elaborate. Memorial folders can include photographs, poems, scripture, collages, and detailed information regarding the life of the deceased. Done with thought and care, the memorial folder can be one of the most significant elements of a funeral service and a personal tribute to honor the life of the departed loved one.

Need help? If you have a computer you may want to purchase the National Management Software's Memorial Folder Program. This easy-to-use program makes designing your memorial folder a snap. The software offers backgrounds, clip art, verses, and poetry. All you do is type in the vital information. Select the type of card or folder you want and print it. Prayer card, acknowledgment, clergy records, and register book designs are also provided. You don't have to lay out the designs yourself, it is done for you. In addition, there is a library of fonts, styles, and beautiful clip art, as well as a collection of religious and poetic verses!

**ONLINE GO TO HYPERLINK**
**http://www.nmsoftware.com/mfp.htm**

## SUGGESTIONS FOR DESIGNING YOUR OWN MEMORIAL FOLDER

**Front cover:**

A picture of the deceased or one of great significance to that person

Commencement line

**Left inside page:**

A collage of pictures

Personal memories, stories or antidotes from the grandchildren, children, spouses and/or friends

Prayer

Poem

Song

Artwork or religious illustration

Agenda/program of the service

Invitation to join the family for a reception after the service

"In lieu of flowers" announcement

**Back cover:**

Personal story or anecdote

Summary of the person's life

List of accomplishments

**Right inside page:**

The name of the deceased

The dates of birth and death

The spouse's name

The children's names

The grandchildren's names

The siblings' names

The date, time, and place of the service

The officiating clergy

Scripture reading and music selections

Reception place and time

The place of internment

## EXAMPLE

### I'm Free

Don't grieve for me, for now I'm free

I'm following the path God laid for me.

I took his hand when I heard him call

I turned my back and left it all.

I could not stay another day.

To laugh, to love, to work or play.

Tasks left undone must stay that way,

I found that peace at close of day.

If my parting has left a void,

Then fill it with remembered joy.

A friendship shared, a laugh, a kiss,

Ah yes, these things I too will miss.

Be not burdened with times of sorrow,

I wish you sunshine of tomorrow.

My life's been full, I've savored much,

Good friends, good times,

a loved one's touch.

Perhaps my time seemed all too brief;

Don't lengthen it now with undue grief.

Lift up your hearts and share with me,

God wanted me now;

He set me free.

### In Loving Memory

*Your name*

*Dates*

**Loving Husband/Wife of**

*Spouse's name*

*Father/Mother of*

*Names of children*

*Brother/Sister of*

*Names of siblings*

**Grandmother/Grandfather of**

*Names of grandchildren*

**Service**

*Date*

*Time*

*Place*

*Officiating clergy*

*Pastor/Reverend/Priest*

*Reception will be held at:*

*Time/place*

**Internment**

*Cemetery*

*City, State*

## YOUR MEMORIAL FOLDER

Using your own ideas or the ones provided on these pages, state what you would like on each page of your memorial folder. The folder will be 4.25" wide by 5.5" long when folded. Include this layout and any pictures you want used in your envelope marked "In the event of my death."

## HOSPICE CARE

With the issuance of the Hospice Care stamp, the Postal Service continues its tradition of raising public awareness of social causes. Hospice is a holistic, team-oriented care program that seeks to treat and comfort terminally ill patients and their families, at home or in a homelike setting. The first American hospice is believed to have been established in 1974 in New Haven, CT. Now more than 2,600 operational or planned hospice programs exist in all 50 states and Puerto Rico. The stamp was designed by veteran stamp designer Phil Jordan to symbolize life's journey to its final stage, the stage where hospice lends its vision for end-of-life care.

**Hospice offers a program of comfort, care and supportive care provided by a team of professional and volunteers. Hospice services include:**

- Medical and nursing care
- Personal care
- Homemaker services
- Social works services
- Grief and other counseling services
- Volunteer assistance
- Spiritual care
- Case management
- Family training in patient's care

# Poems

We thought of you with love today,
But that is nothing new.
We thought about yesterday,
And days before that too.
We think of you in silence,
We often speak your name;
All we have now are memories,
And your picture in a frame.
Your memory is our keepsake,
With which we will never part;
GOD has you in his keep,
We have you in our heart.
It broke our heart to lose you.
But you didn't go alone,
For a part of us went with you...
The day GOD took you home.

*Author Unknown*

The Lord is my shepherd;
I shall not want.
He maketh me to lie down
in green pastures;
He leadeth me beside the still waters.
He restoreth my soul;
He leadeth me in the paths of
righteousness for his name's sake.
Yea, though I walk through the
valley of the shadow of death,
I will fear no evil:
for thou art with me;
Thy rod and thy staff
they comfort me
Thou preparest a table before me in
the presence of mine enemies.
Thou anointest my head with oil;
my cup runneth over.
Surely goodness and mercy shall
follow me all the days of my life.
And I will dwell in the house of the
Lord forever.

*King David (c. 950 BC)*
*Bible, Psalm 23*

### Miss Me But Let Me Go

When I come to the end of the road
And the sun has set for me
I want no rites in a gloom filled room
Why cry for a soul set free?

Miss me a little – but not to long
And not with your head bowed low
Remember the love that we once shared
Miss me – but let me go.

For this is a journey that we all must take
And each must go alone
It's all a part of the master's plan
A step on the road to home.

When you are lonely and sick at heart
Go to the friends we know
And bury your sorrows -
in doing good deeds
Miss me – but let me go.          *Unknown*

I have selected a poem, essay, or memoir that I would like read at my ceremony.

It would honor me if

_____ {person}

would read this selection.

_____
_____
_____

It's often said that life is strange. But compared to what?

*Steve Forbert*

Your candle
burned out long before
Your legend ever did.

*Elton John*
*"Candle In the Wind"*

Because I could not stop for Death,
He kindly stopped for me;
The Carriage held
but just Ourselves
And Immortality.

*Emily Dickinson*

I am ready to meet my Maker. Whether my Maker is prepared for the great ordeal of meeting me is another matter.
**Winston Churchill**

### Remembering…

Go ahead and mention my child,
The one that died you know.
Don't worry about hurting me further.
The depth of my pain doesn't show.
Don't worry about making me cry,
I'm already crying inside.
Help me to heal by releasing
the tears that I try to hide.
I'm hurt when you just keep silent,
PRETENDING he didn't exist.
I'd rather you mention my child,
knowing that he has been missed.
You asked me how I was doing?
I say "pretty good" or "fine."
but healing is something ongoing.
I know it will take a lifetime.

*Elizabeth Dent*

Someday when we meet up yonder
We'll stroll hand and hand again
In a land that knows no parting
Blue eyes crying in the rain.

*Willie Nelson*

If we have been pleased with life, we should not be displeased with death, since it comes from the hand of the same master.

*Michelangelo*

What the caterpillar calls the end of the world, the master calls a butterfly.

*Richard Bach*

To laugh often and much, to win the respect of intelligent people and the affection of children, to earn the appreciation of honest critics and endure the betrayal of false friends, to appreciate beauty, to find the best in others, to leave the world a bit better, whether by a healthy child, a garden patch, or a redeemed social condition; to know even one life has breathed easier because you have lived.
This is to have succeeded!

*Ralph Waldo Emerson*

It's the heart afraid of dying, that never learns to dance; It's the dream afraid of waking, that never takes the chance; It's the one who won't be taken, who cannot seem to give; And the soul afraid of dying, that never learns to live.

*Bette Midler*
*The Rose*

If we could have a lifetime wish
A dream that would come true,
We'd pray to God with all our hearts
For yesterday and You.
A thousand words can't bring you back
We know because we've tried...
Neither will a thousand tears
We know because we've cried...
You left behind our broken hearts
And happy memories too...
But we never wanted memories
We only wanted You.

*Unknown*

**Come To Me**
God saw you getting tired, and a cure was not to be, so he put his arms around you and whispered, "Come to me."
With tearful eyes we watched you, and saw you pass away, and although we loved you dearly, we could not make you stay. A golden heart stopped beating, hard working hands at rest. God broke our hearts to prove to us, he only takes the best.

*Unknown*

**If Tears Could Build A Stairway**

If tears could build a stairway and memories were a lane,
I would walk right up to heaven to bring you home again.
No farewell words were spoken, no time to say goodbye,
You were gone before I knew it, and only God knows why.
My heart still aches in sadness and secret tears still flow,
What it meant to lose you – no one will ever know.

*Unknown*

# Financial Information

You will not want to record your personal financial information in *The Cancer Patient's Workbook* just in case you lose or misplace your workbook. Instead, you should photocopy these two pages, fill in the information on the copies, and include the completed sheets in the envelope you have marked "In the event of my death."

*"When you were born, you cried and the world rejoiced. Live your life in a manner so that when you die the world cries and you rejoice."*

— *Native American Proverb*

## INSURANCE INFORMATION

Life insurance companies require a death certificate.

**Life insurance policy list**

Company: _____

Policy #: _____

Location: _____

Agent: _____

Phone #: _____

Primary beneficiary: _____

Amount: _____

**Accident and health insurance:**

Company" _____

Policy #: _____

Location: _____

Agent: _____

Phone #: _____

Primary beneficiary: _____

Amount: _____

## PROPERTY INSURANCE LIST

Company: _____

Policy #: _____

Location: _____

Agent: _____

Phone #: _____

Primary beneficiary: _____

Amount: _____

Company: _____

Policy #: _____

Location: _____

Agent: _____

Phone #: _____

Primary beneficiary: _____

Amount: _____

## CREDIT CARDS TO BE CANCELLED

Credit card: _____

Account #: _____

Phone #: _____

Credit card: _____

Account #: _____

Phone #: _____

Credit card: _____

Account #: _____

Phone #: _____

Credit card: _____

Account #: _____

Phone #: _____

Credit card: _____

Account #: _____

Phone #: _____

## BANK ACCOUNTS TO BE CANCELLED

Bank: _____

Account #: _____

Type of account: _____

Phone #: _____

Bank: _____

Account #: _____

Type of account: _____

Phone #: _____

Bank: _____

Account #: _____

Type of account: _____

Phone #: _____

Bank: _____

Account #: _____

Type of account: _____

Phone #: _____

Bank: _____

Account #: _____

Type of account: _____

Phone #: _____

## INVESTMENT INFORMATION

Investment: _____

Account #: _____

Agent: _____

Phone #: _____

Investment: _____

Account #: _____

Agent: _____

Phone #: _____

Investment: _____

Account #: _____

Agent: _____

Phone #: _____

Investment: _____

Account #: _____

Agent: _____

Phone #: _____

Investment: _____

Account #: _____

Agent: _____

Phone #: _____

# Legal Stuff

Everyone should give serious thought to their healthcare preferences, patient's rights, and Last Will and Testament. Health and medical issues are a sensitive topic and many points must be taken into consideration, such as the wishes of the patient, the families' feelings, and protection from liability. At the same time, the need to provide the best possible medical care under the circumstances should not be overlooked.

You should make clear your wishes to guide the decisions of others if necessary. There may come a time when you are incapacitated and it is important that your healthcare professionals and family members are not trying to "second guess" what they think you would prefer.

Provided on the next several pages are examples of documents that may assist you. While these documents are legal in most states, they may not be certified in yours. If they are not approved in your state, your doctor or lawyer will be able to provide the acceptable papers.

Make your choices very carefully. It is important to choose family members that you can trust to make sound judgments under pressure. I advise you to discuss your decisions with your family so that there are no hurt feelings at a later date.

The Quicken® Family Lawyer® offers a complete selection of personalized document possibilities to address your unique circumstances. It includes documents covering wills, trusts and estate planning, health care directives, government forms, medicare issues, and much more. It is state-specific and very easy to use. The program costs about $30 and is in most stores that carry software. If you would like to obtain more information or order it

**ONLINE GO TO:**
**http://www.shopmattel.com/product.asp?OID=4140365**

## DIRECTIVE TO PHYSICIANS

Directive made this _____ day of _____, 20_____

I, _____, being of sound mind, willfully and voluntarily make known my desire that my life shall not be artificially prolonged pursuant to the following:

1. If the time comes when I can no longer take part in decisions for my own future, this statement and declaration shall stand as the expression of my wishes. I recognize that death is as much a reality as birth, growth, maturity, and old age – it is but a phase in the cycle of life and is the only certainty. I do not fear death as much as I fear the indignity of deterioration, dependence, and hopeless pain. If there is no reasonable expectation of my recovery from physical or mental disability, I wish to be allowed to die and not be kept alive by artificial means or heroic measures, but wish only that drugs be mercifully administered to me for terminal suffering, even if they hasten the moment of my death.

2. I recognize that my wishes place a heavy burden of responsibility upon you, and I therefore make the following declaration with the intention of sharing this responsibility and the decision with you and of mitigating any feelings of guilt that you may have:

   **DECLARATION**

3. If at any time I should have an incurable injury, disease, or illness certified to be a terminal condition by my physician, and where the application of life-sustaining procedures would serve only to artificially prolong the moment of my death and where any physician determines that my death is imminent whether or not life-sustaining procedures are utilized, I direct that such procedures be withheld or withdrawn, and that I be permitted to die naturally.

4. In the absence of my ability to give directions regarding the use of such life-sustaining procedures, it is my intention that this directive shall be honored by my family and physician as the final expression of my legal right to refuse medical or surgical treatment and accept the consequences from such refusal.

5. I have been diagnosed and notified at least 14 days ago as having a terminal condition by Dr. _____, whose address is _____.

6. I understand the full import of this directive and I am emotionally and mentally competent to make this direction.

Signature _____ Date _____      Witness _____ Date _____

Witness _____ Date _____

### Physician's Directive and Uniform Living Will

These documents direct your doctors not to take extraordinary medical steps to prolong your life if you are suffering from a terminal illness from which you are unlikely to recover. They are similar documents; ask your doctor and lawyer which one is accepted in your state, or whether there is a specific state form that you should use.

## UNIFORM LIVING WILL

To my family, my physician, my lawyer, my clergyman. To any medical facility in whose care I happen to be. To any individual who may become responsible for my health, welfare or affairs. Death is as much a reality as birth, growth, maturity, and old age – it is the one certainty of life. If the time comes when I, _____, can no longer take part in decisions of my own future, let this statement stand as an expression of my wishes while I am still of sound mind. If the situation should arise in which I am in terminal state and there is no reasonable expectation of my recovery, I direct that I be allowed to die a natural death and that my life not be prolonged by extraordinary measures. I do, however, ask that medication be mercifully administered to me to alleviate suffering even though this may shorten my remaining life.

This statement is made after careful consideration and is in accordance with my strong convictions and beliefs. I want the wishes and directions here expressed carried out to the extent permitted by law. Insofar as they are not legally enforceable, I hope that those to whom this will is addressed will regard themselves as morally bound by these provisions. If it is permissible under the laws of the jurisdiction in which I may be hospitalized, I direct that the physicians supervising my care upon a terminal diagnosis to discontinue hydration (water) should the continuation of hydration be judged to result in unduly prolonging a natural death. If it is permissible under the laws of the jurisdiction in which I may be hospitalized, I direct that the physicians supervising my care upon a terminal diagnosis to discontinue feeding should the continuation of hydration be judged to result in unduly prolonging a natural death. I herewith release any and all hospitals, physicians, and others both for myself and for my estate from any and all liability for complying with this declaration, to the fullest extent provided by law. I herewith authorize my spouse, if any, or any relative who is related to me within the third degree to effectuate my transfer from any hospital or other healthcare facility in which I may be receiving care should that facility decline or refuse to effectuate the instructions given herein.

Signed: _____        City of residence _____

Print name: _____        County of residence _____

Witness_____        State of residence: _____

Witness_____

This day personally appeared before me, the undersigned authority, a Notary Public in and for _____ County, _____ State, (Witnesses) who, being first being duly sworn, say that they are the subscribing witnesses to the declaration of _____, the declarant, signed, sealed and published and declared the same as and for his/her declaration, in the presence of both these affiants; and that these affiants, at the request of said declarant, in the presence of each other, and in the presence of said declarant, all present at the same time, signed their names as attesting witnesses to said declaration.

Affiants further say that this affidavit is made at the request of _____, declarant, and in his/her presence, and that _____ at the time the declaration was executed, in the opinion of the affiants, was of sound mind and memory, and over the age of eighteen years.

Taken, subscribed and sworn to before me by _____(witness) and _____ (witness) this _____day of_____, 200 _____.

My commission expires:_____

_____
Notary Public

# Power of Attorney

**General Power of Attorney**

This document authorizes a designated person very broad and extensive powers, including:

- Paying bills
- Handling banking transactions
- Exercising stock rights
- Entering safety deposit boxes
- Entering into contracts

- Handling transactions involving US securities
- Settling claims
- Purchasing life insurance
- Buying, managing, or selling real estate & properties
- Filing tax returns
- Handling government related benefits
- Maintaining business interests

## GENERAL POWER OF ATTORNEY

TO ALL PERSONS, be it known, that I _____ of _____, _____ the undersigned principal, do hereby grant a general power of attorney to _____ of _____ _____ as my attorney-in-fact.

My attorney-in-fact shall have full powers and authority to do and undertake all acts on my behalf that I could do personally including but not limited to the right to sell, deed, buy, trade, lease, mortgage, assign, rent or dispose of any of, my future real or personal property; the right to execute, accept, undertake, and perform all contracts in my name; the right to deposit, endorse, or withdraw funds to or from any of my bank accounts, depositories or safe deposit box; the right to borrow, lend, invest or reinvest funds on any terms; the right to initiate, defend, commence or settle legal actions on my behalf; the right to vote (in person or by proxy) any shares or beneficial interest in any entity; and the right to retain any accountant, attorney, physician or other advisor deemed necessary to protect my interests generally or relative to any foregoing unlimited power.

My attorney-in-fact hereby accepts this appointment subject to its terms and agrees to act and perform in said fiduciary capacity consistent with my best interests as in my attorney's best discretion deems advisable, and I affirm and ratify all acts undertaken.

This power of attorney may be revoked by me at any time, and shall automatically be revoked upon my death, provided any person relying on this power of attorney before or after my death shall have full rights to accept the authority of my attorney-in-fact until in receipt of actual notice of revocation.

This General Power of Attorney shall be governed by the laws of the State of _____.

Signed under seal this _____ day of _____, 200 _____.

STATE OF _____ COUNTY OF _____

On_____ , 20 _____ before me, _____, personally appeared _____ , personally known to me (or proved to me on the basis of satisfactory evidence) to be the person (s) whose name (s) is/are subscribed to the within instrument and acknowledged to me that he/she/they executed the same in his/her/their authorized capacity/capacities, and that by his/her/their signature (s) on the instrument the person (s), or the entity upon behalf of which the person (s) acted, executed the instrument.

WITNESS my hand and official seal.

Signature _____

Affiant_____ Known _____ Produced ID

Type of ID _____

(Seal)

## Medical Power of Attorney

If you feel strongly about avoiding prolonged and expensive medical care in hopeless situations, you may also wish to utilize a Medical Power of Attorney. A Medical Power of Attorney is a document by which you appoint another trusted person (usually a spouse or a child) to act on your behalf in the event you are unable to act for yourself, with regard to the hard decisions that must be made if you are terminally ill.

### MEDICAL POWER OF ATTORNEY

KNOW ALL MEN BY THESE PRESENT THAT I, _____

OF _____ hereby CONSENT and APPOINT_____ as my true and lawful attorney- in-fact, for me and in my name to give medical authorization should I be incapacitated and not able to give same myself, and to bind me thereby in as full and ample a matter as I myself could do, where I personally authorized and signed the same.

I HEREBY AUTHORIZE my said attorney-in-fact to affix my seal to all and every kind of instrument which he/she may think in any way necessary or proper, hereby ratifying and confirming whatever my said attorney-in-fact may do with regard to the foregoing power conferred to him/her.

This POWER OF ATTORNEY shall be in full force and effect from _____ to _____

_____

(Signature)

SIGNED, SEALED, AND DELIVERED IN THE PRESENCE OF:

_____

_____

### WHERE THERE'S A WILL, THERE'S A WAY

Seven out of ten people do not have a will in place at the time of their death. The last will and testament is a document that expresses your wishes as to how you want your property distibuted after your death. If you do not provide a will, the state in which you live will decide how to distribute your property. Because legal wills vary greatly from state to state, a will has not been included in the *Cancer Patient's Workbook*. However, you can purchase a legal will for your home state at your local office supply store. If you have a large estate or special considerations, it is best to retain a lawyer to draft your will.

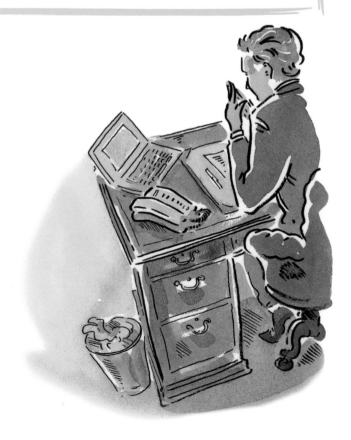

# Treasures & Trash

The definition of treasure is "wealth or riches, stored or accumulated. To regard or treat as precious." Treasures are objects that hold great personal value. We are often astonished to find that our most prized possessions are the small things around our home. The items that remind us of the fun times, family traditions, people we love, or fond memories. The Christmas tree ornament given to you by your favorite aunt, a knickknack you purchased while on a vacation, baseball cards you loved as a boy. Treasures are the gifts made by our children when they were young, the handed-down fishing equipment, old letters and photographs, jewelry, and books.

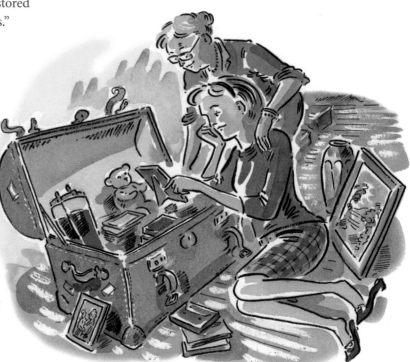

*The familiar possessions that we use and favor around our homes are the belongings that our loved ones will always associate with us.*

For instance, my mother had a huge brandy snifter that she had covered with colored pieces of glass and used as a candle holder. The snifter sat on top of her TV and was lit every night. Before my mom passed away she gave the candleholder to me and it now resides on top of my TV, my most prized possession. My father had a folding yardstick that I played with for endless hours when I was a child. He carried it in his back pocket everywhere he went, measuring everything he could find. I can still picture him with that tape measure, which now resides in the top drawer in my kitchen. No longer an object, but a connection for me to the man who once held it.

Take a walk around your home. Look carefully at those things you possess that hold special meaning to you and are therefore significant to others as well.

*Carefully match those small cherished possessions with whom in your life it would hold the most meaning.*

Record here on these pages what the item is, where you got it, why you love it, and the person you want to have it when you have gone. Let a trusted family member or friend know that this record exists. Do not include items of great monetary value – this is for the little things.

**The gift:** *The old Bible from my mother's family.*

**Location:** *The shelving unit next to the TV in my bedroom. It's fragile and needs to be kept in a dry place.*

**Where it came from:** *It was passed down to my mom when when her father died. There is information inside the Bible but it is so delicate I'm afraid to open it and look. The Bible is well over 100 years old and valuable.*

**What it means to me:** *I've had this Bible for years and when I became a Christian it took on a very special meaning. I have few things that belonged to my parents and this is one of my favorites.*

**Who I'd like to have it and why:** *Mark, I want you to have this Bible because you love things that are old and unusual and you've always been curious about it. I know you will treasure it and make certain it is passed down for generations to come.*

The gift:_____

_____

Location:_____

_____

Where it came from:_____

_____

_____

_____

What it means to me:_____

_____

_____

_____

_____

Who I'd like to have it and why:_____

_____

_____

_____

_____


The gift:_____

_____

Location:_____

_____

Where it came from:_____

_____

_____

_____

What it means to me:_____

_____

_____

_____

_____

Who I'd like to have it and why:_____

_____

_____

_____

_____


The gift:_____

_____

Location:_____

_____

Where it came from:_____

_____

_____

_____

What it means to me:_____

_____

_____

_____

_____

Who I'd like to have it and why:_____

_____

_____

_____

_____


The gift:_____

_____

Location:_____

_____

Where it came from:_____

_____

_____

_____

What it means to me:_____

_____

_____

_____

_____

Who I'd like to have it and why:_____

_____

_____

_____

_____

# Treasures & Trash, cont.

The gift:_____

_____

Location:_____

_____

Where it came from:_____

_____

_____

What it means to me:_____

_____

_____

_____

Who I'd like to have it and why:_____

_____

_____

_____

_____


The gift:_____

_____

Location:_____

_____

Where it came from:_____

_____

_____

What it means to me:_____

_____

_____

_____

Who I'd like to have it and why:_____

_____

_____

_____

_____


The gift:_____

_____

Location:_____

_____

Where it came from:_____

_____

_____

What it means to me:_____

_____

_____

_____

Who I'd like to have it and why:_____

_____

_____

_____

_____


The gift:_____

_____

Location:_____

_____

Where it came from:_____

_____

_____

What it means to me:_____

_____

_____

_____

Who I'd like to have it and why:_____

_____

_____

_____

_____

The gift:_____

_____

Location:_____

Where it came from:_____

_____

_____

What it means to me:_____

_____

_____

_____

Who I'd like to have it and why:_____

_____

_____

_____

_____


The gift:_____

_____

Location:_____

Where it came from:_____

_____

_____

What it means to me:_____

_____

_____

_____

Who I'd like to have it and why:_____

_____

_____

_____

_____


The gift:_____

_____

Location:_____

Where it came from:_____

_____

_____

What it means to me:_____

_____

_____

Who I'd like to have it and why:_____

_____

_____

_____


The gift:_____

_____

Location:_____

Where it came from:_____

_____

_____

What it means to me:_____

_____

_____

Who I'd like to have it and why:_____

_____

_____

_____

# Matters of the Heart

A journal is a book, notebook, or any collection of written thoughts in which one writes about events in more detail, especially and including feelings, opinions, beliefs, hopes, fears, reflections, etcetera. According to new research, the simple act of writing down thoughts and feelings regarding stressful events can improve the health of persons with chronic conditions.

*Research has demonstrated that writing about emotionally traumatic experiences has surprisingly beneficial effects.*

A team of scientists reported in the *Journal of American Medical Association* that a group of asthma and arthritis patients who for several days wrote down their feelings about a stressful event, showed significant improvement in their conditions during a four-month study. In another investigation, researchers found direct physiological evidence: writing increased the level of disease-fighting lymphocytes circulating in the bloodstream. And in yet another study, patients who acknowledged and expressed their anger over their disease achieved a perspective to their ill health that allowed them to cope better. In these and a growing number of studies, it is not simply mind over matter but it is clear that mind matters. The bottom line: standard medical treatment is enhanced with the effective management of emotional distress.

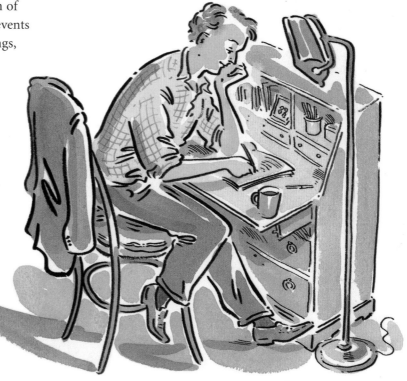

---

Get your thoughts, your anger, and your fear down on paper! It's healthy. Doing so will release the power your emotions hold over you and free you from being consumed by them. In addition, keeping a journal will help you find and heal forgotten pain, detect subconscious feelings and enhance your life by giving you the means to discover the hidden gift that every crisis brings.

Not everyone is comfortable with self-disclosure. Keeping that in mind, I have proved many suggestions to get you started. Pick out a diary or blank notebook; a looseleaf version would allow you to add photocopied pages from this section of the *Cancer Patient's Workbook*.

*In These Days – A Journal* offers suggestions for you to elaborate on these topics, to release anger, to cry out on paper, and/or to journal your innermost thoughts.
*It's All About Me* gives you opportunities to answer simple short questions such as: What's your favorite song? Who is the best actor that ever lived? Who would you pick as the greatest President? What brings you peace?
*Brief Reflections* lets you stretch out a bit, giving you more opportunity to be creative and introspective.
*Memories, Musing and Messages* furnishes you with a structured format to recall your past and express your feelings to those you love.
The personal account of your life's experiences, your wisdom, your regrets, your judgements, your memories and your confessions are the bottom line of who you are. And that, my fellow cancer patient, is worth writing about.

# In These Days – A Journal

*The biggest mistake I have ever made was in not writing down my impressions and thoughts during my battle with cancer. There is a heightened, surreal awareness and intensity of emotions for people who are dealing with the reality of being a cancer patient. Every thought is deeply felt, running the gamut from anger to sadness to childlike hope. The cancer patient's mind is held captive by what he or she feels are earth-shattering revelations, fears, visions, confessions, confirmations, speculations, and meditations.*

*In hindsight, I realize the importance of such a blunder. As a cancer survivor who frequently counsels newly diagnosed patients, I often reflect on how useful the written feelings and thoughts of five years ago would be to me today. How invaluable it would be if I could look back on the reminders of what those days and nights were like. How encouraging to myself and others to recall what I was going through at the time and how far I have managed to come.*

*Significant as that might have been however, the value to me personally would have been the knowledge that much of what I thought and felt would continue to live on in my written words. The assurance and peace of mind, knowing that one day my loved ones could contemplate them, that they might perceive the depth of me, possess a sense of me, and often remember me. Lost for always are the secret reflections of my heart. Gone, too, are the private thoughts of hopes and fears. Vanished forever are my perceptions of what my daily life entailed. Erased by time are the memories of my spiritual rebirth. Seeking to accurately recall the emotions of those days is hopeless. I am left with only thought-provoking bits and pieces and a longing to remember that which I cannot.*

*I urge you to place pen to pad frequently and allow yourself to pour out the private impressions of your soul. There will never be a better time and the value to yourself and your loved ones is infinite.*

*Peace be with you,*

**Joanie Willis**

## HOW TO JOURNAL

- Buy a journal, diary, or notebook to write in.
- Record: date, time, & place.
- Try to journal at least four days a week. A quiet journaling session in the morning may help to soothe, compose, and give you balance throughout the day.
- Always journal when you notice your mind is "racing."
- "Make" time because you'll never "find" time.
- Keep a pen with you. Use a different colored pen or highlighter to mark your most important thoughts.
- Don't lose the opportunity to journal in different locations. Carry your journal with you to; treatment centers, doctors' offices, hospitals, and wherever you travel.
- Do not make your journal a to-do list or record just the events of the day; this is about feelings.
- Write quickly so that revelations about yourself make themselves known. Don't censor yourself. Be free.
- Don't worry about grammar, punctuation, or spelling.
- Be honest. Do not write what you think others want to hear or what you wish you were thinking.
- When you are done with one journal, buy another one!

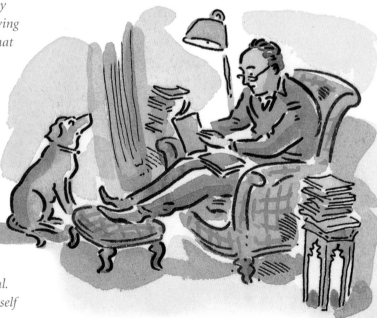

**The Write Way to Wellness**

A Workbook for Healing and Change
*By Kathleen Adams, MA, LPC*

# In These Days, cont.

Paste pictures of your family and friends on this page to look at for encouragement when you need it.

**Paste a picture!**

## IT'S ALL ABOUT ME

MY FAVORITE SONG OF ALL TIME:

_____

THE GREATEST FEMALE SINGER:

_____

THE GREATEST MALE SINGER:

_____

MY FAVORITE BOOK:

_____

MY FAVORITE ACTOR:

_____

MY FAVORITE ACTRESS:

_____

AN EXCELLENT COMEDIAN:

_____

THE FUNNIEST MOVIE I EVER SAW:

_____

THE SADDEST MOVIE I EVER SAW:

_____

MY FAVORITE TV SHOW:

_____

MY FAVORITE NEWSCASTER:

_____

AN ATHLETE I RESPECT AND FOLLOW:

_____

A SPORT I LOVE TO WATCH:

_____

A PRESIDENT I HIGHLY REGARD:

_____

A FOREIGN LEADER I RESPECT:

_____

MY FAVORITE RESTAURANT:

_____

A FOOD I ADORE:

_____

MY FAVORITE DRINK:

_____

THE NICEST CAR I EVER OWNED:

_____

MY FAVORITE ARTIST:

_____

A HOBBY I LOVE:

_____

MY FAVORITE BOARD GAME:

_____

MY FAVORITE CARD GAME:

_____

A TOY I LOVED AS A CHILD:

_____

A TOY I LOVED AS AN ADULT:

_____

A PET I ADORE:

_____

MY FAVORITE BIRD:

_____

MY FAVORITE FLOWER:

_____

MY FAVORITE COLOR:

_____

THE BEST DAY OF THE WEEK:

_____

MY FAVORITE CHARITY:

_____

MY LUCKY NUMBER:

_____

WHAT BRINGS ME PEACE:

_____

A HOLIDAY I LOVE:

_____

A HOLIDAY I HATE:

_____

THE BEST JOB I EVER HELD:

_____

THE WORST JOB I EVER HELD:

_____

AN AWARD I WON:

_____

MY BEST TRAIT:

_____

MY WORST TRAIT:

_____

MY GREATEST VICTORY:

_____

MY GREATEST DISAPPOINTMENT:

_____

WHAT MAKES ME HAPPY:

_____

WHAT MAKES ME ANGRY:

_____

# Brief Reflections

Most of us have never taken the time to sit down and write in a journal. We have been engaged in work, family, and hobbies, relegating writing to the dusty closet of school exercises. Cancer, by virtue of its treatments and their debilitating nature, may leave you with more time on your hands. Transform the hours spent in treatment centers, waiting rooms, and recuperating at home. Use these suggestions for brief reflections to fill the vacant interims, stimulate your mind, and as a springboard to more in-depth, reflective journaling.

**Three things I don't like to think about**

1. _____

_____

2. _____

_____

3. _____

_____

**Things I am grateful for**

_____

_____

_____

_____

_____

**When my children left home I felt...**

_____

_____

_____

_____

_____

**Emotions I can't deal with in others**

_____

_____

_____

_____

_____

**Songs I sing in the shower**

_____

_____

_____

_____

_____

**Emotions I can't deal with in myself**

_____

_____

_____

_____

_____

**Nightmares I have**

_____

_____

_____

_____

_____

Some of the things I love to do

_____
_____
_____
_____
_____
_____

I still have a lot to learn, such as

_____
_____
_____
_____
_____

What scares me the most about having cancer

_____
_____
_____
_____
_____

If I could be anyone...

_____
_____
_____
_____
_____

How cancer has impacted my family

_____
_____
_____
_____
_____

The best day ever

_____
_____
_____
_____
_____

What prevents me from feeling close to others

_____
_____
_____
_____
_____

Once when I was camping

_____
_____
_____
_____
_____

# Memories, Musings, & Messages

*"I will write myself into well-being."*

– Nancy Mair

*"Everything has been thought of before; the challenge is to think of it again."*

– J.W. Goethe

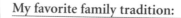

**M**uch can be said about the influence a diagnosis of cancer can have over our thought process. Notions, ideas, and expectations fill our minds regarding the days to come. With apprehension we anticipate the effects of treatments, attempt to mentally forecast their outcome, and worry how we and our families will handle the future. Our minds are consumed with the "what ifs" of tomorrow. Understandably, reflections about the past begin to surface, as well.

*Thoughts of our childhood, parents, experiences, travels, and old friends become a familiar and comfortable safe haven where we can find a fleeting moment of peace.*

We reminisce, get homesick, ponder our values, search our hearts, and dig deeper than we have in years. How we feel and what we think suddenly become significant and something we feel a need to share. We have a lot to say.

The following pages are to encourage you to take an occasional mental "time out" from the realities of the day. Make an effort to compose a written account of your memories, musings and messages. Someday it may be a treasured gift of yourself to your family, and perhaps the best legacy you could ever hope to give.

**My favorite family tradition:**

*The neatest family tradition that I remember as a kid was our Easter 'coffee egg contest'. My mom would take her favorite pot and fill it three quarters full with water. To that she would add a pound of coffee grounds, two onions and two dozen eggs. This concoction would simmer for at least 24 hours filling our home with an aroma I shall never forget. On Easter morning my sister, my mother, my father and I would carefully pick out one of the special colored coffee eggs and gather around in a circle. We would than take turns trying to crack the opponents egg with our own. The game would end when there was only one egg left uncracked. The champion egg and its owner would be declared victorious and the winner would then take possession of everyone else's cracked eggs. The coffee eggs had a great flavor I admit, but at the time, winning seemed so much more important. Give the recipe a try.*

# Memories, Musings, & Messages, cont.

TreeGivers is a unique way to memorialize a loved one before or after their death. The Treegivers program plants trees in memory of individuals or families on public land in every state in the nation. These special trees help repopulate our forests and offer a great way to remember a loved one and help preserve our environment at the same time. You may choose which state the tree is planted in and TreeGivers provides the family or donor with a beautiful personalized commemorative letter and certificate of planting. Over 350,000 trees planted in 50 states since 1981.

TreeGivers,
Forest Lane • P.O. Box 44, Littleton, NH 03561
(800) 862-8733
**ONLINE GO TO**
**http://www.treegivers.com**

---

**STOP**

Complete this chapter. Some pages, such those dealing with financial information, should be photocopied and filled in only on the copies to ensure that it is not lost. Other information may be entered in the workbook, but you should make a second copy

1. Photocopy the chapter or tear the pages out if you prefer.

2. Place in an envelope marked "In the event of my death."

3. Put the envelope in a safe location.

---

## JUST FOR THE FUN OF IT

The following quotes were taken from actual medical records dictated by physicians. They appeared in a column written by Richard Lederer Ph.D., for the *Journal of Court Reporting.*

- By the time he was admitted his rapid heart had stopped and he was feeling better.

- Patient has chest pain if she lies on her left side for over a year.

- On the second day the knee was better and on the third day it had completely disappeared.

- She has had no rigors or shaking chills, but her husband states she was very hot in bed last night.

- The patient has been depressed ever since she began seeing me in 1983.

- The patient is tearful and crying constantly. She also appears to be depressed.

- Discharge status: Alive but without permission.

- The patient will need disposition, and therefore we will get Dr. Blank to dispose of him.

- Healthy-appearing decrepit 69-year-old male, mentally alert but forgetful.

- The patient refused an autopsy.

- The patient has no past history of suicides.

- The patient expired on the floor uneventfully.

- Patient has left his white blood cells at another hospital.

- Patient was becoming more demented with urinary frequency.

- The patient's past medical history has been remarkably insignificant with only a 40-pound weight gain in the past three days.

- She slipped on the ice and apparently her legs went in separate directions in early December.

- The patient left the hospital feeling much better except for her original complaints.

### A few interesting facts:

- Men can read smaller print than women; women can hear better.

- Amount American Airlines saved in 1987 by eliminating one olive from each salad served first class: $40,000.

- Percentage of American men who say they would marry the same woman if they had it to do all over again: 80%.

- Percentage of American women who say they'd marry the same man: 50%.

- Average number of people airborne over the US any given hour: 61,000.

- A duck's quack doesn't echo, and no one knows why.

- The Hawaiian alphabet has 12 letters.

- It is possible to lead a cow upstairs but not downstairs.

- Barbie's measurements if she were life size: 39–23–33.

- The only 15-letter word that can be spelled without repeating a letter is uncopyrightable.

- Intelligent people have more zinc and copper in their hair.

- Every day more money is printed for Monopoly than the US Treasury.

- Coca-Cola was originally green.

- Cost of raising a medium-size dog to the age of eleven: $6,400.

- Average life span of a major league baseball: 7 pitches.

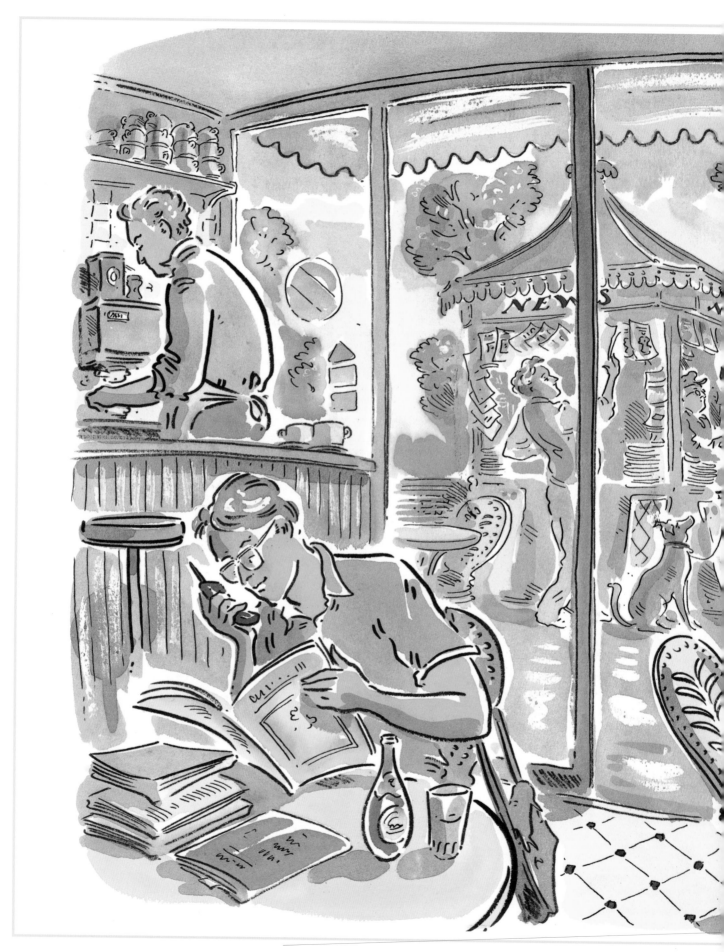

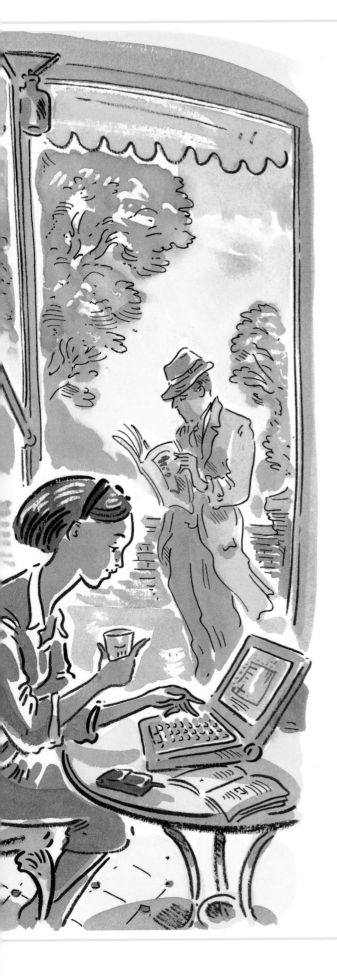

# The New News

*Chapter 7*

# Gathering Information

Fifty years ago the word cancer was rarely spoken and while the disease was prevalent even then, little information was shared between the medical field and news organizations. In the past several years, however, cancer has become a major news story due to promising new research and because, in some form or another, it has touched the lives of so many children and adults in the United States.

The intent of this chapter is to launch you on an ongoing quest for information. While you might think this would be time-consuming and difficult, I can assure you it is not. Before I got cancer I was blind to the impact the disease was having on families, the economy, the healthcare industry, and those in the research field. Shortly after being diagnosed, my eyes opened to the realization that there was information and news on cancer everywhere I turned. I only needed to look.

Inadvertently I became conscious that reports were being run on the nightly news, that every magazine I picked up had an article on nutrition and cancer or the latest treatments being tested, and that the morning paper frequently had something current and exciting to report. All of this came to me without any additional effort on my part. I had always read magazines and newspapers and watched the evening news. But now I started clipping newspaper articles, writing information down on scraps of paper, and saving pages from all sorts of magazines, all of which I promptly misplaced and couldn't find when I needed it. To make matters worse, I ordered health newsletters and cancer pamphlets, and tracked down information on the internet, printing out one report right after another. My kitchen counter, tables, and bookshelves had stacks of information. Some of it was good, some not; some I wanted to keep forever but most I did not.

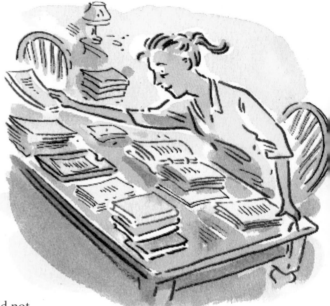

*I realized that the problem was not getting the information, it was in organizing it.*

This chapter allows you to be selective and accumulate the facts and information that you consider to be most important. It will help you organize the information by:
• Furnishing ordering information on health newsletters and magazines that might of benefit.
• Providing a newspaper "clip and paste" section for articles you want for future reference and to discuss with your medical team.
• Showing you how to keep records on relevant nightly news and investigative broadcasts.
• Recording helpful tidbits of information you come across in books, magazines, or treatment rooms, or acquire from doctors, nurses, or other patients.
• Listing websites that provide up-to-date and easy access to the important cancer information available on the Internet.
• Additional brochures and books that may be helpful.

It is my belief that once you have been motivated to educate yourself on your specific cancer, treatment options, and current research, your knowledge will become power and a deterrent to your anxiety and fear.

**One word of caution:**
Information about promising cancer treatments are often released in newspapers or reported on television long before the research studies have been completed or are ready for human trials. Beware of getting your hopes up in regards to what may be premature news. While you should follow up on everything, keep in mind that much of what you find will be in its initial testing stage and inaccessible to you.

# Health Letters & Magazines

Health letters and magazines are an outstanding resource for healthcare information, facts on nutrition, and new research developments. The ones listed to the right are interesting, helpful, and trustworthy. Many of these businesses will send you one free issue, along with a bill for the subscription if you decide to purchase the magazine or newsletter. If you do not want to subscribe, simply write "cancel" on the bill, return it, and keep the free issue. Take a few minutes now to call for information.

---

### FREE FOR THE ASKING

Cancer Care News: Information on support groups, teleconferences, clinical trials, and advocacy, all available free of charge. To order, call (800) 813-HOPE or go online

**http://www.cancercare.org/ patients/informational.htm**

---

**You may come across genuine, authentic-looking healthcare information that is not accurate. Be careful what you believe. Avoid the following:**

• Television shows that have the hidden agenda of selling you a product (infomercials).

• Newspaper reports that are labeled "special advertisements."

• Official-looking health newsletters promoting products.

• Information from any source that cannot be substantiated.

---

HARVARD HEALTH LETTER
P.O. Box 420300
Palm Coast, FL 32142-0300
Call: (800) 829-9045

Subscription price $ _____
# of issues a year _____
Will send a free copy Yes ☐ No ☐
Ordered subscription: Date _____
Canceled subscription: Date _____

**Website: http://www.health.harvard.edu/newsletters**

PREVENTION MAGAZINE
P.O. Box 7305
Red Oak, IA 51591-2305
Call: (800) 813-8070

Subscription price $ _____
# of issues a year _____
Will send a free copy Yes ☐ No ☐
Ordered subscription: Date _____
Canceled subscription: Date _____

**Website: http://www.healthyideas.com/subscribe/**

HEALTH
P.O. Box 56876
Boulder, CO 80323-6876
Call: (800) 274-2522

Subscription price $ _____
# of issues a year _____
Will send a free copy Yes ☐ No ☐
Ordered subscription: Date _____
Canceled subscription: Date _____

**Website: http://www.healthmag.com**

MAYO CLINIC HEALTH LETTER
P.O. Box 53886
Boulder, CO 80323-3886
Call: (800) 876-8633

Subscription price $ _____
# of issues a year _____
Will send a free copy Yes ☐ No ☐
Ordered subscription: Date _____
Canceled subscription: Date _____

**Website: http://www.healthe-store.com**

WELLNESS NEWS LETTER
P.O. Box 420148
Palm Coast, FL 32142-0148
Call: (904) 445-6414

Subscription price $ _____
# of issues a year _____
Will send a free copy Yes ☐ No ☐
Ordered subscription: Date _____
Canceled subscription: Date _____

**Website: http://www.berkleywellness.com/**

MAYO CLINIC WOMEN'S HEALTHSOURCE
P.O. Box 56931
Boulder, CO 80322-6931
Call: (800) 678-5481

Subscription price $ _____
# of issues a year _____
Will send a free copy Yes ☐ No ☐
Ordered subscription: Date _____
Canceled subscription: Date _____

**Website: http://www.mayohealth.org/mayo/product/htm/info_wom.htm**

TUFTS HEALTH AND NUTRITION LETTER
P.O. Box 420235
Palm Coast, FL 32142-0235
Call: (800) 274-7581

Subscription price $ _____
# of issues a year _____
Will send a free copy Yes ☐ No ☐
Ordered subscription: Date _____
Canceled subscription: Date _____

**Website http://healthletter.tufts.edu/**

# Medical Journals

Medical journals are written for a professional audience and, therefore, may be too complicated for many readers or, indeed, may tell them more than they even want to know. However, for those patients who want to research the more technical aspects of study in cancer science and research, especially in their own type of cancer, medical journals may be very rewarding, up to date, and informative. The ones listed have online sites where you can get a good idea of what they have to offer. If you are interested in a complete list of oncology journals go to HYPERLINK

**http://www.sciencekomm.at/ journals/medicine/onco.html**

### CA – A Cancer Journal For Clinicians ACS

1599 Clifton Road, N.E.
Atlanta, GA 30329
Call: (888) ACS-5552

Subscription price $ _____
# of issues a year _____
Will send a free copy Yes ☐ No ☐
Ordered subscription: Date _____
Canceled subscription: Date _____

**Website: http//www.ca-journal.org**

*You do not need a registration number for online access.*
*It is available to anyone who has the use of a computer.*

### The New England Journal of Medicine

10 Shattuck Street
Boston, MA 02115-6094
Call: (800) THE-NEJM

Subscription price $ _____
# of issues a year _____
Will send a free copy Yes ☐ No ☐
Ordered subscription: Date _____
Canceled subscription: Date _____

**Website: http://secure.mms.org/custserv/sub.asp**

*Registration number for online access:_____*

*Please note that a print subscription to the New England Journal of Medicine includes online access.*

### Journal of The National Cancer Institute

Journals Marketing
Oxford University Press
2001 Evans Road
Cary, NC 27513
Call: (800) 852-7323

Subscription price $ _____
# of issues a year _____
Will send a free copy Yes ☐ No ☐
Ordered subscription: Date _____
_____Canceled subscription: Date

**Website: http://www3.oup.co.uk/jnls/list/jnci/subinfo/**

*Registration number for online access:_____*

*Please note that a print subscription to the Journal of the National Cancer Institute includes online access.*

### Cancer

John Wiley & Sons, Inc.
Attn.: Subscription Department
605 Third Avenue
New York, NY 10158
Call: (800) 511-3989

Subscription price $ _____
_____# of issues a year
Will send a free copy Yes ☐ No ☐
Ordered subscription: Date _____
Canceled subscription: Date _____

**Website: http://secure.edoc.com/wiley-bin/cancer-orderform.cgi**

*Registration number for online access: _____*

*Please note that a print subscription to Cancer includes online access.*

# Daily News Clips

An ideal source of easily attainable up-to-date information comes from newspapers and magazines. Make a habit of picking up the newspaper every day and perusing it for information on your type of cancer. Also check for articles on vitamins, nutrition, the immune system, new technologies, cancer prevention, clinical trials, and new treatments and techniques. Clip and paste the articles you find particularly relevant on pages 192–193. I have gotten you started with a few "condensed" news pieces that I found interesting. Carry *The Cancer Patient's Workbook* with you at all times so that you will have the articles for your own personal information, and on hand to show your doctor and share with other cancer patients.

### CRYOSURGERY SUCCESSFUL FOR PROSTATE CANCER PATIENTS WHO HAVE FAILED RADIATION THERAPY

*January, 2000 Urology/MedscapeWire*
Cryosurgery, a technique that uses cold temperatures to freeze and destroy cancerous cells around the prostate gland, is effective for patients whose prostate cancer has recurred after undergoing radiation therapy. This finding was published in a study in the January issue of the journal Urology. Secondary treatment with cryosurgery can stop prostate cancer progression and improve long-term survival.

## NCI CHIEF CALLS FOR FOCUS ON MOLECULAR CANCER RESEARCH

*Washington, DC, Nov. 17, 1999 (Reuters Health)*

Cancer researchers must switch from the thinking of the past 100 years and move toward defining molecular targets, Dr. Richard D. Klausner, director of the National Cancer Institute (NCI), said here Tuesday. "The successful drugs in the future will be directed at molecular targets, whether they are in cancer cells or other cells," he told attendees at the International Conference on Molecular Targets and Cancer Therapeutics: Discovery, Development, and Clinical Validation. The meeting was co-sponsored by the NCI, the American Association for Cancer Research, and the European Organization for Research and Treatment of Cancer. The "molecular revolution" provides researchers with the ability to move beyond the genetics of molecular targeting and view "the pieces of the puzzle" at once, Dr. Klausner said. "We need to understand the function of the target, the pathway it sits on, and the cellular effects altering that target or pathway," he said.

## GE MEDICAL INTRODUCES NEW MRI SYSTEM

*New York, Nov. 17, 1999 (Reuters)*

GE Medical Systems, a unit of General Electric Co. said Wednesday it has introduced a new medical resonance imaging (MRI) system that operates three times faster than any current system.

The new system, GE Signa OpenSpeed, has been cleared by the U.S. Food and Drug Administration and is now commercially available. The company expects to install nearly 100 of the systems worldwide by the end of 2000.

Developed in the 1980s, MRI uses computers and magnetic fields, not radiation, to provide images of the human anatomy.

In addition to traditional MRI imaging capabilities such as knee, spine and brain, the company said the new scanner can be used in pediatric care, and monitoring of stroke therapy.

## MICROWAVE TREATMENT FOR BREAST CANCER TO BE TESTED

*West Palm Beach, Oct. 13, 1999 (Cox News Service)*

An experimental treatment for breast cancer that uses microwaves to zap tumors could make today's gold standard of cancer treatment – surgery, radiation, and drugs – look as primitive as poking holes in the skull to relieve headaches.

Columbia Hospital's Center for Breast Care in West Palm Beach announced Tuesday it is recruiting up to 10 women to take part in the nation's first test of a new technology that pinpoints microwaves to kill breast cancer. Applying technology used in the Gulf War to jam enemy radar and home in on missiles, doctors will heat breast tissue with microwaves, the same energy used to cook TV dinners. "It's been known that heat kills tumors," said Kurt O'Neill, a spokesman for Celsion Corp., the Columbia, Md., company licensed to market the technology. "The problem in the past has been getting heat to the tumor only – and not healthy cells."

# Daily News Clips, cont.

### DI BELLA'S "MIRACLE" CANCER CURE SHORTENS SURVIVAL

*November 15, 1999*
New York (Reuters Health)

The Di Bella therapy, a cancer treatment touted as a cure for up to 100% of patients, actually provides results far worse than standard cancer treatments, study results show. The therapy program was developed in Italy by Dr. Luigi Di Bella, who claims to have treated more than 10,000 patients over the past 20 years. With Di Bella's cooperation, a research team led by Dr. Eva Buiatti, from Azienda USL Firenze in Florence, Italy, reviewed the medical records of 314 patients who received the Di Bella therapy. Compared with patients identified in the Italian cancer registry, who received only standard therapies, patients who received the Di Bella therapy "showed lower survival probability over both the short term and the long term for all the cancer sites considered," Buiatti's team reports in the 11/15/1999 issue of *Cancer*.

**Paste your articles here**

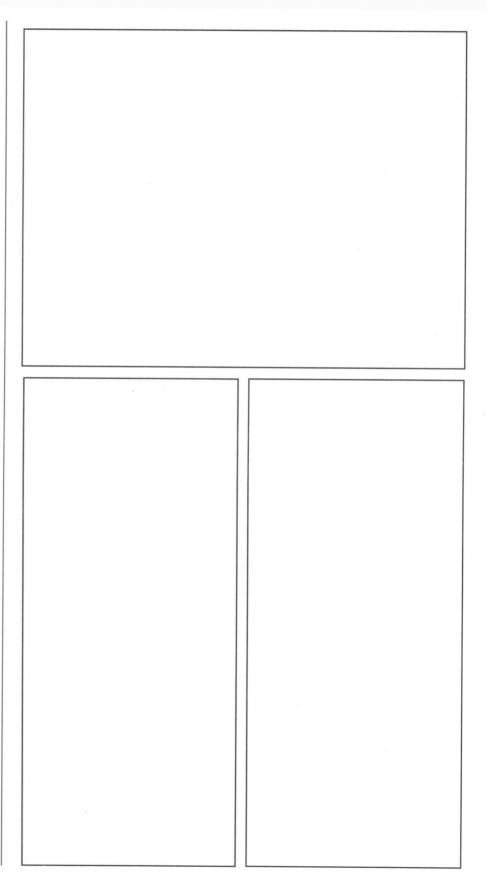

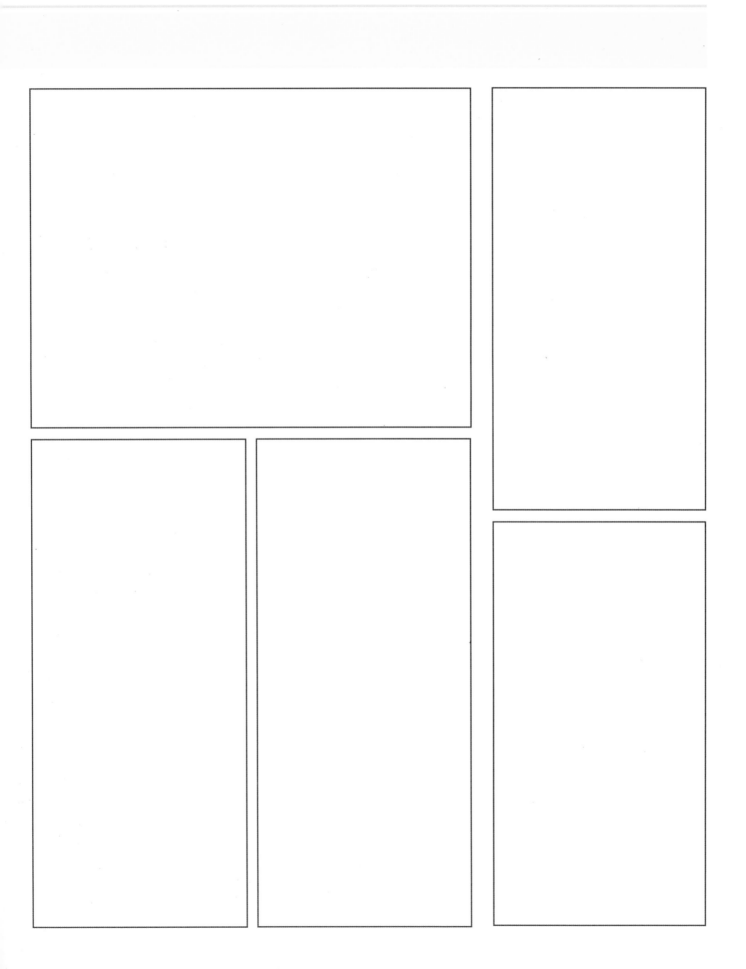

# Television

It is estimated that this year cancer will replace heart disease as the leading cause of death in the United States. Annually, more than a million Americans will be diagnosed and millions more lives will be caught up in the role of becoming primary caregivers. Cancer, its treatments, prevention and search for a cure is very big news. Television's interest is now in widespread reporting on the research of new discoveries and technologies, prevention of cancer, new treatments for cancer, and the optimism of scientists and medical specialists that new avenues of research are bringing us one step closer to making cancer a disease of the past. Take advantage of these up-to-the-minute reports. The media journal on the following pages can be used to track the television programs or news stories you feel are important to you. Listen carefully for the names of doctors, universities, or hospitals where research or clinical trials are underway. Record the names of new drugs and medications. In addition, note the date, time and network in the event you want to follow up later.

## PUBLIC BROADCASTING SERVICE (PBS)

PBS is a private, not-for-profit media enterprise owned and operated by the nation's 348 public television stations. It is a trusted community resource known for providing quality health and medical programs that educate and inform Americans. Check your telephone directory for information on your local station.

---

## MEDIA JOURNAL

Date: _____ Time: _____ Network: _____

Name of doctors, researcher, or investigator: _____
_____

Name of hospital, clinic, or university doing research: _____
_____

Name of lab or pharmaceutical firm, if any: _____
_____

Name of drugs, genes, or new therapies being tested: _____
_____

Subject matter of the broadcast: _____
_____
_____
_____

---

Date: _____ Time: _____ Network: _____

Name of doctors, researcher, or investigator: _____
_____

Name of hospital, clinic, or university doing research: _____
_____

Name of lab or pharmaceutical firm, if any: _____
_____

Name of drugs, genes, or new therapies being tested: _____
_____

Subject matter of the broadcast: _____
_____
_____
_____

---

Date: _____ Time: _____ Network: _____

Name of doctors, researcher, or investigator: _____
_____

Name of hospital, clinic, or university doing research: _____
_____

Name of lab or pharmaceutical firm, if any: _____
_____

Name of drugs, genes, or new therapies being tested: _____
_____

Subject matter of the broadcast: _____
_____
_____

## Media journal

Date: _____ Time: _____ Network: _____

Name of doctors, researcher, or investigator: _____

_____

Name of hospital, clinic, or university doing research: _____

_____

Name of lab or pharmaceutical firm, if any: _____

_____

Name of drugs, genes, or new therapies being tested: _____

_____

Subject matter of the broadcast: _____

_____

_____

Date: _____ Time: _____ Network: _____

Name of doctors, researcher, or investigator: _____

_____

Name of hospital, clinic, or university doing research: _____

_____

Name of lab or pharmaceutical firm, if any: _____

_____

Name of drugs, genes, or new therapies being tested: _____

_____

Subject matter of the broadcast: _____

_____

_____

Date: _____ Time: _____ Network: _____

Name of doctors, researcher, or investigator: _____

_____

Name of hospital, clinic, or university doing research: _____

_____

Name of lab or pharmaceutical firm, if any: _____

_____

Name of drugs, genes, or new therapies being tested: _____

_____

Subject matter of the broadcast: _____

_____

## AMERICAN CANCER SOCIETY BOOKS

A percentage of the purchase price of items you order directly from this link will be donated to the American Cancer Society.

- Kids' First Cookbook
- Consumers Guide to Cancer Drugs
- Healthy Eating Cookbook
- Prostate Cancer
- Colorectal Cancer
- Women and Cancer
- Living Well, Staying Well
- Informed Decisions
- A Portrait of Breast Cancer

**http://www.cancer.org/ bookstore/index_con.html**

## TELEVISION PROGRAMS YOU DON'T WANT TO MISS

Date _____ Time _____

_____

Date _____ Time _____

_____

Date _____ Time _____

_____

Date _____ Time _____

_____

Date _____ Time _____

_____

Date _____ Time _____

_____

Date _____ Time _____

_____

Date _____ Time _____

_____

Date _____ Time _____

_____

Date _____ Time _____

_____

# Helpful Hints & Advice

Record ideas, tips, suggestions, facts and other helpful hints you want available to remember. Keep your workbook handy during doctors visits, support group meetings, in cancer treatment centers, while reading books, magazines or searching the Internet. Information can come from many different sources. If it sounds practical or simply interests you write it down.

### EXAMPLES

**Source:** _A flyer at Dr. Hart's office Aventis Oncology and MAMM magazine send out a free magazine that is devoted to women with breast cancer. To get a free one-year subscription, I can write to: MAMM Magazine, P.O. Box 539, Mount Morris, IL 61054-8410_

**Source:** _American Health Magazine Threats to the immune system are depression lack of sleep, fast food or a lousy diet, periodontal disease, lack of friends or close social ties, stressful job, and lack of exercise._

**Source:** _Pap tests have cut the death rate of cervical cancer by 70%. If I register at this website, http://www.papsmear.org/ I will receive an e-mail reminder to schedule an appointment the date I choose._

**Source:** _Health Magazine Typically a patient is allowed to speak 23 seconds before being interrupted by a doctor. 40% more cancer patients are more worried about the side effects of chemo than of dying. 74% of adults think a doctor should address a patient's spiritual needs._

Source: _____

Source: _____

Source: _____

Source: _____

Source: _____

Source: _____

Source: _____

Source: _____

Source: _____

Source: _____

Source: _____

Source: _____

Source: _____

_____

_____

_____

Source: _____

_____

_____

_____

Source: _____

_____

_____

_____

_____

Source: _____

_____

_____

_____

_____

Source: _____

_____

_____

_____

_____

Source: _____

_____

_____

_____

_____

Source: _____

_____

_____

_____

Source: _____

_____

_____

_____

Source: _____

_____

_____

_____

_____

Source: _____

_____

_____

_____

_____

Source: _____

_____

_____

_____

_____

Source: _____

_____

_____

_____

Source: _____

_____

_____

_____

### WATCH OUT, LADIES!

A study has found that some women lack a specific gene that could make them as much as six times as likely to develop lung cancer if they live with smokers. Secondhand smoke is dangerous to everyone, but if you're female and battling cancer you should ask others not to smoke in your presence.

Source: _____

_____

_____

_____

_____

Source: _____

_____

_____

_____

_____

Source: _____

_____

_____

_____

_____

Source: _____

_____

_____

_____

_____

# The Internet & *the World Wide Web*

The Internet and the World Wide Web has the most complete source of cancer-related information available today. More than 26 million people use the World Wide Web as a reference for medical information and assistance. The WWW can connect you to government agencies, magazines, pharmaceutical companies, research hospitals, news organizations, universities, cancer centers, teaching hospitals, bulletin boards, newspapers, nonprofit organizations, and medical sites of every kind. You can obtain information on nutrition, alternative medicine, drugs, chemotherapy treatments, radiation treatments, food and recipes, exercise, pain control, insurance, work rights, home health care, rehabilitation, Hospice services, family support, children's cancer, common side effects, herbs, vitamins, and current clinical trials. Furthermore, if you own a personal computer you can have access to this data any time of the day or night! The information is all there, but finding it can sometimes be difficult because of the sheer volume of information on the web as well as its exponential growth. I have found the websites listed on pages 202–213, which are related to cancer in general, particular cancers, and many cancer-related subjects, to be particularly helpful. With nearly 450 websites, this list is one of the most complete cancer lists at the time of publication. New websites are created constantly, however, and you may well find discover sites not listed here.

### What to do if you don't own a computer:

- Consider buying one. They can be a great diversion and are not as hard to master as you might think. A laptop would be handy for you to own (or borrow) if you are spending a lot of time on the couch or in bed. A computer would also be great entertainment for a bedridden child who remains at home or in a hospital. Ask a computer-savvy friend to set you up and teach you the basics.

- Use the computer at your local library, nearest college, university, or at work. Don't forget to take along *The Cancer Patient's Workbook.*

- Ask a friend or family member who has a computer to do some research for you.

---

## HELPFUL INTERNET HINTS

- Internet information and advice are never a substitute for professional medical care.
- Your primary online source of information and reference should come from the major institutions and hospitals found under the category "General Cancer Sites."
- Specific cancer websites contain additional information and web links for your particular cancer.
- Some websites may be duplicated because they link to other websites.
- While doing research on the internet, always keep your *Workbook* with you. Jot down those smaller excerpts of information, helpful hints and advice that interest you.
- Make a folder on your computer deskto, and label it "Cancer Information." Copy and paste into the folder all the internet articles and information that you find are important to you.
- Periodically go through your desktop cancer folder and tidy it up, deleting information that is out of date or no longer pertinent, applicable, or important.

- To receive all the information a website offers make certain you scroll to the bottom of the site. Many websites keep the best 'til last. Some of these sites are very rich in content if you look below the desktop storefront. For example, Mother Nature's Online store sells products, but it also includes a complete library and encyclopedia of herbs and vitamins, their descriptions, uses, dangers, interactions with other drugs, and numerous articles about each. Carefully explore each site.
- Use a pencil so that you can erase websites at a later date if you no longer need them.
- Consider maintaining two separate screen names: one for personal use and one devoted to everything cancer-related such as e-mail, newsletters, chat rooms, and favorite cancer websites. This will keep you organized.
- Bookmark (put in "favorite places") your own favorite websites as you rummage around the web.
- If you find a website you think is wonderful and never want to forget, record it on the opposite page.

## GREAT WEBSITES

Website: _____
Usefulness: _____

Website: _____
Usefulness: _____

Website: _____
Usefulness _____

Website: _____
Usefulness: _____

Website: _____
Usefulness: _____

Website: _____
Usefulness: _____

Website: _____
Usefulness: _____

Website: _____
Usefulness: _____

Website: _____
Usefulness: _____

Website: _____
Usefulness: _____

Website: _____
Usefulness: _____

Website: _____
Usefulness: _____

Website: _____
Usefulness: _____

Website: _____
Usefulness: _____

Website: _____
Usefulness: _____

Website: _____
Usefulness: _____

Website: _____
Usefulness: _____

Website: _____
Usefulness: _____

Website: _____
Usefulness: _____

Website: _____
Usefulness: _____

Website: _____
Usefulness: _____

Website: _____
Usefulness: _____

Website: _____
Usefulness: _____

Website: _____
Usefulness: _____

Website: _____
Usefulness: _____

Website: _____
Usefulness: _____

Website: _____
Usefulness: _____

Website: _____
Usefulness: _____

Website: _____
Usefulness: _____

Website: _____
Usefulness: _____

Website: _____
Usefulness: _____

Website: _____
Usefulness: _____

# Fast Facts from the Internet

Below are some examples of information I found while surfing the internet from various cancer sites. The facts cover a variety of cancer topics. Just imagine what you can collect when you customize your research to your particular type of cancer!

- Researchers found that a nasal spray containing the drug midazolam, which is similar to Valium, reduced anxiety in children undergoing painful cancer treatments.

- The top cancer concern among most women surveyed was breast cancer, followed by skin cancer, uterine/cervical cancer, lung cancer, ovarian cancer, and colorectal cancer. Most men were concerned about developing prostate cancer, followed by lung, skin, and colorectal cancer

- Researchers from Finland suggest that past infection with *Chlamydia trachomatis* bacteria is a risk factor for invasive squamous-cell cervical cancer.

- According to the January issue of *Urology,* Johns Hopkins researchers conclude that when patients seek out a surgeon highly experienced in the procedure of prostate removal they are far more likely to remain continent and potent than if the operations were done by a less experienced doctor.

- Canadian researchers report that teenage boys who exercise regularly and those with physically demanding jobs in their 20s may be more likely to develop testicular cancer than their less active counterparts.

- Eating vegetables, particularly cruciferous ones, substantially lowers the risk of prostate cancer according to a report published in the January 5th issue of the *Journal of the National Cancer Institute.* Risk was not affected by fruit.

- US researchers report that by counting the number of underarm lymph nodes after breast tumor surgery, doctors can predict the women's risk of dying from breast cancer over the next 5 years even when cancer has not spread to the nodes.

- Researchers believe that cultural, economic, and genetic factors contribute to African-American women with breast cancer being 67% more likely to die from their illness than white women.

- Using a combination of two chemotherapy drugs – cisplatin and paclitaxel – is just as effective a treatment for advanced ovarian cancer as high doses of a single drug, with fewer serious side effects report US researchers.

- Nearly 60 percent of men who have had cancerous prostates removed are impotent 18 months after surgery.

- The stress of cancer surgery may reduce levels of the immune system's "natural killer" cells which are important to tumor suppression.

- UK researchers estimate that every time a man lights up a cigarette he loses an average of 11 minutes of his life.

- A review published in the *New England Journal of Medicine* found that while 63% of all cancer patients are over 65, they make up just 25% of the people enrolled in cancer studies.

- A study directed by Dr. Nancy Kemeny of Memorial Sloan-Kettering Cancer Center in New York City found that injecting chemotherapy drugs directly into the liver's blood supply can improve the odds of survival in patients with advanced colon cancer that has spread to the liver.

- A study published in the *Journal of the National Cancer Institute* suggests that advanced throat cancer patients are more likely to survive if they have an additional three cycles of chemotherapy during radiation treatment compared with those treated with radiation alone.

- Genentech Inc. announced that it plans to proceed with the third and final stage of clinical trials aimed at developing a new class of drugs that would fight cancer by cutting off the flow of blood to tumors. The experiments may take years before the drugs, called antiangiogenesis agents, prove successful against lung, colon, and rectal tumors.

- Women may take shorter and smaller puffs on cigarettes than men but they enjoy it more, making it harder to quit.

- An experimental pill drug called STI-571 has shown remarkable promise against one form of leukemia in early tests, helping every patient in whom the standard treatment had failed. It could prove to be the first major treatment for the disease in 13 years. "The scientific community is very excited," said Dr. David A. Scheinberg, chief of leukemia at Memorial-Sloan Kettering Cancer Center in New York City.

- Research being done at Johns Hopkins involving the use of a new gel being injected directly into liver tumors is showing promise. Dr. Paul Thuluvath, who directs the Hopkins liver transplant program says, "that doesn't mean this is a cure for

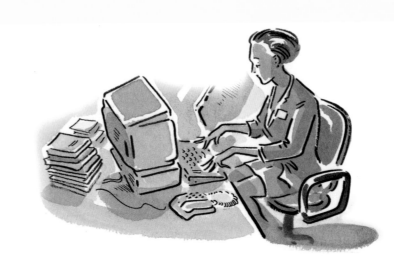

every cancer. It's very promising, at least for small tumors in those with advanced liver disease. We could probably postpone or prolong their life to the degree that we can do a transplantation. That's what it does."

• In the fiscal 2001 budget President Clinton will seek a $27 million increase in funding for research into the possible environmental causes of breast and prostate cancer and other diseases.

• A vasectomy does not increase the risk of prostate cancer, researchers report in the October issue of Cancer Epidemiology, Biomarkers & Prevention.

• Health experts are concerned that women may start skipping annual visits to their gynecologist because of a new low-cost test that can help women over 35 detect early signs of cervical cancer without a doctor's visit.

• Researchers at the Fred Hutchinson Cancer Research Center presented preliminary results from a 3-year study of 168 patients with high-risk blood and immune system cancers that show that those who received stem cell transplants had a survival advantage over those who received standard treatment with bone marrow transplantation. The 2-year survival rate for stem cell transplant recipients was 70% compared with a survival rate of 45% for bone marrow transplant recipients.

• A new study shows that while people with Down syndrome have a high chance of developing childhood leukemia, they have only half the normal lifetime risk of getting other kinds of cancer.

• The tendency to develop moles, linked with fair skin and hair, increase melanoma susceptibility.

Researchers report that melanoma, the most deadly type of skin cancer, is not effected by the use of sunscreen.

• More than 95% of lung cancers belong to the group called bronchogenic carcinoma. Treatments differ for each and it is important to know which type of lung cancer you have. This classification includes: squamous cell carcinoma, adenocarcinoma, small cell (oat cell) carcinoma, and large cell carcinoma.

• People helping people: The Leukemia Society of America will match a newly diagnosed patient with another patient who has been trained. It's a wonderful program called First Connection. Call (800) 955-4572.

• Surprise, surprise: There has been no link between fat and breast cancer. However, a new study reports women who consume two or more alcoholic beverages a day have a 41% higher chance or breast cancer.

• The National Institutes of Health estimate overall annual costs for cancer at $107 billion; $37 billion for direct medical costs (total of all health expenditures); $11 billion for indirect morbidity costs (cost of lost productivity due to illness); and $59 billion for indirect mortality costs (cost of lost productivity due to premature death). Treatment of breast, lung and prostate cancers account for over half of the direct medical costs.

• For Free: Exercise: A Guide from the National Institute on Aging. Order by phone at (800) 222-2225.

• Researchers have reported that acetaminophen – better known as Tylenol – may indeed cut a woman's risk of ovarian cancer in half.

Not enough can be said about Johns Hopkins InteliHealth. More than 150 top healthcare organizations contribute to InteliHealth's online and offline ventures, including government agencies, major nonprofits, other publishers and news media. It has up-to-date complete information on new research, treatments and health information.

InteliHealth is a group of creative, energetic, quality-driven people who are passionate about their mission to promote good health.

**http://www.intelihealth/IH/ihtIH**

# Websites

## General Cancer Information

allHealth Cancer
http://www.allhealth.com/conditions/cancer/0,4264,16,00.html

American Cancer Society
http://www.cancer.org/

BioOncology Online
http://www.biooncology.com/biooncology/index.htm

CancerBACUP
http://www.cancerbacup.org.uk/index.shtml

Cancer Care, Inc.
http://www.cancercare.org

CancerNet – A service of the National Cancer Institute
http://cancernet.nci.nih.gov/index.html

Cancer News on the Net
http://www.cancernews.com/quickload.htm

Cancer Research Foundation of America
http://www.preventcancer.org/

Cancer Survivors On Line
http://www.cancersurvivors.org/

Cancer Treatment Information Center
http://canceranswers.com/

CanSearch Websites
http://www.cansearch.org/canserch/canserch.htm

CNN – Health – Cancer
http://www.cnn.com/HEALTH/indepth.health/cancer/index.html

Dana-Farber Cancer Institute
http://www.dana-farber.net/IE4index.shtml

Disease Centers
http://pharminfo.com/disease/disdb_mnu.html#onc

Duke University Medical Center – Departments
http://www.mc.duke.edu/depts/

InteliHealth – Home to Johns Hopkins Health Information: Cancer
http://www.intelihealth.com/IH/ihtIH/WSIHW000/8096/8096.html?k=CancerZoneFR48

Johns Hopkins Oncology Center
http://www.hopkins.cancercenter.jhmi.edu/

Mayo Clinic Health Oasis: Information on Cancer
http://www.mayohealth.org/mayo/common/htm/canhpage.htm

MD Anderson Cancer Center
http://www.mdanderson.org/ Medicine Online
http://www.meds.com/index.html

Medscape Oncology Home Page
http://www.medscape.com/Home/Topics/oncology/oncology.html

Memorial Sloan-Kettering Cancer Center
http://www.mskcc.org/patients_n_public/

National Cancer Institute
http://rex.nci.nih.gov/

National Comprehensive Cancer Center Network
http://www.nccn.org/

National Hospice Organization
http://www.nho.org/general.htm

Noah Cancer Care Inc.
http://www.noah.cuny.edu/providers/cancare.html#Tips

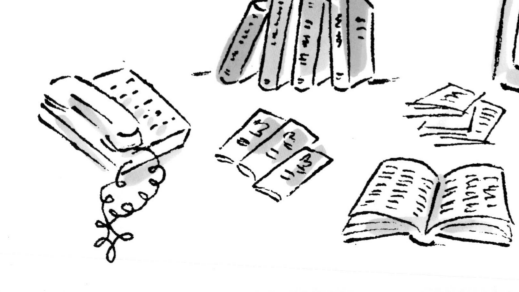

PDQ – A SERVICE OF THE NATIONAL CANCER INSTITUTE
http://cancernet.nci.nih.gov/pdq.html

R.A. BLOCH CANCER FOUNDATION, INC.
http://www.blochcancer.org/

TAUSSIG CANCER CENTER
http://www.ccf.org/cc/c_cancer.html

## GENERAL MEDICAL INFORMATION
THE AMERICAN MEDICAL ASSOCIATION
http://www.ama-assn.org

DRKOOP.COM.
http://www.drkoop.com/

HEALTHANSWERS
http://www.healthanswers.com/

HEALTHFINDER
http://www.healthfinder.gov/

KIDSHEALTH
http://www.kidshealth.org/

MEDICONSULT.COM
http://www.mediconsult.com/

NATIONAL INSTITUTES OF HEALTH
http://www.nih.gov/

NATIONAL LIBRARY OF MEDICINE'S MEDLINE PLUS
http://www.nlm.nih.gov/medlineplus/

PDR.NET
http://www.pdr.net/

REUTERS HEALTH INFORMATION
http://www.reutershealth.com/

THRIVE@NEWSSTAND
http://www.thriveonline.com/

WEBMD
http://www.webmd.org/

## ADULT AMUSEMENT SITES
BEST HUMOR SITES
http://www.startingpage.com/html/humor.html

BEST JOKES SITES
http://startpage.com/html/jokes.html

BOXERJAM
http://www.boxerjam.com/

BRAINBLITZ.COM
http://www.brainblitz.com/

CANDYSTAND
http://www.candystand.com/home.htm

CHESSED
http://www.chessed.com/

CLICK TO PLAY
http://www.clicktoplay.com/

GAMESVILLE
http://www.gamesville.com/

JAEGER'S WEB PAINTBALL GAME
http://www.mv.com/ipusers/paintball/game/

MSN GAMING ZONE
http://go.msn.com/2/5/0/

MSNBC CROSSWORD PUZZELS
http://www.msnbc.com/comics/xword_class_files/crossword.asp

ONE ON ONE FREE BASKETBALL GAME
http://basketball-game.com/

PHATGAMES.NET
http://www.phatgames.net/

TRIVALBLITZ
http://www.thefreesite.com/triviablitz.htm

## ALTERNATIVE AND COMPLEMENTARY MEDICINE
ACUPUNCTURE.COM
http://www.acupuncture.com/

ALTERNATIVE AND COMPLEMENTARY MEDICINE CENTER
http://www.alternativemedicine.net/

ALTERNATIVE HEALTH NEWS ONLINE
http://www.altmedicine.com/

ARTICLES ON HEALTH
http://aimthisway.com/aimthisway/aronheal.html

NATIONAL CENTER FOR COMPLEMENTARY AND ALTERNATIVE MEDICINE
http://nccam.nih.gov/nccam

THE NATIONAL COUNCIL FOR RELIABLE HEALTH INFORMATION
http://www.ncahf.org/

## BONE MARROW TRANSPLANTS
BLOOD & MARROW TRANSPLANT
http://www.bmtnews.org/

# Websites, cont.

BONE MARROW DONORS WORLDWIDE
http://www.bmdw.org/

BONE MARROW TRANSPLANTS
http://www.bmtnews.org/bmt/bmt.book/toc.html

NATIONAL MARROW DONOR PROGRAM
http://www.marrow.org/

## CHILDREN'S FUN SITES
CRAYOLA
http://www.crayola.com/

DISNEY GAMES
http://disney.go.com/home/channels/games/today/html/index.html

DR. SEUSS'S SEUSSVILLE
http://www.randomhouse.com/seussville/

FUN STUFF FOR KIDS
http://ww2.med.jhu.edu/peds/neonatology/fun.html

KIDLAND
http://www.kidland.com/

LEGO
http://www.lego.com/

## CLINICAL TRIALS
CANCER CLINICAL TRIALS DIRECTORY
http://www.fda.gov/oashi/cancer/trials.html

CANCERTRIALS-A SERVICE OF THE NATIONAL CANCER INSTITUTE
http://cancertrials.nci.nih.gov/

CENTERWATCH CLINICAL TRIALS LISTING SERVICE
http://www.centerwatch.com/

CLINICAL TRIALS LISTING BY DISEASE CATEGORY
http://www.centerwatch.com/studies/LISTING.HTM#Section12

CLINICAL TRIALS AT THE CANCER TREATMENT CENTERS OF AMERICAS
http://www.cancercenter.com/home/294/

## DEATH AND BEREAVEMENT
CHOICE IN DYING
http://www.choices.org/

COMPASSIONATE FRIENDS
http://www.needsyou.org/comp.htm

DEATH AND DYING GREIF SUPPORT
http://www.death-dying.com/

GRIEFNET
http://www.griefnet.org/

## DOCTORS AND HOSPITALS
AMERICAN MEDICAL ASSOCIATION DOCTOR FINDER
http://www.ama-assn.org/aps/amahg.htm

BEST DOCTORS.COM
http://www.bestdoctors.com/

GOOD HOUSEKEEPING-318 TOP SPECIALISTS FOR WOMEN
http://goodhousekeeping.women.com/gh/eatwell/health/
tools/39docs16.htm

HOSPITAL WEB (LOCATE HOSPITALS IN THE UNITED STATES
http://neuro-www2.mgh.harvard.edu/hospitalwebusa.html

U.S.NEWS – BEST HOSPITALS FOR CANCER CARE
http://www.usnews.com/usnews/nycu/health/hosptl/tophosp.htm

U.S.NEWS BEST HMO'S
http://www.usnews.com/usnews/nycu/health/hetophmo.htm

## EXERCISE
BREAST CANCER SURVIVOR'S REHABILATATION EXERCISE VIDEO
http://www.breastfit.com/index.html

EXERCISE: A GUIDE FROM NIA AND NASA
http://weboflife.arc.nasa.gov/exerciseandaging/cover.html

EXERCISE AND FITNESS
http://www.oznet.ksu.edu/ext_f&n/NUTLINK/pages/
EXERCISE.HTM

FIT FACTS
http://www.acefitness.org/fitfacts

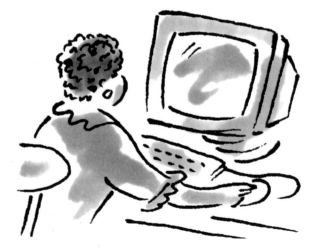

FITNESS LINK
http://www.fitnesslink.com/

GLOBAL FITNESS
http://www.global-fitness.com/

## FOOD, NUTRITION, AND RECIPES

CANCER / CANCER PREVENTION – INFORMATION FROM AICR – ONLINE
http://www.aicr.org/

EAT 5 A DAY FOR BETTER HEALTH
http://www.healthyfood.org/

THE FOOD PYRAMID
http://www.ganesa.com/food/index.html

LIVING AND RAW FOODS: THE LIVING AND RAW FOODS FAQ
http://www.rawfoods.com/faq.html

MEALS FOR YOU – RECIPES
http://www.mymenus.com/

NUTRITION NEWS
http://www.health-alliance.com/nutritionnews.html

TUFTS UNIVERSITY NUTRITION NAVIGATOR
http://www.navigator.tufts.edu/

US FOOD AND DRUG ADMINISTRATION
http://www.ama-assn.org/

## HOME HEALTH CARE AND CAREGIVERS

CAREGUIDE
http://www.careguide.com/

FAMILY CAREGIVER ALLIANCE
http://www.caregiver.org/

NATIONAL ASSOCIATION FOR HOME CARE
http://www.nahc.org/

NATIONAL FAMILY CAREGIVERS ASSOCIATON
http://www.nfcacares.org/

VISITING NURSE ASSOCIATIONS OF AMERICA
http://www.vnaa.org/

## LEGAL HELP AND GOVERNMENT SITES

ADMINISTRATION ON AGING
http://www.aoa.dhhs.gov/

DEPARTMENT OF VETERENS AFFAIRS
http://www.va.gov/

DISABLED AMERICAN VETERANS NATION HEADQUARTERS
http://www.dav.org

HCFA-MEDICARE, MEDICAID AND CHILDREN'S HEALTH INSURANCE AGENCY
http://www.hcfa.gov/

SOCIAL SECURITY ONLINE
http://www.ssa.gov/

## MEDICAL TERMINOLOGY

LIST AND GLOSSARY OF MEDICAL TERMS
http://allserv.rug.ac.be/~rvdstich/eugloss/EN/lijst.html

MEDICAL AND SURGICAL GLOSSARY
http://www.mtdesk.com/swg.shtml

MEDICAL TERMINOLOGY AND CANCER
http://spade39.ncl.ac.uk/medterm/

PATIENT'S GUIDE GLOSSARY
http://www3.bc.sympatico.ca/me/patientsguide/glos_a.htm

## MEDICINES AND DRUGS

CancerBACUP-CHEMOTHERAPY DRUGS
http://www.cancerbacup.org.uk/info/cancer-treatments.htm

FOOD AND DRUG ADMINISTRATION
http://www.fda.gov/default.htm

MEDICINENET.COM
http://medicinenet.com/Script/Main/AlphaIdx.asp?li=MNI&d=61&p=A_PHARM

NONPRESCRIPTION MEDICINES
http://www.fda.gov/opacom/what'sright/index.html

PATIENTSUPPORT.COM COMMON CHEMOTHERAPY DRUGS
http://patientsupport.com/Drugs/CommonDrugs.asp

PHARMINFONET
http://pharminfo.com/pin_hp.html

## MISCELLANEOUS CANCER-RELATED WEBSITES

ALCOHOLICS ANONYMOUS
http://www.alcoholics-anonymous.org/

CANCER HOPE NETWORK
http://www.cancerhopenetwork.org/

CHEMOTHERAPY SIDE EFFECTS
http://cancernet.nci.nih.gov/chemotherapy/chemoside.html#anchor1297603

COMPLETE LIST OF ONCOLOGY JOURNALS
http://www.sciencekomm.at/journals/medicine/onco.html

# Websites, cont.

ESTATE PLANNING
http://www.savewealth.com/planning/estate/index.html

FUNERALS; A CONSUMER GUIDE
http://www.ftc.gov/bcp/conline/pubs/services/funeral.htm

HAIR LOSS
http://bigjohn.bmi.net/mcaron/hair.html

IMPOTENCE
http://www.healthlinkusa.com/
161feat.htm

INSURANCE GLOSSARY
http://www.life-line.org/life/glossary/glossarya.html

INSURANCE GUIDE FOR CONSUMERS
http://www.hiaa.org/cons/cons.htm MEALS ON WHEELS
http://www.projectmeal.org/

MEDICALERT
http://www.medicalert.org/

GILLETTE WOMEN'S CANCER CONNECTION
http://www.gillettecancerconnect.org/

NATIONAL ASSOCIATION FOR CONTINENCE
http://www.nafc.org/

NATIONAL LOSS OF LIMB INFORMATION CENTER
http://www.amputee-coalition.org/

ONLINE LIST OF PET FACILITIES
http://www.nuc.ucla.edu/html_docs/PET/petcenters.html

OUTLOOK-LIFE BEYOND CHILDHOOD CANCER
http://www.outlook-life.org/

PATIENT ADVOCATES FOR ADVANCED CANCER TREATMENTS
http://www.osz.com/paact/

PET SCAN FREQUENTLY ASKED QUESTIONS
http://www.usc.edu/schools/medicine/academic_departments/radiology/uscpet/PETfaqs.html

PORTS AND CATHETERS
http://www.mededcon.com/cvct_c.htm

TREATING CANCER WITH RADIATION THERAPY
http://www.astro.org/patients/treating_cancer/what_happens_before.html

UNDERSTANDING ADJUVANT CHEMOTHERAPY
http://www.cancerguide.org/adjuvant.html

UNDERSTANDING BLOOD TESTS
http://www.bmtnews.org/bmt/bmt.book/appendix.a.html

UNDERSTANDING PATHOLOGY REPORTS
http://www.cancerguide.org/pathology.html

VIATICAL SETTLEMENTS (ACCELERATED INSURANCE BENEFITS)
http://www.ftc.gov/bcp/conline/pubs/services/viatical.htm

WHAT IS A CAT SCAN?
http://www.imaginiscorp.com/ct-scan/

WHAT IS AN OPEN MRI?
http://www.washingtonopenmri.com/openmri.htm

WHAT IS GAMMA KNIFE RADIOSURGERY?
http://www.nwhgammaknife.com/aboutframes/frameset.html

YOU ARE NOT ALONE
http://www.yana.org/organizations.htm

## NCI'S CLINICAL TRIALS COOPERATIVE GROUP, COMMUNITY CLINICAL ONCOLOGY PROGRAM (CCOP), CANCER CENTERS PROGRAM, AND COMPREHENSIVE CANCER CENTERS

CANCER CENTERS PROGRAM
http://www.nci.nih.gov/cancercenters/centerslist.html

CLINICAL CANCER CENTERS
http://rex.nci.nih.gov/massmedia/backgrounders/clin_cancer_cents.htm

CLINICAL TRIALS COOPERATIVE GROUP
http://cancernet.nci.nih.gov/clinpdq/nci/NCI's_Clinical_Trials_Cooperative_Group_Program.html#1

COMMUNITY ONCOLOGY AND PREVENTION TRIALS RESEARCH
http://dcp.nci.nih.gov/corb/

COMPREHENSIVE CANCER CENTERS
http://rex.nci.nih.gov/massmedia/backgrounders/nciccc.HTM

SEARCH FOR CANCER CENTERS BY GEOGRAPHICAL REGION
http://cancertrials.nci.nih.gov/finding/centers/html/map.html

## ONLINE CANCER SUPPORT GROUPS, CHAT ROOMS, AND BULLETIN BOARDS

ALLHEALTH CHATS
http://www.ivillage.com/allhealth/chat/weekglance/

CANCER CHATS-LINKS
http://www.geocities.com/HotSprings/1505/cancerchats.html

DRKOOP.COM HEALTH CHATS
http://www.drkoop.com/community/chat/general.asp

MEDICONSULT.COM SUPPORT GROUPS
http://www.mediconsult.com/mc/mcsite.nsf/conditionnav/supportgroup

ONCOCHAT
http://www.oncochat.org/

## ONLINE HEALTH NEWSLETTERS

SUBSCRIBE TO CANCER INFORMATION AND SUPPORT INTERNATIONAL
http://www.cancer-info.com/

SUBSCRIBE TO HEALTHANDAGE NEWSALERT
http://www.healthandage.com/fpatient.htm

SUBSCRIBE TO HOUSECALL FROM MAYO CLINIC
http://www.mayohealth.org/mayo/common/htm/hsecall.htm

SUBSCRIBE TO INTELIHEALTH FROM JOHNS HOPKINS
http://www.intelihealth.com/IH/ihtIH/WSIHW000/408/7046.html?
k=menuEMailFR8096

SUBSCRIBE TO MEDINEWSLETTER
http://www.mediconsult.com/mc/mcsite.nsf/newsletter

SUBSCRIBE TO LATELY AT MEMORIAL-SLOAN KETTERING CANCER CENTER
(MSKCC)
http://www.mskcc.org/patients_n_public/outreach_and_education/
lately_mskcc/subscribe.cfm

SUBSCRIBE TO NUTRITIONAL NEWS FOCUS
http://www.nutritionnewsfocus.com/archive/a1/NuFrEldrly.html

## ONLINE PHARMACIES

DRUGSTORE.COM
http://www.drugstore.com

ECKERD ONLINE
http://www.eckerd.com/

PLANTETRX.COM
http://www.planetrx.com/

WALGREENS
http://www.walgreens.com/

## PAIN MANAGEMENT

AMERICAN CHRONIC PAIN ASSOCIATION
http://www.theacpa.org/

AMERICAN PAIN FOUNDATION
http://www.painfoundation.org/

CANCER PAIN AT PAIN.COM
http://www.pain.com/cancerpain/default2.cfm

MANAGEMENT OF CANCER PAIN
http://www.drugguide.com/documents/articles/management.htm

THE NATIONAL FOUNDATION FOR THE TREATMENT OF PAIN
http://www.paincare.org/

PAIN.COM
http://www.pain.com/cancerpain/default2.cfm

## STOP SMOKING

AMERICAN CANCER SOCIETY – TOBACCO INFORMATION
http://www.cancer.org/tobacco/index.html

AMERICAN LUNG ASSOCIATION
http://www.lungusa.org/

CHECK YOUR SMOKING
http://www.heartscreen.com/smoking_info.html

HOW TO QUIT SMOKING-US DEPT. OF HEALTH AND HUMAN SERVICES
http://www.hoptechno.com/book43.htm

QUITNET
http://www.quitnet.org/qn_main.jtml?nosession=true

QUIT SMOKING ONLINE GROUPS
http://www.geocities.com/HotSprings/Spa/8122/

## TRANSPORTATION SERVICES

AIRLIFELINE
http://www.airlifeline.org/

CORPORATE ANGLE NETWORK, INC
http://www.corpangelnetwork.org/

DREAMLINE, FREE TRAVEL FOR CHILDREN WITH CANCER
http://www.bobiverson.com/dreamline.htm

# Websites, cont.

MERCY MEDICAL AIRLIFT
http://www.mercymedical.org/

NATIONAL PATIENT AIR TRANSPORT HELPLINE
http://www.npath.org/

## UP-TO-THE-MINUTE HEALTH NEWS
ABCNEWS.COM-HEALTH
http://abcnews.go.com/sections/living/

AMERICAN CANCER SOCIETY-NEWS TODAY
http://www2.cancer.org/zine/index.cfm

CBS NEWS-HEALTH
http://www.cbs.com/now/section/0,1636,204-311,00.shtml

CNN.COM-HEALTH
http://www.cnn.com/HEALTH/

INTELIHEALTH-TOP NEWS
http://www.intelihealth.com/IH/ihtIH/WSIHW000/333/
7228.html?k=NEWSbyTopicFR408

MAYO HEALTH OASIS
http://www.mayohealth.org/

MSNBC-HEALTH
http://www.msnbc.com/tools/nm/nm9no.asp?p=/news/
HEALTH_Front.asp

REUTERS HEALTH INFORMATION
http://www.reutershealth.com/frame_eline.html

TODAY ON MEDSCAPE
http://www.medscape.com/

USA TODAY HEALTH-INDEX OF RECENT CANCER STORIES
http://www.usatoday.com/life/health/archive.htm#cancer

YOUR HEALTH DAILY
http://www.yourhealthdaily.com/

## VITAMINS AND HERB INFORMATION AND ONLINE STORES
GNC
http://www.gnc.com/

HENA'S HERB GARDEN
http://www.herblore.com/

HERBAL ENCYCLOPEDIA
http://www.wic.net/waltzark/herbindex.htm

HERBAL INFORMATION CENTER
http://www.kcweb.com/herb/herbmain.htm

HERBS HERBAL
http://www.herbsherbals.com/index2.html

MOTHER NATURE
http://www.mothernature.com/

PURITAN PRIDE
http://www.puritan.com

VITAMINS.COM
http://www.vitamins.com/

VITAMIN SHOPPE
http://www.vitaminshoppe.com/

## SPECIFIC CANCERS

### ADRENAL CANCER
ANDRENAL CANCER
http://www.femaleurology.com/adrenalcancer

ADRENAL GLAND DISORDERS AND TREATMENTS
http://www.adrenal.com/

ENDCOCRINE WEB.COM.
http://www.endocrineweb.com/

### ANAL CANCER
ANAL CANCER
http://www.cancer-info.com/analcanc.htm

ANAL CANCER-MEDNEWS
http://imsdd.meb.uni-bonn.de/cancernet/100022.html

### BILE DUCT CANCER
EXTRAHEPATIC BILE DUCT CANCER
http://www.meb.uni-bonn.de/Cancernet/101191.html

RECURRENT EXTRAHEPATIC BILE DUCT CANCER
http://rarediseases.info.nih.gov/ord/wwwprot/menu/dx01194.html

### BLADDER CANCER
BLADDER CANCER
http://www.tirgan.com/bladder.htm

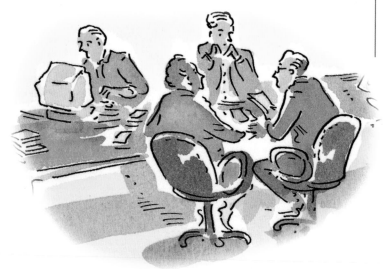

BLADDER CANCER
http://www.2rui.com/html/bladder_cancer.html

BLADDER CANCER LINKS
http://www.cancerlinks.org/bladder.html#BLADDER

TCC BLADDER CANCER
http://www.urologyconsultants.com/tcc.htm

UNDERSTANDING BLADDER CANCER
http://telescan.nki.nl/bladder2.html

WELLNESS WEB-BLADDER CANCER
http://www.wellweb.com/index/qbladcan.htm

## BRAIN TUMORS

AMERICAN BRAIN TUMOR ASSOCIATION
http://www.abta.org

BRAIN CANCER LINKS
http://www.cancerlinks.org/brain.html#BRAIN

BRAIN TUMOR INFORMATION
http://member.aol.com/lsdpout/brtmr.htm

BRAIN TUMOR SOCIETY HOME PAGE
http://www.tbts.org/

NATIONAL BRAIN TUMOR ASSOCIATION
http://www.braintumor.org/

PEDIATRIC BRAIN TUMOR FOUNDATION
http://www.ride4kids.org/

WELLNESS WEB-BRAIN CANCER
http://www.wellweb.com/index/qbrainca.htm

## BREAST CANCER

BREAST CANCER
http://www.cancernews.com/breast.htm

BREAST CANCER
http://msn.directhit.com/fcgi-bin/RedirURL.fcg?url=
http://www.mskcc.org/document/WICBREAS.htm
&qry=breast+cancer&rnk=3&src=MSN_SRCH

BREAST CANCER-DOCTORS GUIDE TO THE INTERNET
http://www.cancerhelp.com/ed

BREAST CANCER FUND EVENTS
http://www.breastcancerfund.org/index.html

BREAST CANCER LINKS
http://www.cancerlinks.org/breast.html#BREAST

BREAST CANCERINFO.COM
http://www.erinet.com/fnadoc/brest.htm

INFO BREAST CANCER
http://www.infobreastcancer.cyberus.ca/

NATIONAL ALLIANCE OF BREAST CANCER ORGANIZATIONS
http://www.nabco.org/

SUSANLOVEMD.COM
http://www.susanlovemd.com/

THE SUSAN G. KOMEN BREAST CANCER FOUNDATION
http://www.komen.org/

WELLNESS WEB-BREAST CANCER
http://www.wellweb.com/BREAST/BRHOMEPG.htm

## CERVICAL CANCER

CANCER OF THE CERVIX
http://www.gyncancer.com/cervix.html

CERVICAL CANCER LINKS
http://www.cancerlinks.org/cervical.html#CERVICAL

GYNECOLOGICAL ONCOLOGY
http://www.wvhealth.wvu.edu/clinical/oncology/index.htm

NATIONAL CERVICAL CANCER COALITION
http://www.nccc-online.org/

WELLNESS WEB-CERVICAL CANCER
http://www.wellweb.com/index/QCERVICA.HTM

## CHILDHOOD CANCERS

CANDLELIGHTERS CHILDHOOD CANCER FOUNDATION
http://www.candlelighters.org/

CHILDHOOD BRAIN TUMOR ORGANIZATION
http://www.mnsinc.com/cbtf/index.html#links

CHILDREN'S HOSPICE INTERNATIONAL
http://www.chionline.org/

THE CHILDREN'S ORGAN TRANSPLANT ASSOCIATION
http://www.unitedway.bartholomew.in.us/irisonline/
Childrens_Organ_Transplant_Association_COTA.html

FAMILIES WITH CHILDREN CANCER HOME PAGE
http://www.interlog.com/~fcc/

HOLE IN THE WALL GANG CAMP
http://www.holeinthewallgang.org/index2.html

HOSPITAL TOUR FOR KIDS
http://ww2.med.jhu.edu/peds/neonatology/fun.html

MAKE-A-WISH FOUNDATION OF AMERICA
http://www.wish.org/

NATIONAL CHILDHOOD CANCER FOUNDATION
http://www.nccf.org/

NATIONAL CHILDREN'S LEUKEMIA FOUNDATION
http://www.leukemiafoundation.org/

# Websites, cont.

NATIONAL BRAIN TUMOR ASSOCIATION
http://www.braintumor.org/

PEDIATRIC BRAIN TUMOR FOUNDATION
http://www.ride4kids.org/

WELLNESS WEB-BRAIN CANCER
http://www.wellweb.com/index/qbrainca.htm

PEDIATRIC ONCOLOGY GROUP
http://www.pog.ufl.edu/

RONALD McDONALD HOUSE CHARITIES
http://www.mcdonalds.com/community/rmhc/index.html

SPECIAL LOVE FOR CHILDREN WITH CANCER
http://www.speciallove.org/

STARLIGHT FOUNDATION INTERNATIONAL
http://www.starlight.org/

ST. JUDE CHILDREN'S RESEARCH HOSPITAL
http://www.stjude.org/

SUNSHINE FOUNDATION
http://enetis.net/~dkendall/sunshine.htm

## COLON AND RECTAL CANCER
A PATIENTS GUIDE TO RECTAL CANCER
http://www.mdanderson.org/focus/colon/guide.htm

COLON CANCER ALLIANCE
http://www.ccalliance.org/

COLON CANCER LINKS
http://www.cancerlinks.org/colon.html#COLON

COLON CANCER ONLINE
http://www.meds.com/colon/colon.html

COLON CONNECTIONS
http://rattler.cameron.edu/colon/

COLON POLYPS, COLON CANCER
http://www.maxinet.com/mansell/polyp.htm

COLORECTAL CANCER
http://www.wehealny.org/healthinfo/coloncancer/treat.html

COLORECTAL CANCER
http://www.mskcc.org/document/WICcolon.htm

COLORECTAL CANCER LINKS
http://www.cancerlinks.org/colorectal.html#COLORECTAL

WELLNESS WEB-COLON CANCER
http://www.wellweb.com/index/qcolonca.htm

## ENDOCRINE CANCER
THE ENDOCRINE SOCIETY HOME PAGE
http://www.endo-society.org/index.htm

ENDOCRINE WEB.COM.
http://www.endocrineweb.com/

## ENDOMETRIAL CANCER
ENDOMETRIAL CANCER
http://members.xoom.com/mariok123/ec/ec.htm

ENDOMETRIAL CANCER LINKS
http://www.cancerlinks.org/endometrial.html#ENDOMETRIAL

## ESOPHAGEAL CANCER
ESOPHAGEAL CANCER-CANCERLINKSUSA.COM
http://www.cancerlinks.org/esophagus.html#ESOPHAGUS

UNDERSTANDING CANCER OF THE ESOPHAGUS
http://msn.directhit.com/fcgi-bin/RedirURL.fcg?url=
http://www.cancerbacup.org.uk/info/oesophagus.htm&qry=
esophagus+cancer&rnk=1&src=MSN_SRCH

WHAT YOU NEED TO KNOW ABOUT CANCER OF THE ESOPHAGUS-NCI
http://rex.nci.nih.gov/WTNK_PUBS/esoph/index.htm

## EYE CANCER
EYE CANCER LINKS
http://www.cancerlinks.org/eye.html#EYE

THE EYE CANCER NETWORK
http://www.eyecancer.com/

## GALL BLADDER CANCER
GALL BLADDER CANCER
http://www.cancer-info.com/gallblad.htm

## GASTROINTESTINAL TRACT
GASTROINTESTINAL CANCER
http://www.graylab.ac.uk/cancerweb/further/gastro.html

ONCOLINK: GASTRIC CANCER
http://www.oncolink.upenn.edu/disease/gastric/index.html

TUMORS OF THE GASTROINTESTINAL TRACT
http://www.bioscience.org/atlases/tumpath/gitract/resource.htm

## GYNECOLOGICAL CANCERS
FEMALE GENITAL CANCER LINKS
http://www2.kumc.edu/kci/cancerlinks/female.htm

GYNECOLOGICAL CANCER INQUIRY
http://members.aol.com/GynCancer/

GYNECOLOGICAL ONCOLOGY
http://www.wvhealth.wvu.edu/clinical/oncology/index.htm

VAGINAL CANCER LINKS
http://www.cancerlinks.org/vaginal.html#VAGINAL

VULVAR CANCER LINKS
http://www.cancerlinks.org/vulvar.html#VULVAR

WOMEN'S CANCER CENTER
http://wccenter.com/

## HEAD AND NECK
AMERICAN ORAL CANCER CLINIC
http://www.tonguecancer.com/

CANCER OF THE LARYNX-CANCERLINKS
http://cancerlinksusa.com/larynx/

HEAD AND NECK CANCER
http://www.upmc.edu/HealthMed/Services/Cancer/HeadNeck/

HEAD AND NECK CANCERS-CANCER NET LINKS
http://cancer.miningco.com/msubh-n.htm

MDACC - HEAD AND NECK
http://www.mdanderson.org/centers/headneck/

SUPPORT FOR PEOPLE WITH ORAL AND HEAD AND NECK CANCER
http://www.spohnc.org/

VOICE BOX CANCER
http://www.tonguecancer.com/voice_box_cancer.htm

## KAPOSI'S SARCOMA
THE BODY-KAPOSI'S SARCOMA
http://www.thebody.com/treat/kaposis.html

HIV CLINICAL TRIALS SEARCH
http://hivinsite.ucsf.edu/tsearch KAPOSI'S SARCOMA
http://www.noah.cuny.edu/cancer/nci/cancernet/201271.html

SARCOMA CANCER LINKS
http://www.cancerlinks.org/sarcoma.html#SARCOMA

## KIDNEY CANCER
AMERICAN FOUNDATION FOR UROLOGIC DISEASE
http://www.afud.org

KIDNEY CANCER ASSOCIATION
http://www.nkca.org/index.stm

KIDNEY CANCER HEALTH AND MEDICAL INFORMATION
http://www.mediconsult.com/mc/mcsite.nsf/conditionnav/kidney~
sectionintroduction

UNDERSTANDING CANCER OF THE KIDNEY
http://www.cancerbacup.org.uk/info/kidney.htm

## LEUKEMIA
GRANNYBARB AND ART'S LEUKEMIA LINKS:
http://www.acor.org/leukemia/frame.html

LEUKEMIA CANCER LINKS
http://www.cancerlinks.org/leukemia.html#LEUKEMIA

LEUKEMIA SOCIETY OF AMERICA
http://www.leukemia.org/

NATIONAL CHILDREN'S LEUKEMIA FOUNDATION
http://www.leukemiafoundation.org/

## LIVER CANCER
LIVER CANCER IN CHILDREN
http://www.livertx.org/livercancerlinks.html

LIVER CANCER LINKS
http://www.cancerlinks.org/liver.html#LIVER

LIVER CANCER NETWORK
http://www.livercancer.com/

LIVER DISEASE
http://www.mediconsult.com/mc/mcsite.nsf/conditionnav/liver~sec
tionintroduction

## LUNG CANCER
ALLIANCE FOR LUNG CANCER ADVOCATES
http://www.alcase.org/

AMERICAN LUNG ASSOCIATION
http://www.lungusa.org/

LUNG CANCER LINKS
http://www.cancerlinks.org/lung.html#LUNG

LUNG CANCER ONLINE
http://www.lungcanceronline.org/

LUNG CANCER STAGING
http://www.erinet.com/fnadoc/images/pathol~1/lungca~1/
stage.htm

MERCK MANUAL GERIATRICS-LUNG CANCER
http://www.merck.com/pubs/mm_geriatrics/50x.htm

NON-SMALL CELL LUNG CANCER
http://www.meds.com/pdq/nonsmallcell_pat.html

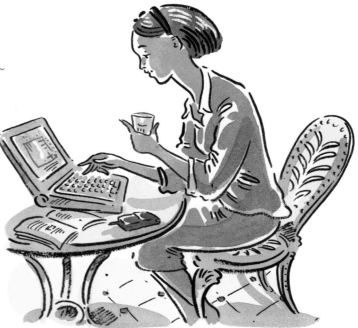

# Websites, cont.

NON-SMALL CELL LUNG CANCER
http://members.aol.com/Chester878/info.html

WELLNESS WEB – LUNG CANCER NSC
http://www.wellweb.com/index/QLUNGNONSMALL.HTM

## LYMPHEDEMA

LYMPHEDEMA
http://www.geocities.com/~akoffman/msub17.html

LYMPHEDEMA  E-SUPPORT GROUP
http://www.acor.org/listserv.html?to_do=
interact&listname=LYMPHEDEMA

LYMPHEDEMA RESEARCH FOUNDATION
http://www.lymphaticresearch.org/

NATIONAL LYMPHEDEMA NETWORK
http://www.lymphnet.org/

## LYMPHOMA

CURE FOR LYMPHOMA FOUNDATION
http://www.cfl.org

LYMPHOMA CANCER LINKS
http://www.cancerlinks.org/lymphoma.html#LYMPHOMA

LYMPHOMA INFORMATION NETWORK
http://www.lymphomainfo.net/

LYMPHOMA RESEARCH FOUNDATION
http://www.lymphoma.org/

NON-HODGKINS LYMPHOMA
http://www.westvirginia.net/~sigley/NHL_Web_site_explain.htm

## MESOTHELIOMA

MEDICINE NET– MESOTHELIOMA
http://www.medicinenet.com/Script/Main/Art.asp?li=MNI&d=171
&f=406&ArticleKey= 12308

MESOTHELIOMA INFORMATION NEWSLETTER
http://www.mesothelioma-facts.com/

MESOTHELIOMA WEB
http://www.mesotheliomaweb.org/

## MYELOMA

THE INTERNATIONAL MYELOMA FOUNDATION
http://www.myeloma.org/

MULTIPLE MYELOMA RESEARCH
http://myeloma.med.cornell.edu/

MULTIPLE MYELOMA RESEARCH FOUNDATION
http://www.ghgroup.com/myelomafoundation/

MYELOMA CANCER LINKS
http://www.cancerlinks.org/myeloma.html#MYELOMA

## OVARIAN CANCER

GILDA RADNER FAMILIAL OVARIAN CANCER REGISTRY
http://rpci.med.buffalo.edu/clinic/gynonc/grwp.html

GYNECOLOGICAL ONCOLOGY
http://www.wvhealth.wvu.edu/clinical/oncology/index.htm

NATIONAL OVARIAN CANCER COALITION
http://www.ovarian.org/main.html

OVARIAN CANCER DIAGNOSIS
http://www.jeffersonhealth.org/diseases/gyn_onc/ovdiag.htm

OVARIAN CANCER LINKS
http://www.cancerlinks.org/ovarian.html#OVARIAN

## PANCREATIC CANCER

JOHNS HOPKINS PANCREATIC CANCER
http://www.path.jhu.edu/pancreas

PANCREATIC CANCER ACTION NETWORK
http://www.pancan.org/

PANCREATIC CANCER LINK PAGE
http://www.1mainst.com/cancer/

PANCREATIC CANCER LINKS
http://www.cancerlinks.org/pancreas.html#PANCREATIC

WHAT YOU NEED TO KNOW ABOUT CANCER OF THE PANCREAS
http://www.sterner.org/~dsterner/pancreas/95-1560/95-1560.htm

## PENILE CANCER

PENILE CANCER
http://imsdd.meb.uni-bonn.de/cancernet/201082.html

PENILE CANCER
http://www.noah.cuny.edu/cancer/nci/cancernet/201082.html

## PITUITARY CANCER

PITUITARY CANCER
http://www.noah.cuny.edu/cancer/nci/cancernet/201273.html

PITUITARY TUMOR
http://imsdd.meb.uni-bonn.de/cancernet/101273.html

PITUITARY TUMOR NETWORK ASSOCIATION
http://www.pituitary.com/

## PROSTATE CANCER

FLORIDA UROLOGICAL INSTITUTE
http://www.fla-urological.com/proscanc.html

PROSTATE CANCER HOME PAGE
http://www.cancer.med.umich.edu/prostcan/prostcan.html

PROSTATE CANCER INFOLINK
http://www.comed.com/Prostate/

PROSTATE CANCER LINKS
http://www.cancerlinks.org/prostate.html#PROSTATE

PROSTATE CANCER PDQ
http://www.wellweb.com./PROSTATE/pdq.htm

PROSTATE DICTIONARY
http://www.comed.com/Prostate/Glossary.html

US TOO INTERNATIONAL, INC. PROSTATE CANCER SUPPORT GROUPS
http://www.ustoo.com/

VIRGIL'S PROSTATE-ONLINE
http://prostate-online.com/

WELLNESS WEB-PROSTATE CANCER
http://www.wellweb.com/PROSTATE/prostate.htm

## SARCOMAS

SARCOMA CANCER LINKS
http://www.cancerlinks.org/sarcoma.html#SARCOMA

WELLNESS WEB-SARCOMA
http://www.wellweb.com/index/QSARCOMA.HTM

## SKIN

AMERICAN ACADEMY OF DERMATOLOGY
http://www.aad.org

INTRODUCTION TO SKIN CANCER
http://www.maui.net/~southsky/introto.html

MELANOMA CANCER LINKS
http://www.cancerlinks.org/melanoma.html#MELANOMA

MELANOMA.COM
http://www.melanoma.com/

NATIONAL CANCER INSTITUTE: MELANOMA
http://cancernet.nci.nih.gov/wyntk_pubs/melanoma.htm

SKIN CANCER – CONSUMER ZONE
http://www.skin-cancer.com/consumer/con_indx.htm

WELLNESS WEB-SKIN CANCER
http://www.wellweb.com/index/QSKINCAN.HTM

## SMALL INTESTINES

SMALL INTESTINE CANCER
http://www.noah.cuny.edu/cancer/nci/cancernet/201175.html

SMALL INTESTINE CANCER LINKS
http://www2.kumc.edu/kci/cancerlinks/intestine.htm

## STOMACH

STOMACH CANCER
http://www2.kumc.edu/kci/cancerlinks/stomach.htm

WELLNESS WEB-STOMACH CANCER
http://www.wellweb.com/INDEX/QSTOMACH.HTM

WHAT YOU NEED TO KNOW ABOUT STOMACH CANCER
http://www.cancerlinksusa.com/stomach/wynk.htm

## TESTICULAR CANCER

TESTICULAR CANCER LINKS
http://www.cancerlinks.org/testicular.html#TESTICULAR

THE TESTICULAR CANCER RESOURCE CENTER
http://www.acor.org/TCRC/

TESTICULE
http://prostate.urol.jhu.edu/diseases/testicle/testicle.html

## THYROID

AMERICAN THYROID CLINIC,
http://www.thyroidcancer.com/

CANCER OF THE THYROID
http://www.thyroid.org/patient/brochur1.htm

THYROID CANCER
http://www.endocrineweb.com/thyroidca.html

THYROID CANCER-CANCER WEB
http://www.graylab.ac.uk/cancernet/201252.html

THYROID CANCER LINKS
http://www.cancerlinks.org/thyroid.html#THYROID

# Other Resources

## NATIONAL CANCER INSTITUTE PUBLICATIONS

These booklets are free from NCI's Cancer Information Service and are a rich source of information for patients and their families. Placing your order is simple and can be done in one of two ways. Call (800)4-CANCER, which will connect you to the regional office of the Cancer Information Service, or go online to use the National Cancer Institute publication locator, a fast and easy way to order those of interest to you. Their web address is **http://publications.nci.nih.gov/ default.asp** The limit is 20 publications per order.

• Anticancer Drug Information Sheets
• Chemotherapy and You: A Guide to Self-help During Treatment
• Eating Hints: Recipes and Tips for Better Nutrition During Cancer Treatments
• Radiation Therapy and You: A Guide to Self-help During Treatments

• Taking Time: Support for People with Cancer and the People Who Care about Them
• What You Need to Know: A Series of Booklets Detailing Specific Types of Cancer
• Advanced Cancer: Living Each Day.
• What are Clinical Trials All About?
• Facing Forward: A Guide for Cancer Survivors.
• Questions and Answers about Pain Control
• When Cancer Recur: Meeting the Challenge Again
• What You Need to Know about Bladder Cancer
• Questions and Answers about Bone Cancer
• What You Need to Know about Brain Tumors
• Breast Cancer Risk Assessment Tool
• Genetic Testing for Breast Cancer Risk: It's Your Choice
• Mammograms...Not Just Once but for a Lifetime!
• Questions and Answers about Breast Calcifications
    • The Picture of Health: How to Increase Breast Cancer Screening in your Community
    • The Facts about Breast Cancer and Mammography
    • Understanding Breast Cancer Treatment: A Guide for Patients

• Understanding Breast Changes: A Health Guide for All Women
• What You Need to Know about Breast Cancer
• Having a Pelvic Exam and Pap Test
• Pap Test: A Healthy Habit for Life!
• The Pap Test: It Can Save Your Life!
• What You Need to Know about Cervical Cancer
• Managing Your Child's Eating Problems during Cancer Treatment
• Talking with Your Child about Cancer
• Young People with Cancer: A Handbook for Parents
• We Need You to Make a Difference: Prostate, Lung, Colorectal, and Ovarian Cancer Screening Trial
• What You Need to Know about Cancer of the Colon and Rectum
• What You Need to Know about Esophagus Cancer
• What You Need to Know about Hodgkin's Disease
• What You Need to Know about Kidney Cancer
• What You Need to Know about Cancer of the Larynx
• What You Need to Know about Leukemia
• Questions and Answers about Liver Cancer
• We Need You to Make a Difference: Prostate, Lung, Colorectal, and Ovarian Cancer Screening Trial
• What You Need to Know about Lung Cancer
• What You Need to Know about Melanoma
• What You Need to Know about Moles and Dysplastic Nevi
• What You Need to Know about Multiple Myeloma
• What You Need to Know about Non-Hodgkin's Lymphoma

- What You Need to Know about Oral Cancers
- What You Need to Know about Cancer of the Pancreas
- Understanding Prostate Changes: A Health Guide for All Men
- What You Need to Know about Prostate Cancer
- What You Need to Know about Skin Cancer
- What You Need to Know about Stomach Cancer
- Question and Answers about Thyroid Cancer
- What You Need to Know about Cancer of the Uterus
- Bone Marrow Transplantation and Peripheral Blood Stem Cell Transplantation
- Clinical Trials: A Blueprint for the Future
- Get Relief from Cancer Pain
- Helping Yourself during Chemotherapy: 4 Steps for Patients
- Taking Part in Clinical Trials: What Cancer Patients Need to Know
- Questions and Answers about Metastatic Cancer
- The Immune System – How It Works
- Understanding the Immune System
- Understanding Gene Testing
- Helping Yourself during Chemotherapy: 4 Steps for Patients
- 5–A–Day: Time to Take Five: Eat 5 Fruits and Vegetables Every Day
- Action Guide for Healthy Eating
- Cancer at a Crossroads
- Clearing the Air: A Guide to Quitting Smoking
- Dangerous Game: The Truth about Spit Tobacco
- Down Home Healthy Cookin'
- Eat Five Fruits and Vegetables Everyday
- Why Do You Smoke?

## CANCER CARE BRIEFS AND PUBLICATIONS

I am a firm believer that the best things in life are free, and the help that Cancer Care, Inc. provides confirms my convictions. Their online service

**(http://www.cancercare.org/ patients/informational.htm)**

provides access to:

**The Cancer Care Library:** Numerous articles on sexuality, breast cancer detection, and many other relevant and informative topics.

**Cancer Care Briefs:** Simple, yet comprehensive, one-to two-page briefs provide tips on a range of topics, from managing your HMO to structuring your healthcare team to finding information on the Internet.

**Media Stories and Links to Media Websites** – a constantly updated library of media stories concerning cancer and cancer-related topics, as well as several other cancer-related media websites.

In addition to the information you can download from their website, Cancer Care will send you free of charge the following publications if you call (800) 813-HOPE:

- *A Helping Hand: The Resource Directory for People with Cancer* This 144-page invaluable guide is an absolute must-have for all those with cancer. It is the first nationwide directory of free services and resources for people with cancer and their families, and it is remarkably helpful and easy to follow.
- *Learning about Lung Cancer: It Helps to Understand* This 44-page publication has extensive information on lung cancer symptoms, stages, recommended treatments and treatment side effects, tips on managing cancer pain, how to assess clinical trials, how to eat well during treatment, and how to find help and support.
- *Lung Cancer Information* An easy-to-read collection of Cancer Care Briefs with titles such as:
  What Is Lung Cancer?
  What Are the Symptoms of Lung Cancer and How Is It Diagnosed?
  What Are the Different "Stages" of Lung Cancer and What Is the Recommended Treatment?
  Your Lung Cancer Health Team: Your Doctor Is Only the Beginning
  "Doctor, Can We Talk?" Tips for Communicating with Your Doctor, Nurse, or Health Care Team if You Have Lung Cancer
  Lung Cancer and Clinical Trials: How Do I Decide if a Clinical Trial Is Right for Me?
- *Learning about Pancreatic Cancer: It Helps to Understand* A 60-page publication with extensive information on pancreatic cancer symptoms; stages; recommended treatments and their side effects; and important tips on managing cancer pain, assessing clinical trials, eating well during treatment, and getting the proper and necessary help and support.
- *Treatment Choices in Prostate Cancer* This 42-page booklet and accompanying video provide important information to help you take the right attitude toward the disease and make informed decisions about your treatment plan. You will find detailed information on prostate cancer, such as risk factors, role of testosterone, diagnosis, staging, treatment choices, and frequently asked questions.

# In Conclusion

## A personal letter to my fellow cancer patient

I hate that you have cancer. To be honest, I hate that I have had it, too. I hate the disease. I hate that people are forced to deal with it and I hate it that you have had reason to purchase this cancer workbook. I'm sorry for your pain. I'm sorry for your anxiety and for that of your loved ones, and for your suffering, both physical and mental. I wish that I could tell you in person how truly grieved I am. Over twenty-seven hundred people will be diagnosed with cancer today. Twenty-seven hundred. The very thought of it makes me weep. My desire to be with each and every one of you is hampered by the shear numbers of the newly diagnosed. This book is the product of my longing to get to you somehow, some way. To share with you what I know and have learned, to provide you with research skills, to encourage you to take the bull by the horns, and to steer you away from cancer's many pitfalls.

❋

I would like to get a little personal now and give you some things to think about: a bit of advice, a few warnings, suggestions, and helpful hints from someone who has been there and done that – a couple of times.

Different people are driven by different dynamics and no two will approach a crisis in the same way. The diagnosis of cancer brings out the unexpected in us and in those around us. I've seen and experienced a lot in the last six years. I have watched families and friends rise to the occasion by surrounding a patient with unrelenting love and support. I have seen just the opposite, as well. Friends that didn't call because of their own fears and spouses who have abandoned their partners to deal alone with that which they could not. I have sat by powerlessly and observed as cancer patients have fallen into the trap of depression. I've seen many emerge brand-new from the trauma and the darkness. I have watched as patients who could barely stand up, shuffled slowly across the floor of a doctor's office to place their arms around a crying stranger. I have been witness to families fighting over nothing at all. I've observed the power of determined cancer patients who have made getting well their priority. I've watched other patients become bitter and resentful as their priority has become everything but their

health. I've been honored to observe such bravery in the halls of hospitals and in treatment rooms that it has changed my life forever. I have seen the best in others and myself and I have seen the worst, as well.

Most patients will encounter problems at some level with family, friends, feelings, unfamiliar thoughts, or difficult circumstances. Emotionally you may feel as if you are up to your neck in uncharted waters but there are a few basics that I believe can help you stay afloat. First and foremost, do not expect others suddenly to alter their personalities because you are ill. Chances are if you have not been able to get emotional support, open communication, and an intimate connection with someone preceding cancer, you will not suddenly be able to obtain it now. If you are telling a companion your innermost private thoughts and he or she isn't connecting, be smart; and go where you have always gone in the past to relate your feelings. Remember that not everyone has the gift of knowing what to say. Not all people know how to show compassion or empathize and because you are ill doesn't mean that those things will automatically change. For the most part, your loved ones will love you in the way that they always have. Some will listen to you for five hours as you fall apart and some will make you a chocolate shake. Take it for what it is: their attempt at comfort. Do not put expectations on others – you are setting them up for failure. During this time it will be easy to feel let down by those you had hoped would instantly understand you, and resentment can rush in. Don't allow that. Treasure everything that is done for you by those who want to show their love their way.

Don't get angry if friends and family members cannot grasp the impact that the recurring fear holds over you each time you have a diagnostic test. They can not possibly understand the experience of having one's fate being decided by a CT scan or blood test. Realize, too, that the longer you stay in remission the more relaxed about your tests everyone else may become. They may feel that the importance of the tests have diminished. You'll feel differently.

Whatever you are thinking has been thought by someone else with cancer. You are not crazy. Don't hide from these thoughts and don't be hard on yourself, either. Remember, just because a particular family member or friend cannot

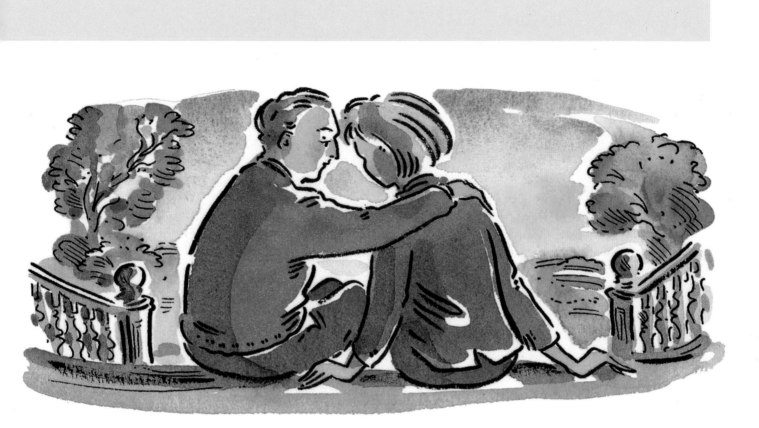

understand where you are coming from doesn't mean that where you are coming from isn't understandable. Join a support group!

Beware of mentally hibernating. That is a dangerous thing to do and can lead to depression. After months and months of dealing with the crisis of cancer, you may become sick and tired of being sick and tired. You especially get weary of talking out loud about your illness to people who you are sure are just as weary of hearing about it. If you have fears, worries, anxiety and questions that plague your mind, you need to keep talking. The day will come when you feel you have said it all. Until then…

Watch out for guilt; there seems to be tons of it circulating around those with cancer. Any number of things can cause you to feel self-condemnation: the fact that you require so much care and are costing your family a bundle of money; the realization that someone will have to take time out of their busy day to get you to the doctors. You blame yourself that your children are worried. You feel self-recrimination for thinking that you have become a burden. You even feel guilty that you are depressed and not your normal upbeat

self. GET OVER IT! These thoughts are self-defeating. You did not ask for this disease and no matter how much your loved ones are having to go through, they are not the ones going through cancer, you are. So be thankful for ever single thing that others do for you. Remember that you would do the same for them and discard the guilt!

Be careful that you don't assume the role of super-patient. There is no right or wrong way to have and fight the disease of cancer; you will find the best way for you. Live one day at a time. If you're happy, show it. If you're hurting, talk about it. Don't let the expectations of others dictate how you get through these days. However you handle this crisis is the best way for you to handle this crisis.

Watch out for resentment! It is like drinking poison and expecting someone else to die from it. Do not hold on to unforgivness, anger, hurt, hostility, rage, or sadness. If something needs to be settled, for crying out loud, settle it. Find a minister, mentor, trusted friend, or a counselor to help you with your issues. There is a lot on your plate right now but this can't wait. Forgiving someone is not for their benefit, it is for yours.

# In Conclusion, cont.

Take your pride and throw it out the window. Offer an apology to every person that you know deep in your heart deserves one. If apologies come your way, accept them.

Spend time loving your children. Tell them you are proud of them, that you cherish them, that they have enriched your life. Remember that they are scared, too.

Don't be a martyr. People will eventually see through it. Self-pity isn't all that bad as long as you immerse yourself in it, cry like a banshee, and move on. Don't wonder "why me?" It's counterproductive. The only answers you can come up with to a question like that are negative ones.

Nothing can play games with your mental state the way fatigue can. Cancer and its treatments will "take it out of you" and your exhaustion can leave you very vulnerable and touchy. Rest every chance you get. Don't overdo, trying to prove something to yourself or others. Keep in mind that if you suddenly feel like you're a "victim," you may be just bone-weary.

Dig a hole sixty feet deep. Bury all thoughts that pertain to feeling useless because you can't do what you use to do. Of course you can't, you are dealing with cancer. Let others help you. It will make them feel valuable and will nurture you.

Face the reality that you may never get back to the way you were before cancer. Grieve the loss and accept yourself. Don't allow the frustration of who you have become overpower the fact that you are alive. Bear in mind what is important here. If you can afford to lay off work while you are going through treatments and recuperating, do it. If it would drive you crazy to be stuck at home, then keep working. This is your life and you know what is best for you.

Watch out for the green-eyed devil. There is much to be jealous of. Basic things such as taking one's health for granted, carefree laughter, mobility, energy, holding a job, eating, having hair, the ability to exercise, a full night's sleep, a blank mind, a pain-free day and confidence in the future. The list goes on and on. Jealousy leads to resentfulness so don't think about "what everybody else has." It won't do you a bit of good.

If you can't stop thinking about your cancer and it is driving you insane, try thinking about someone else. The best thing I ever did during my bouts with cancer was to focus on helping patients who had just been diagnosed. I personally think that the act of giving during that time is what saved me.

Read this paragraph twice. It's that important. People who have never had cancer can NOT understand every single thing you are going through. They can listen to you, console you, hand you a pain pill, cry with you, worry about you, rub your legs, and even be more frightened for you than you are yourself, but they cannot know what it is like to have cancer. At some point you will feel "let down" if you don't continually bear that in mind. Remember, I said read that again.

When you get into remission (and I pray that you will), your friends and family will expect you to move on. Don't let that upset you. You may need to contemplate the impact that cancer has had on your life and to analyze what the victory of defeating this disease has cost you. That will likely take time.

In addition, you may find it almost impossible to believe that you are actually in remission. You may become acutely aware of every headache, sniffle, eye twitch, back ache, or twinge of pain. This awareness may bring on intense fear and thoughts that the cancer has returned. These feelings are completely normal. If the pain doesn't go away or if it intensifies after a few days, call your doctor for reassurance. Be gentle with yourself during this period of healing. The extreme highs and lows can be an open door to depression. Don't expect to bounce right back. Take your time, you have tomorrow.

Well, there it is, a bit of advice, a few warnings, suggestions, and helpful hints. I'm not terribly proud to admit it but I am intimately acquainted with everythng I've written about in this letter. These attributes have been part and parcel of my cancer experience. I've laid bare my imperfections and shortcomings in hopes that it might in some way be of help to you.

If I could change one thing in the world, I would change that you have ever heard the words "you have cancer". I hate that you have cancer, I really do. I am going to fight this disease in any way that I can. You fight it in any way that you can. Maybe together we can win.

In the meantime, I'll be praying for you.
*Joanie Willis*

## A Little Help from My Friends

*I could use your help. When I began writing* **The Cancer Patient's Workbook** *I had several goals in mind. To keep it simple, to make cancer less intimidating, to be as upbeat as possible, to focus on a variety of issues, to furnish information that a patient could actually use and to satisfy the need for a medical record-keeping journal. With over 100 different types of cancer I know that I can not possibly have considered every single issue, found every great internet site, posed every question for a doctor, or found every interesting bit of information out there. Please, if you know of something you believe would be suitable for this workbook and might benefit another cancer patients, please write to me care of Dorling Kindersley Publishing, Inc.*

*One last thing: If this workbook has helped you, you can safely assume that it will help others. In hospitals, doctors' offices, and treatment rooms across the country there are newly diagnosed patients who don't have a clue as to what is happening to them. If you observe patients you believe could use a book such as this, recommend it to them. Keep in mind that this may be a perfect opening to help someone and, in turn, to help yourself. Thanks and God Bless,*

*Joanie*

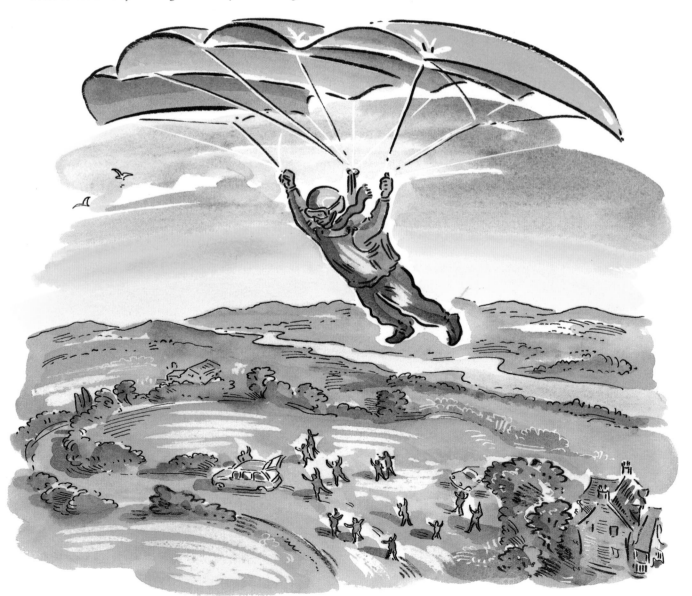

# Bibliography

**The Juicing Book,** by Stephen Blauer (Avery Publishing Group Inc., 1989)

**Food – Your Miracle Medicine,** by Jean Carper (HarperCollins Publishers, 1993)

**The Food Pharmacy,** by Jean Carper (Bantam Books, 1988)

**Miracle Cures,** by Jean Carper (HarperCollins Publishers, 1997)

**Stop Aging Now,** by Jean Carper (HarperCollins Publishers, 1995)

**Anatomy of an Illness,** by Norman Cousins (Bantam Doubleday Dell Publishers, 1979)

**Everyone's Guide to Cancer Therapy,** by Malin Dollinger, M.D., Ernest H. Rosenbaum, M.D., and Greg Cable (Somerville House Books Limited, 1991)

**Making the Chemotherapy Decision,** by David Drum (Lowell House, 1996)

**Making the Right Choice,** by Richard A. Evans, M.D. (Avery Publishing Group, 1995)

**Cancer Clinical Trials,** by Robert Finn (O'Reilly & Associates, Inc., 1999)

**The People's Pharmacy Guide to Home and Herbal Remedies,** by Joe Graedon and Teresa Graedon, Ph.D. (St. Martin's Press, 1999)

**The Healing Foods,** by Patricia Hausman & Judith Benn Hurley (Rodale Press, 1989)

**Foods That Heal,** by Dr. Bernard Jensen (Avery Publishing Group Inc., 1988)

**What to Eat if You Have Cancer,** by Maureen Kean, and Daniella Chace (Contemporary Books, Inc., 1996)

**The Juiceman's Power of Juicing,** by Jay Kordich (William Morrow & Co., Inc., 1992)

**Herbal Defense,** by Robyn Landis with Karta Purkh Singh (Warner Books, 1997)

**The Chemotherapy Survival Guide,** by Judith McKay, R.N. and Nancee Hirano, R.N., M.S.N. (New Harbinger Publication, Inc, 1993)

**Nature's Medicines** by Gale Maleskey and the Editors of Prevention Health Books (Rodale Press, Inc., 1999)

**Choices,** by Marion Morra & Eve Potts (William Morrow & Co., Inc., 1994, rev. ed.)

**American Cancer Society – Informed Decisions,** by Gerald P. Murphy, M.D., Lois B. Morris, and Dianne Lange (Viking Penguin, 1997)

**The Antioxidant Miracle,** by Lester Packer, Ph.D., and Carol Colman (John Wiley & Sons, Inc., 1999)

**The Complete Idiot's Guide to Vitamins and Minerals,** by Alan H. Pressman, D.C., Ph.D., C.C.N., with Sheila Buff (Alpha Books, 1997)

**Healing Foods,** by Miriam Polunin (Dorling Kindersley Publishing, Inc., 1997)

**Preventions' Healing with Vitamins,** by the Editors of Prevention Magazine Health Books (Rodale Press, Inc., 1996)

**Readers Digest Foods That Harm, Foods That Heal** (The Readers Digest Association, Inc., 1997)

**The Rodale Herb Book** (Rodale Press Book Division, 1974)

**The Survivor Personality,** by Al Siebert, Ph.D. (Berkley Publishing Group, 1996)

**The Essential Guide to Vitamins and Minerals,** by Elizabeth Somer, M.A., R.D., and Health (Media of AmericaHarperPerennial, 1995)

**Medicinal Herbs in the Garden, Field & Marketplace,** by Lee Sturdivant and Tim Blakley (San Juan Naturals, 1999)

**Nutrition, Health & Disease,** by Gary Price Todd, M.D. (Schiffer Publishing, Ltd., 1985)

**Cancer Free,** by Sidney J. Winawer, M.D., and Moshe Shike, M.D. (Simon & Schuster, 1995)

**The Activist Cancer Patient,** by Beverly Zakarian (John Wiley & Sons, Inc., 1996)

Many books have been written on cancer and how to live with it. I would like to suggest the following titles in addition to the ones I have listed in the bibliography. These books are informative, engaging, and examine the many different aspects of cancer.

**Making the Radiation Therapy Decision,** by David Brenner, Arthur C. Upton, and Eric Hall (Lowell House, 1995)
*The latest facts on cancer treatments, radiation versus other therapies, and radiation therapy's side effects are included in a guide which covers different types of radiation therapies and their physical and psychological effects.*

**Cancer Doesn't Have to Hurt:** How to Conquer the Pain Caused by Cancer and Cancer Treatment, by Pamela J. Haylock and Carol P. Curtiss (Hunter House, 1997)
*Explains cancer pain and how to manage it through various medical options, explores its emotional effects on sufferers and caregivers, and offers practical tips on how to find and afford effective treatment.*

**The Human Side of Cancer:** Living with Hope, Coping with Uncertainty, by Jimmie C. Holland and Sheldon Lewis (HarperCollins, 2000)
*This book tackles the emotional issues of cancer head-on.*

**Dr. Susan Love's Breast Book** (Perseus Press, 1995, rev. ed.)
*Dr. Susan Love's Breast Book has been considered the bible of breast-care books since it first appeared in 1990.*

**The Encyclopedia of Popular Herbs**: From the Herb Research Foundation, by Robert S. McCaleb, Evelyn Leigh, Krista Morien, and Wendy Smith (Prima Publishing, 2000)
*This book combines both traditional uses with current scientific research.*

**Beating Cancer with Nutrition:** Clinically Proven and Easy-to-Follow Strategies to Dramatically Improve Quality and Quantity of Life and Chances for a Complete Remission, by Patrick Quillin with Noreen Quillin (Nutrition Times Press, 1998, rev. ed.)
*The impact of healthful diet on cancer survivorship is the subject of innumerable laboratory and clinical studies. This book explains the crucial discoveries and how you can use these for optimal success.*

**Love, Medicine and Miracles:** Lessons Learned about Self-Healing from a Surgeon's Experience with Exceptional Patients, by Bernie S. Siegel (HarperPerennial Library, 1990)
*Bernie Siegel's book is an upbeat, positive approach and plan in dealing with any life-altering diagnosis.*

**The Complete Cancer Survival Guide:** Everything You Must Know and Where to Go for State-of-the-art Treatment of the 25 Most Common Forms of Cancer, by Peter Teeley and Philip Bashe (Main Street Books, 2000)
*Teeley, a survivor of stage-three colon cancer, teaches every patient how to get the most out of the medical system and maximize your own chances of survival.*

**Visiting Nurse Associations of America Caregiver's Handbook.** (Dorling Kindersley Publishing, Inc., 1998)
*Aimed at the home-based caregiver, this handbook offers indispensable advice on providing quality care, necessary equipment, coping emotionally, and financial support.*

**American Cancer Society Consumers' Guide to Cancer Drugs,** by Gail M. Wilkes, Terri B. Ades, and Irwin H. Krakoff (Jones & Bartlett Publishers, 2000)
*This authoritative cancer drug guide from the American Cancer Society offers over 500 information-packed pages in a remarkably portable size.*

# Index

# Index

# Acknowledgments

No one survives a battle of cancer alone and I am eternally grateful to all my family, friends, neighbors, and Sanibel residents for helping me survive these last 6 years.

I especially want to remember my parents, Arthur and Merilyn Clark, who by their love infused my spirit with the will to fight, I treasure your memory and miss you every day. To my husband, Jimmy, who had the unsung job of holding our family together, financially and emotionally, by means of your quiet strength and commitment to us, I adore, admire, and love you. To my precious sons, Andy and Mark, you gave me the purpose to live and the strength to hope; you are the very breath of my life. To my little sister "One Clark girl to another." We did it! Thank you for getting me through this. No words can express how much I love you Patty. I am grateful to my mother-in-law, Sue for bringing me into her family and loving me like one of her own. I miss you. To Jim, Susan, Tony, Jeanne, Alex and the extended Willis family, I cherish you all.

How grateful I am to you Leslie, for all that you've done and your willingness to be "Jesus with skin on" until I could see Him on my own. Your devotion to me has been matched by none and I love you. To my precious friend Lisa, cancer introduced us and love binds us. I'm so glad I have you to share my thoughts, fears and pain with. I love you sweetie. To the Mayerons and the Mucky Duck girls and crew, what can I say. You were always more than just bosses and coworkers, you were my dearest friends. I appreciate your help and support and love you all for it.

My gratitude to Merri for the difficult task of juicing and for always being there, Ellen for making me her "little miracle" and keeping my hopes up, Dr. Fisher and Caroline for peaceful reassurance, and to Joy for laughter. Thank you also to Joni and Marty for the raffle and health tips, to Curly for the fresh veggies, and to Karen for your organizational skills and the many months of planned meals. To all the loving members of the Sanibel Community Church, thank you for prayer and for enriching my life.

No words can express my gratitude to Libby, Rupert, Patty, Leslie, Peter, and Caroline for taking the time to help, encourage, and support me with the Cancer Patient's Workbook.

To my editor, Jill Hamilton. You are wonderful! Thanks for walking me through this process on a daily basis, for being terrific at your job, but mostly for becoming my friend. To Dorling Kindersley Publishing, LaVonne Carlson, and Tina Vaughan: I thank you on behalf of all cancer patients for your desire to provide a workbook that assists newly diagnosed cancer patients. To the entire design team, including Diana Catherines, artists Paul Cox and Mary Ross, the Dorling Kindersley design team of Mandy Earey, Michelle Baxter, Dirk Kaufman, Clare Legemah, and Soo Jin Park thank you for the vision, talent, and effort that have made this workbook so very special to those who find themselves in need of it. Thanks too to Crystal Coble, Jonathan Bennett, Laurel Given, Andrew Sicco, and SooJin for editorial, design, and production assistance, and to Nanette Cardon for the index.

I owe my thanks to Diane Blum and Debbie Haber of CancerCare for their input and advice and to Richard Bloch, Dr. Creagan, Al Siebert, and the American Cancer Society for allowing me the use of their material.
I am forever indebted and grateful to the many doctors, nurses, researchers and biologists who have dedicated their lives to fighting the disease of cancer. A very special thank you to my caring, compassionate and expert team of doctors: Dr. Lowell Hart and Dr. Peter Blitzer. Thank you as well to your loving staff of nurses, receptionists, and technicians who helped get me through some very tough times. May God bless your work and all of your lives.
To my community, I thank you all you for the beautifully cooked meals, the special attention you gave my boys, the hours of driving me to and from the doctors and treatments, for cleaning my house, buying raffle tickets, sending cards and financially subsidizing myself and my family. It has meant more to me than you will ever know. I am grateful as well to the Fossil Club of Sanibel for paying many of my medical bills and to the many business on the island for donating prizes and for their support. To those of you that I do know well and to the hundreds of you that I have never had the honor to meet, please accept my heartfelt gratitude.

In honor of all those lost to the disease of cancer, including my mom, Kathy Fowler, Jan Sutherland, Dee Stewart, Jennifer Clements, Fred Carlson, Patrick Hanley, Sharon Schlagel, Robin Grinstead, Janie Mullins, Helen Ganer Veronika Aronoff, and Jacque Trueheit, your lives inspired me with the deepest heartfelt need to bring help and healing to others. I love each one of you and though I mourn your loss, I know heaven rejoices in your triumphant return.

To you Lord Jesus, I give my heart, my love, my life, and my spirit in gratitude. Thank You Lord, for the peace, joy, and blessings you have bestowed on me, for your healing touch, for giving me purpose, for changing me, and for life…eternal.